Heart Failure with Preserved Ejection Fraction

Editors

CAROLYN S.P. LAM
BURKERT PIESKE

HEART FAILURE CLINICS

www.heartfailure.theclinics.com

Consulting Editors
MANDEEP R. MEHRA
JAVED BUTLER

Founding Editor
JAGAT NARULA

July 2014 • Volume 10 • Number 3

ELSEVIER

1600 John F. Kennedy Boulevard • Suite 1800 • Philadelphia, Pennsylvania, 19103-2899

http://www.theclinics.com

HEART FAILURE CLINICS Volume 10, Number 3
July 2014 ISSN 1551-7136, ISBN-13: 978-0-323-31164-9

Editor: Adrianne Brigido
Developmental Editor: Susan Showalter

Heart Failure Clinics (ISSN 1551-7136) is published quarterly by Elsevier Inc., 360 Park Avenue South, New York, NY 10010-1710. Months of publication are January, April, July, and October. Business and editorial offices: 1600 John F. Kennedy Boulevard, Suite 1800, Philadelphia, PA 19103-2899. Periodicals postage paid at New York, NY, and additional mailing offices. Subscription prices are USD 235.00 per year for US individuals, USD 382.00 per year for US institutions, USD 80.00 per year for US students and residents, USD 280.00 per year for Canadian individuals, USD 442.00 per year for Canadian institutions, USD 300.00 per year for international individuals, USD 442.00 per year for international institutions, and USD 100.00 per year for Canadian and foreign students/residents. To receive student and resident rate, orders must be accompanied by name of affiliated institution, date of term, and the *signature* of program/residency coordinator on institution letterhead. Orders will be billed at individual rate until proof of status is received. Foreign air speed delivery is included in all *Clinics* subscription prices. All prices are subject to change without notice. **POSTMASTER:** Send address changes to *Heart Failure Clinics*, Elsevier Health Sciences Division, Subscription Customer Service, 3251 Riverport Lane, Maryland Heights, MO 63043. **Customer Service: 1-800-654-2452 (US and Canada). From outside of the US and Canada, call 314-447-8871. Fax: 314-447-8029. For print support, E-mail: JournalsCustomerService-usa@elsevier.com. For online support, E-mail: JournalsOnlineSupport-usa@elsevier.com.**

Reprints. For copies of 100 or more of articles in this publication, please contact the Commercial Reprints Department, Elsevier Inc., 360 Park Avenue South, New York, NY 10010-1710. Tel.: 212-633-3874; Fax: 212-633-3820; E-mail: reprints@elsevier.com.

Heart Failure Clinics is covered in *MEDLINE/PubMed (Index Medicus).*

Contributors

CONSULTING EDITORS

MANDEEP R. MEHRA, MD
Professor of Medicine, Harvard Medical
School; Medical Director, BWH Heart and
Vascular Center; Executive Director, Center for
Advanced Heart Disease, Brigham and
Women's Hospital, Boston, Massachusetts

JAVED BUTLER, MD, MPH
Professor of Medicine, Director, Heart Failure
Research, Emory Clinical Cardiovascular
Research Institute, Emory University, Atlanta,
Georgia

EDITORS

CAROLYN S.P. LAM, MBBS, MRCP, MS
Associate Professor, Yong Loo Lin School of
Medicine, National University of Singapore;
Consultant Cardiologist and Clinical Director,
Women's Heart Health Clinic, National
University Heart Centre, National University
Health System, Singapore

BURKERT PIESKE, MD
Professor Head, Department of Cardiology,
Medical University Graz, Graz, Austria

AUTHORS

MADS J. ANDERSEN, MD, PhD
Post Doctoral Fellow, Division of
Cardiovascular Diseases, Department of
Medicine, Mayo Clinic, Rochester, Minnesota;
Department of Cardiology, Aarhus University
Hospital, Aarhus, Denmark

CHARLOTTE ANDERSSON, MD, PhD
Framingham Heart Study, Framingham;
Section of Preventive Medicine and
Epidemiology, Boston University School of
Medicine, Boston, Massachusetts;
Department of Cardiology, Gentofte Hospital,
Hellerup, Denmark

BARRY A. BORLAUG, MD
Associate Professor of Medicine, Division of
Cardiovascular Diseases, Department of
Medicine, Mayo Clinic, Rochester,
Minnesota

ROSS T. CAMPBELL, MB ChB
BHF Cardiovascular Research Centre,
University of Glasgow, Glasgow, Scotland,
United Kingdom

**JOHN G.F. CLELAND, MD, FRCP, FACC,
FESC**
Professor, National Institute of Health
Research (UK) Senior Investigator, National
Heart & Lung Institute, NIHR Cardiovascular
Biomedical Research Unit, Royal Brompton
and Harefield Hospitals NHS Trust, Imperial
College, London, United Kingdom

RAHUL C. DEO, MD, PhD
Division of Cardiology, Department of
Medicine, Cardiovascular Research Institute,
University of California, San Francisco,
San Francisco, California

RIET DIERCKX, MD
Department of Cardiology, Castle Hill Hospital,
Hull and York Medical School, University of
Hull, Kingston-upon-Hull, United Kingdom

**ROBERT N. DOUGHTY, MD, FRCP, FRACP,
FCSANZ**
Department of Medicine, National Institute for
Health Innovation, University of Auckland;
Greenlane Cardiovascular Service, Auckland
City Hospital, Auckland, New Zealand

FRANK EDELMANN, MD
Clinic for Cardiology and Pneumology, DZHK
(German Center for Cardiovascular Research),
University of Göttingen, Göttingen,
Germany

JAMES C. FANG, MD, FACC
Professor of Medicine, Chief, Division of
Cardiovascular Medicine, Department of
Medicine, University of Utah Health Sciences
Center; Cardiology Section, Veterans Affairs
Salt Lake City Health Care System, Salt Lake
City, Utah

DEEPAK K. GUPTA, MD
Instructor of Medicine, Vanderbilt Heart and
Vascular Institute; Department of Medicine,
Vanderbilt University Medical Center,
Nashville, Tennessee

MARK J. HAYKOWSKY, PhD
Faculty of Rehabilitation Medicine, Alberta
Cardiovascular and Stroke Research Centre
(ABACUS), Mazankowski Alberta Heart
Institute, University of Alberta, Edmonton,
Alberta, Canada

JAMES L. JANUZZI Jr, MD
Director, Cardiac Intensive Care Unit; Roman
DeSanctis Endowed Clinical Scholar,
Massachusetts General Hospital; Hutter Family
Professor of Medicine, Harvard Medical
School, Boston, Massachusetts

DANIEL H. KATZ, BA
Division of Cardiology, Department of
Medicine, Feinberg Cardiovascular Research
Institute, Northwestern University Feinberg
School of Medicine, Chicago, Illinois

DALANE W. KITZMAN, MD
Cardiology Section, Department of Internal
Medicine, Wake Forest School of Medicine,
Winston-Salem, North Carolina

ÁRPÁD KOVÁCS, MD
Division of Clinical Physiology, Faculty of
Medicine, Institute of Cardiology, University of
Debrecen, Debrecen, Hungary

ALAN S. MAISEL, MD
Professor of Medicine, Director, Coronary Care
Unit and Heart Failure Program, Cardiology
Section (9111-A), VA San Diego Healthcare
System, San Diego, California

JOHN J.V. MCMURRAY, MD
BHF Cardiovascular Research Centre,
University of Glasgow, Glasgow, Scotland,
United Kingdom

LÁSZLÓ NAGY, MD
Division of Clinical Physiology, Faculty of
Medicine, Institute of Cardiology, University of
Debrecen, Debrecen, Hungary

JOSE NATIVI-NICOLAU, MD
Assistant Professor of Medicine, Division of
Cardiovascular Medicine, Department of
Medicine, University of Utah Health Science
Center; Cardiology Section, Veterans Affairs
Salt Lake City Health Care System, Salt Lake
City, Utah

ZOLTÁN PAPP, MD, PhD, DSc
Division of Clinical Physiology, Faculty of
Medicine, Institute of Cardiology, University of
Debrecen, Debrecen, Hungary

PIERPAOLO PELLICORI, MD
Department of Cardiology, Castle Hill
Hospital, Hull and York Medical School,
University of Hull, Kingston-upon-Hull,
United Kingdom

KATRINA K. POPPE, PhD
Department of Medicine, National Institute for
Health Innovation, University of Auckland,
Auckland, New Zealand

**A. MARK RICHARDS, MB ChB, MD, PhD,
FRACP, FRCP**
Professor, Cardiac Department,
Cardiovascular Research Institute, National
University Heart Centre, National University of
Singapore, Singapore, Singapore; Department
of Medicine, Christchurch Heart Institute,
University of Otago, Christchurch,
Christchurch, New Zealand

JOHN J. RYAN, MD
Assistant Professor of Medicine, Division of
Cardiovascular Medicine, Department of
Medicine, University of Utah Health Science
Center, Salt Lake City, Utah

KEVIN S. SHAH, MD
Resident Physician, Department of Internal
Medicine, University of California, San Diego,
San Diego, California

SANJIV J. SHAH, MD
Associate Professor of Medicine; Director, Heart Failure with Preserved Ejection Fraction Program, Division of Cardiology, Department of Medicine, Feinberg Cardiovascular Research Institute, Northwestern University Feinberg School of Medicine, Chicago, Illinois

SCOTT D. SOLOMON, MD
Professor of Medicine, Division of Cardiology, Department of Medicine, Brigham and Women's Hospital, Harvard Medical School, Boston, Massachusetts

RICHARD W. TROUGHTON, MB ChB, PhD, FRACP
Professor, Department of Medicine, Christchurch Heart Institute, University of Otago, Christchurch, Christchurch, New Zealand

RAMACHANDRAN S. VASAN, MD
Framingham Heart Study, Framingham; Section of Preventive Medicine and Epidemiology; Section of Cardiology, Boston University School of Medicine, Boston, Massachusetts

ROLF WACHTER, MD
Clinic for Cardiology and Pneumology, DZHK (German Center for Cardiovascular Research), University of Göttingen, Göttingen, Germany

Contents

Heart failure with preserved ejection fraction (HFPEF) is a common condition, and the prevalence is projected to increase further. Studies differ in the reported incidence and mortality associated with this condition, although there is agreement that between a third and one-half of all patients with heart failure have HFPEF. Although several consensus statements and guidelines have been published, some recent randomized clinical trials have reported low mortality, raising doubts about whether all patients diagnosed with HFPEF have HFPEF or whether the condition is heterogeneous in its cause and prognosis. The overall reported prognosis of patients with HFPEF remains poor.

Heart failure with preserved ejection fraction (HFPEF) is frequently associated with multiple disorders complicating both the clinical management and the understanding of the underlying mechanisms. This review focuses on the causes and pathophysiology of HFPEF and overviews how cellular and molecular changes related to various comorbidities may influence the age-dependent and gender-dependent hemodynamic alterations of diastolic ventricular function.

Heart failure with preserved ejection fraction (HFpEF) constitutes a growing health care burden worldwide. Although definitions vary somewhat among guidelines, in general the presence of typical heart failure symptoms and signs in combination with a preserved left ventricular ejection fraction ($\geq$50%) and functional and/or structural left ventricular changes makes the diagnosis likely. This review focuses on the current understanding of diagnostic criteria, as presented in current guidelines and consensus recommendations, and on new insights from recent papers. The role of comorbidities that often contribute to symptoms and hamper the HFpEF diagnostics is also reviewed.

Heart failure with preserved ejection fraction (HFpEF) is a heterogeneous syndrome, with several underlying etiologic and pathophysiologic factors. The heterogeneity of

and chronic heart failure (HF). Plasma concentrations of the cardiac natriuretic peptides (NPs) are valuable aids in each of these elements of care. However, most data are derived from cohorts with undifferentiated HF or HF with reduced ejection fraction (HFREF), and the performance and best application of NPs in HF with preserved ejection fraction (HFPEF) is less certain. This review outlines the evidence for use of NPs in the evaluation and management of HFPEF.

phenotype patients precisely and create better definitions of HFpEF based on biomarkers.

Jose Nativi-Nicolau, John J. Ryan, and James C. Fang

Heart failure with preserved ejection fraction (HFpEF) is a clinical syndrome characterized by decreased exercise capacity and fluid retention in the setting of preserved left ventricular systolic function and evidence of abnormal diastolic function. Therapeutic strategies include pharmacologic agents, pacing, baroreflex modification, diet, and exercise. Despite symptomatic and hemodynamic improvements with some therapies, large clinical trials have not demonstrated a clear improvement in clinical outcomes. The current management of patients with HFpEF is directed to symptomatic relief of congestion with diuretics and risk factor modification. In this article, we summarize the available evidence base for potential targets of therapy.

HEART FAILURE CLINICS

Foreword

Heart Failure with Preserved Ejection Fraction: A Bouillabaisse

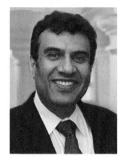 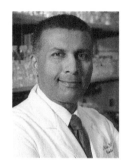

Mandeep R. Mehra, MD   Javed Butler, MD, MPH
Consulting Editors

Bouillabaisse, a traditional fish stew, accurately depicts the phenotypic mixture that has often been stirred together in our understanding of heart failure with preserved ejection fraction (HFpEF). Variably referred to as "diastolic heart failure" or "heart failure with normal ejection fraction," it became apparent early on that this nomenclature was a misfit and either allowed only a high specificity in diagnosis (those with clinical heart failure and clearly discernable diastolic dysfunction) or was too sensitive (where any normal ejection fraction patient with dyspnea was categorized as having the disease). This conundrum led to lumping of noncardiac causes of dyspnea or functional intolerance (severe obesity) into this basket diagnosis or distinct pathology characterized erroneously as heart failure ("angina equivalent"). Recognition that diastolic compliance abnormalities were not an absolute character of this particular syndrome and that ejection fraction was not always "normal" led to a more apt generalized naming of this syndrome as HFpEF.

We now recognize that this syndrome may arise from a primary myocardial defect, or also equally important, represent a mismatch between the coupling of the heart with its adjoining vasculature. In other situations structural aberrations in electrical activity, such as a chronotropic insufficiency, may be important participants in the expression of the clinical syndrome. As such, clinical trials that are initiated after the basic pathologic aberrations of hypertension, atrial arrhythmias, and fluid congestion have been adequately controlled have fallen short in providing incremental disease-modifying impact. Steadily, renin angiotensin aldosterone directed therapy has not been convincingly shown to alter the natural history of this distinct expression of heart failure. Similarly, treatment designed to influence lusitropy has found its way to the graveyard. Thus, a fascination with this disease state has led to the creation of scholarly camps in the "diastolic dysfunction" and "nondiastolic dysfunction" groups, neither yielding adequate therapeutic reward.

Going back to the drawing board, one can characterize HFpEF as a specific syndrome where the left atrium typically bears the brunt of a chronic elevation in intracardiac filling pressures at rest or in response to exercise, where the systemic vasculature demonstrates a reduced arterial compliance, and where the systolic blood pressure is elevated "pound for pound" at any given measure of arterial elastance. The sum total of these aberrations is expressed by an increase in circulating natriuretic peptides. We are steadily moving toward a more comprehensive appreciation and application of diagnostic and therapeutic principles in HFpEF and in this vein the timely and scholarly compendium of articles weaved together under the expert editorship of Drs Lam and Pieske

Heart Failure Clin 10 (2014) xiii–xiv
http://dx.doi.org/10.1016/j.hfc.2014.05.001
1551-7136/14/$ – see front matter © 2014 Elsevier Inc. All rights reserved.

heartfailure.theclinics.com

represents a unified front forward in this war on the global epidemic of heart failure.

Mandeep R. Mehra, MD
Harvard Medical School
BWH Heart and Vascular Center
Center for Advanced Heart Disease
Brigham and Women's Hospital
75 Francis Street, A Building
3rd Floor, Room AB324
Boston, MA 02115, USA

Javed Butler, MD, MPH
Heart Failure Research
Emory Clinical Cardiovascular
Research Institute
Emory University
1462 Clifton Road Northeast, Suite 504
Atlanta, GA 30322, USA

E-mail addresses:
MMEHRA@partners.org (M.R. Mehra)
javed.butler@emory.edu (J. Butler)

Preface

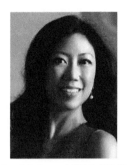

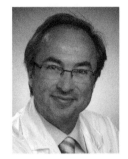

Carolyn S.P. Lam, MBBS, MRCP, MS   Burkert Pieske, MD

Editors

Heart failure with preserved ejection fraction (HFPEF) currently represents one of the greatest unmet needs in Cardiology. Barely 25 years ago, we did not believe that heart failure could exist in the presence of an apparently normal ejection fraction. We now know not only that HFPEF exists and can be diagnosed, but also that it currently constitutes half the heart failure population in many parts of the world and will become the predominant type of heart failure in future. Furthermore, it is a highly morbid and deadly disease. Most significantly, our attempts to extrapolate proven therapies in heart failure with reduced ejection fraction to this population have uniformly failed to improve outcomes in HFPEF, and in fact, this is a syndrome still in search of a cure.

The controversies surrounding HFPEF is reflected in the transition of nomenclature used to refer to it, from diastolic heart failure to heart failure with normal systolic function, heart failure with normal ejection fraction, and now heart failure with preserved ejection fraction. This evolution also reflects our increasing understanding of this important syndrome.

This issue therefore aims to summarize the current state of understanding in HFPEF. We are grateful to our colleagues, all well-known experts in this field, for their valuable contributions. We trust that the perspectives shared will be useful to clinicians, investigators, and researchers alike to better cope with this still underrecognized syndrome.

Carolyn S.P. Lam, MBBS, MRCP, MS
National University Health System
Tower Block Level 9
1E Kent Ridge Road
Singapore 119228

Burkert Pieske, MD
Department of Cardiology
Medical University Graz
Graz, Austria

E-mail addresses:
carolyn_lam@nuhs.edu.sg (C.S.P. Lam)
burkert.pieske@medunigraz.at (B. Pieske)

http://dx.doi.org/10.1016/j.hfc.2014.05.002

Epidemiology of Heart Failure with Preserved Ejection Fraction

Charlotte Andersson, MD, PhD[a,b,c],*,
Ramachandran S. Vasan, MD[a,b,d]

KEYWORDS

• Epidemiology • Heart failure • Preserved ejection fraction • Mortality • Prognosis

KEY POINTS

• Heart failure with preserved ejection fraction (HFPEF) is a common disease, especially among the elderly and in women.
• With an increasing prevalence of hypertension, obesity, atrial fibrillation, and diabetes, and the growing elderly segment of the general population, the prevalence of HFPEF is projected to increase in the future.
• HFPEF presents a diagnostic challenge and studies differ widely in the reported incidence and mortality associated with this condition.
• There is agreement that between a third and one-half of patients with heart failure have HFPEF.
• Prognosis is overall poor. Patients with HFPEF have substantial comorbidity, high rates of repeated hospitalizations, and a high mortality.

INTRODUCTION

Heart failure with preserved ejection fraction (HFPEF) can be defined as a clinical syndrome in which the heart is unable to deliver the requisite amount of oxygen to the tissues commensurate with their metabolic needs, or does so but only at the expense of increased left ventricular (LV) filling pressures, despite a normal ejection fraction. Other terms used for this condition include backward heart failure and diastolic heart failure. The reported prevalence of HFPEF is increasing, in part because of a greater awareness of the diagnosis, refined echocardiographic techniques, and also because of changes in demographics (such as aging of the population) and higher burden of lifestyle-related risk factors (such as obesity and diabetes). For many years, HFPEF has remained a clinically illusive concept with lack of both national and international consensus on criteria for its diagnosis.[1,2] There are no clinical symptoms or signs that have a high sensitivity or specificity for the diagnosis of HFPEF, and the pathophysiologic mechanisms underlying the

This work was supported in part by N01-HC-25195. Dr C. Andersson was supported by an independent research grant from the Danish Agency For Science, Technology, and Innovation (the Danish Medical Research Council, grant no. FSS - 11-120873).

The authors have nothing to disclose.

[a] Framingham Heart Study, Mt Wayte Avenue 73, Suite 2, Framingham, MA 01702-5827, USA; [b] Section of Preventive Medicine and Epidemiology, Boston University School of Medicine, 801 Massachusetts Avenue, Suite 470, Boston, MA 02118, USA; [c] Department of Cardiology, Gentofte Hospital, Niels Andersens vej 65, Hellerup 2900, Denmark; [d] Section of Cardiology, Boston University School of Medicine, 801 Massachussetts Avenue, Suite 470, Boston, MA 02118, USA

* Corresponding author. Framingham Heart Study, Mt Wayte Avenue 73, Suite 2, Framingham, MA 01702-5827.

E-mail address: ca@heart.dk

condition are not well established. Moreover, patients with HFPEF often have concomitant comorbidities that may either mask or confound the diagnosis.

The current American Heart Association/American College of Cardiology and European Society of Cardiology guidelines both recommend that a diagnosis of HFPEF should be based on the presence of the following features: (1) signs and symptoms consistent with a diagnosis of heart failure; (2) absence of depressed ejection fraction (ie, an LV ejection fraction [LVEF] $\geq$50%); and (3) objective measures showing an impaired LV diastolic function.[3,4] Furthermore, the clinical findings should not be explainable by other conditions, such as a primary volume overload state or chronic pulmonary disease. The diagnostic criteria are still subject to variability between hospitals and across studies. No single noninvasive measure of LV diastolic function is optimally accurate and sensitive for establishing a diagnosis of LV diastolic dysfunction (the third criterion). Therefore, the guidelines concur that LV diastolic function should be measured by more than one technique in these patients, if feasible. In addition, guidelines are not specific regarding the combination of symptoms and signs that adequately and accurately establishes a clinical diagnosis of heart failure.

Most symptoms and clinical findings, especially those that are present in milder states of HFPEF (such as reduced exercise capability or mild ankle edema) are inherently nondiscriminatory and may be caused by a variety of clinical conditions, including chronic pulmonary disease, physical deconditioning, obesity, and/or renal disease. Symptoms and signs of more severe heart failure (like paroxysmal nocturnal dyspnea and pulmonary edema) are more specific, but have a lower sensitivity. The Framingham Heart Study heart failure criteria are among the most commonly used and are widely accepted for an initial evaluation of suspected heart failure. They are based on an algorithm that combines different objective signs for diagnosing heart failure (**Box 1**) and are intended for epidemiologic settings. Because there is no gold standard for the clinical diagnosis, validation of different algorithms and measures to diagnose HFPEF is challenging. As an illustrative example, in the recent placebo-controlled randomized trial of spironolactone (the Aldo-DHF trial) only 1 of 422 patients died during 12 months of follow-up, which is lower than the mortality expected in patients with HFPEF based on prior reports from other observational and clinical trials. The observed low mortality of these patients in some series has led some investigators to

---

Box 1
Framingham criteria for congestive heart failure (2 major, or 1 major plus 2 minor criteria are required)

Major:

Paroxysmal nocturnal dyspnea

Neck vein distension

Rales

Radiographic cardiomegaly

Acute pulmonary edema

Third sound gallop

Increased central venous pressure

Increased circulation time ($\geq$25 seconds)

Hepatojugular reflux

Pulmonary edema, visceral congestion, or cardiomegaly on autopsy

Weight loss greater than or equal to 4.5 kg in 5 days in response to treatment of heart failure

Minor:

Bilateral ankle edema

Nocturnal cough

Dyspnea on ordinary exertion

Hepatomegaly

Pleural effusion

Decrease in vital capacity by 33% of maximal value recorded

Tachycardia ($\geq$120 beats per minute)

---

question the diagnosis of HFPEF with the added speculation that some of these patients may not have heart failure.[1,5] The most common heart failure symptoms for inclusion in the Aldo-DHF trial were fatigue (59%) and nocturia (80%), which are not specific enough for a diagnosis of heart failure (compared with the more exhaustive Framingham criteria).[6] Supporting the notion that HFPEF may be overdiagnosed, Caruana and colleagues[5] reported that, in a sample of consecutively referred patients with suspected heart failure and normal systolic function but without atrial fibrillation or valve disease, an alternative diagnosis (such as obesity, reduced pulmonary capacity, or coronary artery disease) was present in most patients even though they had demonstrable LV diastolic dysfunction. The investigators therefore concluded that few if any patients satisfied the criteria for a diagnosis of pure diastolic heart failure.[5] The echocardiographic findings suggestive of heart failure were recently compared with clinical findings based on the

Framingham criteria in 216 consecutive patients admitted with suspected heart failure to a cardiology unit at an academic hospital in Spain.[7] The investigators concluded that the Framingham criteria were very sensitive (92%) and moderately specific (72%) for diagnosing heart failure. The absence of positive Framingham criteria conclusively ruled out heart failure with reduced ejection fraction (HFREF), and almost conclusively ruled out HFPEF.[7] The recent guidelines suggesting a combination of echocardiography (showing normal LVEF and LV diastolic dysfunction) and clinical signs and symptoms of heart failure (preferably in accordance with the Framingham criteria) therefore seem both appropriate and necessary to make a correct clinical diagnosis of HFPEF.

Despite limitations and inconsistency in the diagnosis of HFPEF, numerous reports in the literature have provided valuable data regarding the condition. This article summarizes these epidemiologic studies. However, HFPEF still receives less attention than HFREF (both in clinical care and in published guidelines), perhaps because there is no clear mortality benefit associated with any pharmacologic treatment of the former.

Risk Factors

It is challenging to elucidate the relative contributions of one or more risk factors to the overall burden of HFPEF in the community. The prevalence of risk factors varies between individuals with HFPEF, and these risk factors likely interact (conjointly and synergistically) to augment the risk of developing HFPEF.[8] Overall, the most important risk factors for developing HFPEF include hypertension,[9] older age, and female sex.[10,11] The prevalence of HFPEF in community-based settings increases rapidly with advancing age, especially in women, approaching 10% in women aged 80 years or more in a recent Portuguese survey.[12] Other comorbidities frequently associated in patients with HFPEF and likely contributing to disease risk include coronary artery disease, atrial fibrillation,[13] obesity,[14] and diabetes.[15] Reports of large-scale trials or clinical databases with patients with HFPEF have shown that hypertension is present in 50% to 90% of patients with preserved ejection fraction, which is higher than its prevalence in the general population, and also higher than in patients with HFREF.[16-20] Although high blood pressure is causally related to HFPEF incidence, a history of hypertension has been associated with a neutral or paradoxic survival benefit after the onset of heart failure.[21] Nonetheless, a history of hypertension has been associated with high mortality, especially among patients with a restrictive LV filling pattern (the ultimate consequence of hypertension and cardiac hypertrophy).[22]

In a general community, Lee and colleagues[23] sought to clarify the cause of incident heart failure according to preserved (defined as LVEF $\geq$45%) or reduced ejection fraction (LVEF<45%) in the Original and Offspring cohorts of the Framingham Heart Study. Using a hierarchical schema for attributing heart failure sequentially to different causes (weighting coronary insufficiency highest, followed by valve disease, followed by hypertension), hypertension was the primary cause of HFPEF in 36% of the cases; 37% and 11% of the cases were attributable to coronary artery disease and valve disease, respectively, whereas the remaining 16% were unclassified. Several studies have supported the notion that global myocardial ischemia may cause diastolic dysfunction and HFPEF.[24-26] The active part of the myocardial relaxation has been shown to be the most energy-consuming step of the cardiac cycle. As a result, ischemia initially affects LV diastolic function.[27] Thus, especially in the presence of key risk factors such as diabetes and hypertension, patients with stable coronary artery disease may develop HFPEF.[28] A contributing reason for the high risk of HFPEF among the elderly and among women could be that these demographic subsets often have microvascular heart disease (compared with younger men who more often develop macrovascular heart disease and as a result have a greater occurrence of HFREF).[29] This finding was recently confirmed in an analysis of the Framingham Heart Study Original and Offspring cohorts, in which men and women had similar risks of developing HFPEF, whereas men were at higher risk of developing HFREF, and this excessive this risk was mainly related to interim myocardial infarction.[30] Similar findings were recently reported in the Prevention of Renal and Vascular End-stage Disease (PREVEND) community-based cohort study (although women were reported to be at higher risk of HFPEF compared with men in this study).[31] The incidence of HFPEF increases rapidly with age.[32] For example, in a large Danish cohort study of consecutively hospitalized patients with heart failure between 2002 and 2003, the prevalence of HFPEF was significantly higher among elderly patients compared with younger patients (53% vs 36% in patients less than and equal to or more than 85 years of age).[33]

Other conditions associated with an increased risk of HFPEF include sleep apnea,[34] chronic obstructive pulmonary disease,[35] renal

Table 1
Echocardiographic features and mortality of some recent clinical trials

	TOPCAT[62]	PARAMOUNT[63]	RELAX[20]	I-PRESERVE[17,64]	CHARMES[65,66]	Aldo-DHF[6]	PEP-CHF[18]
N	935	292	216	745	312	422	850
Definition of diastolic heart failure	LVEF ≥45%, HF hospitalization, or BNP ≥100, or NT-proBNP ≥360 pg/mL	LVEF ≥45%, NT-proBNP >400 pg/mL	LVEF ≥50%, NT-proBNP >400, pVo_2 <60% of predicted	LVEF ≥45%, recent HF hospitalization, or other objective signs of HF	LVEF >40%	LVEF ≥50%, echocardiographic diastolic dysfunction or AF, pVo_2 ≤25	LVEF >40%, HF by clinical criteria
Age (y)	70 ± 10	71 ± 9	69 (62–77)	72 ± 7	66 ± 11	67 ± 8	75 (72–79)
Women (%)	49	56	48	62	34	52	56
LV Structure							
EDD (cm)	4.80 ± 0.58	4.64 ± 0.48	4.6 (4.3–5.1)	4.8 ± 0.6	5.4 ± 0.7	4.65 ± 0.62	4.6 (4.2–5.1)
EDVi (mL/m²)	49.9 ± 15.5	61.4 ± 15.4	NA	49 ± 14	NA	NA	NA
MWT (cm)	1.18 ± 0.20	0.91 ± 0.16	NA	0.93 ± 0.15	NA	NA	1.3 (1.2–1.5)
LVMI (g/m²)	111 ± 31	79.1 ± 22.2	78 (62–94)	NA	117 ± 42	109 ± 28	NA
RWT	0.49 ± 0.10	0.38 ± 0.08	NA	0.40 ± 0.08	NA	NA	NA
LV Geometry							
Normal (%)	14	72	NA	46	NA	NA	NA
Concentric remodeling (%)	34	14	NA	25	NA	NA	NA
Concentric hypertrophy (%)	43	7	NA	29	NA	NA	NA
Eccentric hypertrophy (%)	9	7	NA	0	NA	NA	NA
LV Systolic Function							
EF (%)	59.6 ± 8.0	57.7 ± 7.9	60 (56–65)	64 ± 9	50 (18–65)	67 ± 8	65 (56–66)

LV Diastolic Function							
LAVi (mL/m²)	29.8 ± 12.5	35.9 ± 13.5	44 (36–59)	NA	41.3 ± 14.7	28.0 ± 8.4	NA
LA diameter (cm)	4.3 ± 0.6	3.7 ± 0.5	NA	NA	NA	NA	4.5 (4.1–4.8)
E/A ratio	1.2 ± 0.7	1.1 ± 0.62	1.5 (1.0–2.1)	1.05 ± 0.74	1.1 ± 0.7	0.91 ± 0.33	0.7 (0.6–0.9)
TDI E′ septal (cm/s)	6.1 ± 2.2	5.8 ± 2.0	6 (5–8)	7.2 ± 2.9	NA	5.9 ± 1.3	NA
TDI E′ lateral (cm/s)	8.2 ± 3.2	7.5 ± 2.8	NA	9.1 ± 3.4	NA	NA	NA
E/E′ ratio (septal)	15.6 ± 6.8	15.9 ± 7.3	16 (11–24)	NA	NA	12.8 ± 4.0	NA
E/E′ ratio (lateral)	11.8 ± 5.9	12.7 ± 7.4	NA	10.0 ± 4.5	NA	NA	NA
Diastolic dysfunction, any (%)	66	92	NA	69	67	100	NA
None (%)	34	8	31	33	NA	0	NA
Grade 1 (%)	22	31	NA	29	22	77	NA
Grade 2 (%)	34	43	NA	36	37	21	NA
Grade 3 (%)	10	18	NA	4	7	2	NA
Pulmonary pressure	2.8 ± 0.5 (TR [m/s])	2.5 ± 0.4 (TR [m/s])	41 (33–53) (RVSP [mm Hg])	37 ± 13 (RVSP [mm Hg])	NA	NA	NA
Mortality in placebo group	176 out of 1723 (10.2%)[a]	NA	0 out of 103 (0%)	436 out of 2061 (21%)	170 out of 1509 (11.3%)[a]	0 out of 209 (0%)	53 out of 426 (12.4%)
Length of follow-up	Mean 3.3 y	12 wk	24 wk	Mean 49.5 mo	Mean 36.6 mo	12 mo	Mean 2.1 y
Annual mortality (%)[b]	3.1	NA	0	5.1	3.7	0	5.8

Continuous variables are expressed as means (±standard deviation) or median (interquartile range).

Abbreviations: AF, atrial fibrillation; HF, heart failure; pVo_2, partial pressure of Oxygen in venous blood. Mortalities derived from www.clinicaltrialresults.org/Slides/AHA%202013/Pfeffer_TOPCAT.ppt.

[a] Refers to cardiovascular mortality only.

[b] Calculated as mortality in placebo group divided by average length of follow-up.

Adapted from Shah AM, Shah SJ, Anand IS, et al. Cardiac structure and function in heart failure with preserved ejection fraction: baseline findings from the echocardiographic study of the treatment of preserved cardiac function heart failure with an aldosterone antagonist trial. Circ Heart Fail 2014;7:104–15; with permission.

Table 2
Echocardiographic features of some recent population-based studies

	Olmsted County[67]	CHS[68]	He et al,[69] 2009	ARIC/Jackson[70]	NY Heart Failure Registry[71]	French Registry[57]	Northwestern Registry[72]
N	244	167	128	85	619	368	402
Definition of diastolic heart failure	LVEF ≥50%	LVEF ≥55%	LVEF >55%	LVEF ≥50%	LVEF ≥50%	LVEF ≥50%	LVEF ≥50%
Age (y)	76 (22–99)[a]	76 ± 7	72 ± 10	61 (57–67)	72 ± 14	76 ± 10	65 ± 10
Women (%)	55	57	45	85	73	53	62
LV Structure							
EDD (cm)	NA	5.1 ± 0.8	4.7 ± 0.6	4.4 (4.1–4.7)	4.70 ± 0.76	5.0 ± 0.8	4.63 ± 0.63
EDVi (mL/m²)	56.4 ± 14.4	69 ± 22	53 ± 16	NA	NA	NA	40.6 ± 11.0
MWT (cm)	NA	0.9 ± 0.2	1.2 ± 0.2	1.2 (1.1–1.4)	NA	NA	1.19 ± 0.28
LVMI (g/m²)	102 ± 29	98 ± 34	118 ± 36	NA	66 (53–85)	NA	103 ± 38
RWT	0.45 ± 1.0	0.36 ± 0.11	NA	0.57 (0.51–0.62)	NA	NA	0.51 ± 15
LV Geometry							
Normal (%)	31	NA	NA	5	NA	NA	12
Concentric remodeling (%)	27	NA	NA	20	NA	NA	28
Concentric hypertrophy (%)	26	NA	NA	73	NA	NA	48
Eccentric hypertrophy (%)	16	NA	NA	2	NA	NA	12

LV Systolic Function							
EF (%)	62 ± 6	72 ± 7	64 ± 5	67 (59–75)	59.8 ± 7.3	63 ± 8	61 ± 6
LV Diastolic Function							
LAVi (mL/m^2)	NA	NA	NA	NA	NA	NA	34 ± 14
LA diameter (cm)	NA	NA	3.9 ± 0.5	3.4 (3.1–3.8)	NA	4.1 ± 0.7	NA
E/A ratio	1.3 ± 1.2	0.75 ± 1.2	1.1 ± 0.8	0.94 (0.79–1.12)	NA	NA	1.4 ± 0.7
TDI E' septal (cm/s)	6.0 ± 2.1	NA	8 ± 2	NA	NA	NA	7.0 ± 2.7
TDI E' lateral (cm/s)	8.2 ± 3.2	NA	NA	NA	NA	NA	9.3 ± 3.9
E/E' ratio (septal)	18.4 ± 9.7	NA	10	NA	NA	NA	17 ± 9
Diastolic dysfunction, any (%)	NA	NA	NA	27	NA	NA	91
Pulmonary pressure	NA	NA	NA	NA	47 ± 17 (PASP [mm Hg])	NA	3.0 ± 0.6 (TR [m/s])
Mortality	NA	NA	NA	26 out of 85 (31)	4.2	57	48 out of 402 (12)
Length of follow-up	NA	NA	NA	Median 13.7 y	In-hospital mortality	5 y	Mean 12.5 mo
Annual mortality (%)[b]	NA	NA	NA	2.3	NA	11.4	11.5

Continuous variables are expressed as means (±standard deviation) or median (interquartile range).

[a] Data presented as mean (range).

[b] Calculated as mortality divided by average length of follow-up.

Adapted from Shah AM, Shah SJ, Anand IS, et al. Cardiac structure and function in heart failure with preserved ejection fraction: baseline findings from the echocardiographic study of the treatment of preserved cardiac function heart failure with an aldosterone antagonist trial. Circ Heart Fail 2014;7:104–15; with permission.

dysfunction,[31] dyslipidemia/cardiac steatosis,[36] rheumatoid arthritis and other systemic inflammatory diseases,[37–40] and select medications (especially antineoplastic therapy),[41] although the exact and independent role of these contributing conditions to the risk of HFPEF remains to be determined.

Subclinical Disease Measures and Biomarkers Relating to HFPEF

HFPEF may have a long preclinical phase, and the identification of subclinical disease by echocardiography (LV hypertrophy and diastolic dysfunction) and biomarkers can help identify those at high risk of HFPEF. LV diastolic dysfunction measured by transthoracic echocardiography was shown to be a common and independent predictor of overt HFPEF in an asymptomatic sample of middle-aged to elderly individuals in the Olmsted County Heart Function Study (24% and 39% had diastolic dysfunction at baseline and after 4 years, respectively).[42] A separate report from Framingham confirmed this association.[43] Moreover, echocardiographic LV hypertrophy in asymptomatic middle-aged and elderly individuals was recently shown to be an independent long-term predictor of HFPEF in the Framingham Heart Study, with age-adjusted and sex-adjusted 10-year incidence rates of heart failure corresponding with 0.77 (0.33–1.21) per 100 persons among those with normal left ventricle, 1.57 (0.37–2.72) among those with concentric hypertrophy, and 2.11 (1.03–3.14) among those with eccentric hypertrophy.[44] A recent study based on the Dallas Heart Study cohort further showed that, among asymptomatic individuals with hypertrophy, those with a particularly malignant subtype were characterized by increased circulating levels of troponin T and N-terminal probrain natriuretic peptide (NT-proBNP).[45] As discussed in detail by Cheng and colleagues,[46] there are several other circulating novel biomarkers that are associated with incident HFPEF and are informative about the clinical course of disease, including growth differentiation factor-15, cystatin C, resistin, and galectin-3.

PREVALENCE AND INCIDENCE OF HFPEF

Although the incidence of HFPEF seems to be stable, its prevalence may have increased over the last couple of decades. The proportion of HFPEF among all heart failure cases lies somewhere between 44% and 72%, with a suggestion of a temporal increase in the proportion of HFPEF cases in recent years.[32] In 2010, a total of 1,023,000 people were discharged with a primary diagnosis of heart failure from US hospitals.[47] This number was unchanged compared with the year 2000 and was higher than the numbers diagnosed in the 1990s.[47] Among patients admitted with decompensated heart failure to Mayo Clinic Hospitals in Olmsted County, Minnesota, the proportion of patients with HFPEF increased from approximately 38% in 1987 to 54% in 2001; an increase that was solely explained by an increase in numbers of admissions for HFPEF and not by a decrease in numbers of individuals with HFREF.[48] During the same time period, the proportion of patients with heart failure who had hypertension, diabetes, or atrial fibrillation increased.[48] This finding is consistent with the current global increases in the prevalence of hypertension, obesity, diabetes, and atrial fibrillation, and underscores the importance of HFPEF as a potential growing global public health problem.[49] A similar increasing trend in the prevalence of HFPEF was recently shown in a survey of 275 hospitals in the Get With the Guidelines–Heart Failure report from January 2005 to October 2010.[50] Based on data from a sample of individuals in Olmsted County, Rogers and colleagues[51] reported that age-adjusted incidence rates of overall heart failure between 1979 and 2000 were not declining in either men or women.

WORLDWIDE/REGIONAL INCIDENCE AND MORTALITY

In 2009, 1 in 9 death certificates (corresponding with 275,000 individuals) in the United States had heart failure registered as a primary or contributing cause of death.[47] A common belief has been that HFPEF is something you die with and not die of.[52] Individuals with HFPEF often have a significant burden of comorbidities. However, even after adjustment of comorbid conditions, the mortalities associated with HFPEF are higher compared with background populations of similar age. For example, data from the Framingham Heart Study suggested that individuals with HFPEF and HFREF had a comparable 4-fold increase in relative risk of death compared with age-matched controls.[53] Moreover, the survey from the Olmsted County showed that mortality of HFPEF did not improve between 1987 and 2001, as opposed to improvement in the outcomes for HFREF.[48] The most common causes of death in HFPEF have been suggested to be noncardiovascular, perhaps supporting the notion that HFPEF is not something that patients necessarily die of, but more likely something that they die with.[54] However, some uncertainty remains in this area. A recent review of contemporary epidemiologic and clinical randomized trials concluded that most deaths were of cardiovascular causes (51%–60% for epidemiologic studies, and >70% in clinical randomized trials).[55] Campbell and colleagues[56] compared the mortality of patients from clinical HFPEF trials with patients from clinical trials of other cardiovascular diseases and similarly concluded that, although having comparable prevalence of comorbidities, age, and gender, those with HFPEF had significantly worse outcomes compared with patients from other cardiovascular trials, suggesting that the high mortality seen for patients with HFPEF cannot completely be explained by comorbidity burden.

Mortalities for HFPEF have varied in different reports, probably as a consequence of differences in diagnostic criteria and clinical settings (population-based vs In-hospitalization settings vs clinical trials). **Tables 1** and **2** summarize selected characteristics and mortality of some of the most recent clinical trials and population-based samples. The echocardiographic characteristics showed larger differences between the different samples. There were low to very low mortalities in these clinical trials, compared with those reported in community-based or hospitalization settings. The Meta-Analysis Global Group in Chronic Heart Failure (MAGGIC) recently evaluated mortalities in 41,972 patients, of whom 10,347 (24.7%) had HFPEF, from 18 observational and clinical trial studies.[16] There were 121 (95% confidence intervals, 117–126) deaths per 1000 person-years in the HFPEF group and 141 (138–144) deaths per 1000 person-years in the HFREF group. When excluding randomized clinical trials, mortalities were more similar for HFPEF and HFREF: 146 (138–154) versus 159 (154–165) deaths per 1000 person-years, respectively.[16] In a French cohort of patients hospitalized for the first time with heart failure, 5-year survival rates were not significantly different in patients with preserved and reduced ejection fractions (43% vs 46%; $P = .95$).[57] Comparable high mortalities were also found in a Canadian survey of patients hospitalized with heart failure: 30-day mortalities were 5.3% versus 7.1% ($P = .08$), and 1-year mortalities of 25.5% versus 22.2% ($P = .08$) for patients with HFPEF and HFREF, respectively.[40] However, 1 meta-analysis based on prospective observational studies showed that the mortality of HFPEF was only 50% that of HFREF.[58] Perhaps prognosis in HFPEF and HFREF are more similar once patients have been hospitalized.[55]

Comprehensive studies of worldwide trends in incidence, prevalence, and heart failure–related mortality are lacking, but HFPEF seems to be an increasingly common disease in several parts of the westernized world. For example, heart failure is now a common disease with significant impacts on the health care systems in several parts of Africa because of the rapid adoption of westernized living habits (ie, sedentary lifestyle, consumption of fast food and salt, with increasing prevalence of hypertension and obesity), despite coronary artery disease still being uncommon in the African continent.[59]

CLINICAL CORRELATION

Patients with HFPEF seem to have comparable hospitalization rates with patients with HFREF.[10] Because approximately 50% of all patients with heart failure have preserved ejection fraction, about half of the total burden of heart failure costs is presumably arise from HFPEF. In 2010, there were 1801 million physician office visits with heart failure as the primary diagnosis.[47] The number of emergency room visits as a result of heart failure was 668,000 and the number of outpatient visits was 293,000 in 2009.[47] Further, most hospitalizations among patients with heart failure (>50%) are for noncardiac causes that were not included in the statistics discussed earlier.[60] Although heart failure hospitalization rates seem to have declined during the past decade (age-adjusted, sex-adjusted, and race-adjusted rates were reported to be 2845 per 100,000 person-years in 1998, and 2007 per 100,000 person-years in 2008 [$P<.001$] among Medicare beneficiaries),[61] the clinical and community burden of heart failure is still high and is expected to increase because of the growing number of elderly individuals. The recent American Heart Association's Heart Disease and Stroke Statistics projections predicted an increase of almost 120% in total cost of heart failure in the United States in 2030 compared with 2013 (from US $32 to 70 billion).[47]

SUMMARY

HFPEF still poses a diagnostic challenge and mortalities associated with the condition vary widely between clinical trials, epidemiologic cohort studies, and hospitalization settings, partly because of differences in diagnostic criteria. In community-based surveys the prevalence of HFPEF approaches 10% for people more than 80 years of age, and incidence rates seem stable in the face of a growing prevalence. The overall prognosis of patients with HFPEF remains poor. Thus, prevalence as well as costs related to HFPEF is expected to increase in the United States as well as internationally. Given that HFPEF poses a considerable societal burden, efforts are warranted to reduce its burden through better control of modifiable risk factors like hypertension, diabetes, and obesity.

REFERENCES

1. Cleland JG, Pellicori P. Defining diastolic heart failure and identifying effective therapies. JAMA 2013; 309:825–6.

2. Vasan RS, Levy D. Defining diastolic heart failure: a call for standardized diagnostic criteria. Circulation 2000;101:2118–21.

3. McMurray JJ, Adamopoulos S, Anker SD, et al. ESC guidelines for the diagnosis and treatment of acute and chronic heart failure 2012: The Task Force for the Diagnosis and Treatment of Acute and Chronic Heart Failure 2012 of the European Society of Cardiology. Developed in collaboration with the Heart Failure Association (HFA) of the ESC. Eur Heart J 2012;33:1787–847.

4. Yancy CW, Jessup M, Bozkurt B, et al. 2013 ACCF/AHA guideline for the management of heart failure: executive summary: a report of the American College of Cardiology Foundation/American Heart Association Task Force on practice guidelines. Circulation 2013;128:1810–52.

5. Caruana L, Petrie MC, Davie AP, et al. Do patients with suspected heart failure and preserved left ventricular systolic function suffer from "diastolic heart failure" or from misdiagnosis? A prospective descriptive study. BMJ 2000;321:215–8.

6. Edelmann F, Wachter R, Schmidt AG, et al. Effect of spironolactone on diastolic function and exercise capacity in patients with heart failure with preserved ejection fraction: the Aldo-DHF randomized controlled trial. JAMA 2013;309:781–91.

7. Maestre A, Gil V, Gallego J, et al. Diagnostic accuracy of clinical criteria for identifying systolic and diastolic heart failure: cross-sectional study. J Eval Clin Pract 2009;15:55–61.

8. Maurer MS, King DL, El-Khoury Rumbarger L, et al. Left heart failure with a normal ejection fraction: identification of different pathophysiologic mechanisms. J Card Fail 2005;11:177–87.

9. Vasan RS, Levy D. The role of hypertension in the pathogenesis of heart failure. A clinical mechanistic overview. Arch Intern Med 1996; 156:1789–96.

10. Fonarow GC, Stough WG, Abraham WT, et al. Characteristics, treatments, and outcomes of patients with preserved systolic function hospitalized for heart failure: a report from the OPTIMIZE-HF Registry. J Am Coll Cardiol 2007;50:768–77.

11. Vasan RS, Benjamin EJ, Levy D. Prevalence, clinical features and prognosis of diastolic heart failure: an epidemiologic perspective. J Am Coll Cardiol 1995;26:1565–74.

12. Ceia F, Fonseca C, Mota T, et al. Prevalence of chronic heart failure in southwestern Europe: the EPICA study. Eur J Heart Fail 2002;4:531–9.

13. Maisel WH, Stevenson LW. Atrial fibrillation in heart failure: epidemiology, pathophysiology, and rationale for therapy. Am J Cardiol 2003;91:2D–8D.

14. Kenchaiah S, Evans JC, Levy D, et al. Obesity and the risk of heart failure. N Engl J Med 2002;347: 305–13.

15. Fang ZY, Prins JB, Marwick TH. Diabetic cardiomyopathy: evidence, mechanisms, and therapeutic implications. Endocr Rev 2004;25:543–67.

16. Meta-analysis Global Group in Chronic Heart Failure (MAGGIC). The survival of patients with heart failure with preserved or reduced left ventricular ejection fraction: an individual patient data meta-analysis. Eur Heart J 2012;33:1750–7.

17. Massie BM, Carson PE, McMurray JJ, et al. Irbesartan in patients with heart failure and preserved ejection fraction. N Engl J Med 2008;359:2456–67.

18. Cleland JG, Tendera M, Adamus J, et al. The Perindopril in Elderly People with Chronic Heart Failure (PEP-CHF) study. Eur Heart J 2006;27:2338–45.

19. Chinali M, Joffe SW, Aurigemma GP, et al. Risk factors and comorbidities in a community-wide sample of patients hospitalized with acute systolic or diastolic heart failure: the Worcester Heart Failure Study. Coron Artery Dis 2010;21:137–43.

20. Redfield MM, Chen HH, Borlaug BA, et al. Effect of phosphodiesterase-5 inhibition on exercise capacity and clinical status in heart failure with preserved ejection fraction: a randomized clinical trial. JAMA 2013;309:1268–77.

21. Guder G, Frantz S, Bauersachs J, et al. Reverse epidemiology in systolic and nonsystolic heart failure: cumulative prognostic benefit of classical cardiovascular risk factors. Circ Heart Fail 2009;2: 563–71.

22. Andersson C, Gislason GH, Weeke P, et al. The prognostic importance of a history of hypertension in patients with symptomatic heart failure is substantially worsened by a short mitral inflow deceleration time. BMC Cardiovasc Disord 2012;12:30.

23. Lee DS, Gona P, Vasan RS, et al. Relation of disease pathogenesis and risk factors to heart failure with preserved or reduced ejection fraction: insights from the Framingham Heart Study of the National Heart, Lung, and Blood Institute. Circulation 2009;119:3070–7.

24. Mogelvang R, Sogaard P, Pedersen SA, et al. Tissue Doppler echocardiography in persons with hypertension, diabetes, or ischaemic heart disease: the Copenhagen City Heart Study. Eur Heart J 2009;30:731–9.

25. Hoffmann S, Jensen JS, Iversen AZ, et al. Tissue Doppler echocardiography improves the diagnosis of coronary artery stenosis in stable angina

pectoris. Eur Heart J Cardiovasc Imaging 2012;13: 724–9.

26. Garcia-Fernandez MA, Azevedo J, Moreno M, et al. Regional diastolic function in ischaemic heart disease using pulsed wave Doppler tissue imaging. Eur Heart J 1999;20:496–505.

27. Nagueh SF, Rao L, Soto J, et al. Haemodynamic insights into the effects of ischaemia and cycle length on tissue Doppler-derived mitral annulus diastolic velocities. Clin Sci (Lond) 2004;106: 147–54.

28. Lewis EF, Solomon SD, Jablonski KA, et al. Predictors of heart failure in patients with stable coronary artery disease: a PEACE study. Circ Heart Fail 2009;2:209–16.

29. Vaccarino V. Ischemic heart disease in women: many questions, few facts. Circ Cardiovasc Qual Outcomes 2010;3:111–5.

30. Ho JE, Lyass A, Lee DS, et al. Predictors of new-onset heart failure: differences in preserved versus reduced ejection fraction. Circ Heart Fail 2013;6: 279–86.

31. Brouwers FP, de Boer RA, van der Harst P, et al. Incidence and epidemiology of new onset heart failure with preserved vs. reduced ejection fraction in a community-based cohort: 11-year follow-up of PREVEND. Eur Heart J 2013;34:1424–31.

32. Hogg K, Swedberg K, McMurray J. Heart failure with preserved left ventricular systolic function; epidemiology, clinical characteristics, and prognosis. J Am Coll Cardiol 2004;43:317–27.

33. Mogensen UM, Ersboll M, Andersen M, et al. Clinical characteristics and major comorbidities in heart failure patients more than 85 years of age compared with younger age groups. Eur J Heart Fail 2011;13:1216–23.

34. Bitter T, Faber L, Hering D, et al. Sleep-disordered breathing in heart failure with normal left ventricular ejection fraction. Eur J Heart Fail 2009;11:602–8.

35. Ather S, Chan W, Bozkurt B, et al. Impact of noncardiac comorbidities on morbidity and mortality in a predominantly male population with heart failure and preserved versus reduced ejection fraction. J Am Coll Cardiol 2012;59:998–1005.

36. Rijzewijk LJ, van der Meer RW, Smit JW, et al. Myocardial steatosis is an independent predictor of diastolic dysfunction in type 2 diabetes mellitus. J Am Coll Cardiol 2008;52:1793–9.

37. Myasoedova E, Crowson CS, Nicola PJ, et al. The influence of rheumatoid arthritis disease characteristics on heart failure. J Rheumatol 2011;38: 1601–6.

38. Davis JM 3rd, Roger VL, Crowson CS, et al. The presentation and outcome of heart failure in patients with rheumatoid arthritis differs from that in the general population. Arthritis Rheum 2008;58: 2603–11.

39. Roman MJ, Salmon JE. Cardiovascular manifestations of rheumatologic diseases. Circulation 2007; 116:2346–55.

40. Bhatia RS, Tu JV, Lee DS, et al. Outcome of heart failure with preserved ejection fraction in a population-based study. N Engl J Med 2006;355:260–9.

41. Maxwell CB, Jenkins AT. Drug-induced heart failure. Am J Health Syst Pharm 2011;68:1791–804.

42. Kane GC, Karon BL, Mahoney DW, et al. Progression of left ventricular diastolic dysfunction and risk of heart failure. JAMA 2011;306:856–63.

43. Lam CS, Lyass A, Kraigher-Krainer E, et al. Cardiac dysfunction and noncardiac dysfunction as precursors of heart failure with reduced and preserved ejection fraction in the community. Circulation 2011;124:24–30.

44. Velagaleti RS, Gona P, Pencina MJ, et al. Left ventricular hypertrophy patterns and incidence of heart failure with preserved versus reduced ejection fraction. Am J Cardiol 2014;113:117–22.

45. Neeland IJ, Drazner MH, Berry JD, et al. Biomarkers of chronic cardiac injury and hemodynamic stress identify a malignant phenotype of left ventricular hypertrophy in the general population. J Am Coll Cardiol 2013;61:187–95.

46. Cheng JM, Akkerhuis KM, Battes LC, et al. Biomarkers of heart failure with normal ejection fraction: a systematic review. Eur J Heart Fail 2013; 15:1350–62.

47. Go AS, Mozaffarian D, Roger VL, et al. Executive summary: heart disease and stroke statistics–2013 update: a report from the American Heart Association. Circulation 2013;127:143–52.

48. Owan TE, Hodge DO, Herges RM, et al. Trends in prevalence and outcome of heart failure with preserved ejection fraction. N Engl J Med 2006;355: 251–9.

49. Lim SS, Vos T, Flaxman AD, et al. A comparative risk assessment of burden of disease and injury attributable to 67 risk factors and risk factor clusters in 21 regions, 1990–2010: a systematic analysis for the Global Burden of Disease Study 2010. Lancet 2012;380:2224–60.

50. Steinberg BA, Zhao X, Heidenreich PA, et al. Trends in patients hospitalized with heart failure and preserved left ventricular ejection fraction: prevalence, therapies, and outcomes. Circulation 2012;126:65–75.

51. Roger VL, Weston SA, Redfield MM, et al. Trends in heart failure incidence and survival in a community-based population. JAMA 2004;292:344–50.

52. Murad K, Kitzman DW. Frailty and multiple comorbidities in the elderly patient with heart failure: implications for management. Heart Fail Rev 2012; 17:581–8.

53. Vasan RS, Larson MG, Benjamin EJ, et al. Congestive heart failure in subjects with normal versus

reduced left ventricular ejection fraction: prevalence and mortality in a population-based cohort. J Am Coll Cardiol 1999;33:1948–55.

54. Henkel DM, Redfield MM, Weston SA, et al. Death in heart failure: a community perspective. Circ Heart Fail 2008;1:91–7.

55. Chan MM, Lam CS. How do patients with heart failure with preserved ejection fraction die? Eur J Heart Fail 2013;15:604–13.

56. Campbell RT, Jhund PS, Castagno D, et al. What have we learned about patients with heart failure and preserved ejection fraction from DIG-PEF, CHARM-preserved, and I-PRESERVE? J Am Coll Cardiol 2012;60:2349–56.

57. Tribouilloy C, Rusinaru D, Mahjoub H, et al. Prognosis of heart failure with preserved ejection fraction: a 5 year prospective population-based study. Eur Heart J 2008;29:339–47.

58. Somaratne JB, Berry C, McMurray JJ, et al. The prognostic significance of heart failure with preserved left ventricular ejection fraction: a literature-based meta-analysis. Eur J Heart Fail 2009;11:855–62.

59. Ntusi NB, Mayosi BM. Epidemiology of heart failure in sub-Saharan Africa. Expert Rev Cardiovasc Ther 2009;7:169–80.

60. Dunlay SM, Redfield MM, Weston SA, et al. Hospitalizations after heart failure diagnosis a community perspective. J Am Coll Cardiol 2009;54:1695–702.

61. Chen J, Normand SL, Wang Y, et al. National and regional trends in heart failure hospitalization and mortality rates for Medicare beneficiaries, 1998-2008. JAMA 2011;306:1669–78.

62. Shah AM, Shah SJ, Anand IS, et al. Cardiac structure and function in heart failure with preserved ejection fraction: baseline findings from the echocardiographic study of the treatment of preserved cardiac function heart failure with an aldosterone antagonist trial. Circ Heart Fail 2014;7:104–15.

63. Solomon SD, Zile M, Pieske B, et al. The angiotensin receptor neprilysin inhibitor LCZ696 in heart failure with preserved ejection fraction: a phase 2 double-blind randomised controlled trial. Lancet 2012;380:1387–95.

64. Zile MR, Gottdiener JS, Hetzel SJ, et al. Prevalence and significance of alterations in cardiac structure and function in patients with heart failure and a preserved ejection fraction. Circulation 2011;124:2491–501.

65. Persson H, Lonn E, Edner M, et al. Diastolic dysfunction in heart failure with preserved systolic function: need for objective evidence: results from the CHARM Echocardiographic Substudy-CHARMES. J Am Coll Cardiol 2007;49:687–94.

66. Yusuf S, Pfeffer MA, Swedberg K, et al. Effects of candesartan in patients with chronic heart failure and preserved left-ventricular ejection fraction: the CHARM-Preserved Trial. Lancet 2003;362:777–81.

67. Lam CS, Roger VL, Rodeheffer RJ, et al. Cardiac structure and ventricular-vascular function in persons with heart failure and preserved ejection fraction from Olmsted County, Minnesota. Circulation 2007;115:1982–90.

68. Maurer MS, Burkhoff D, Fried LP, et al. Ventricular structure and function in hypertensive participants with heart failure and a normal ejection fraction: the Cardiovascular Health Study. J Am Coll Cardiol 2007;49:972–81.

69. He KL, Burkhoff D, Leng WX, et al. Comparison of ventricular structure and function in Chinese patients with heart failure and ejection fractions >55% versus 40% to 55% versus <40%. Am J Cardiol 2009;103:845–51.

70. Gupta DK, Shah AM, Castagno D, et al. Heart failure with preserved ejection fraction in African-Americans - The Atherosclerosis Risk in Communities (ARIC) Study. JACC Heart Fail 2013;1:156–63.

71. Klapholz M, Maurer M, Lowe AM, et al. Hospitalization for heart failure in the presence of a normal left ventricular ejection fraction: results of the New York Heart Failure Registry. J Am Coll Cardiol 2004;43:1432–8.

72. Katz DH, Beussink L, Sauer AJ, et al. Prevalence, clinical characteristics, and outcomes associated with eccentric versus concentric left ventricular hypertrophy in heart failure with preserved ejection fraction. Am J Cardiol 2013;112:1158–64.

Causes and Pathophysiology of Heart Failure with Preserved Ejection Fraction

Árpád Kovács, MD, Zoltán Papp, MD, PhD, DSc*,
László Nagy, MD

KEYWORDS

- Heart failure with preserved ejection fraction • Ventricular-arterial uncoupling • Exercise intolerance
- Comorbidities • Myocardial stiffness

KEY POINTS

- The pathophysiology of heart failure with preserved ejection fraction (HFPEF) is driven by interactions among age-dependent and gender-dependent characteristics of ventricular-arterial coupling and various predisposing comorbidities and risk factors.
- Ventricular diastolic dysfunction is central in the pathogenesis of HFPEF caused by an increased ventricular stiffness and is responsible for limited exercise tolerance.
- At tissue, cellular, and molecular levels, concentric myocardial hypertrophy, alterations in extracellular matrix and fibrosis, expressional changes, and posttranslational modifications of titin leading to increased cardiomyocyte passive stiffness ($F_{passive}$) as well as perturbations of intracellular Ca^{2+} handling have been implicated.
- Further phenotyping of patients with HFPEF and preclinical studies in animal models of HFPEF may bring further insights into the pathogenesis of the complex syndrome of HFPEF.

INTRODUCTION

Clinical experience of the last 2 decades has shown that the prognosis of heart failure (HF) has improved when the ejection fraction (EF) is reduced (HFREF), but not when the EF is preserved (HFPEF). A distinction between the pathophysiologic background for these syndromes is also supported by their pathomorphologic phenotypes: mainly eccentric left ventricular (LV) remodeling in HFREF versus concentric remodeling in HFPEF.[1–3] Nevertheless, diverse patterns of ventricular remodeling in patients with HFPEF were also shown mirroring the clinical and pathophysiologic heterogeneity of this syndrome. These findings suggest that although concentric LV remodeling is common among patients with HFPEF, many of them show normal LV dimensions or may even have an eccentric pattern.[4]

The typical patient with HFPEF is an elderly woman with a clinical history of systolic hypertension (HT), diabetes mellitus (DM), and obesity.[5] One of the initial signs of HFPEF is decreased exercise tolerance during physical stress.[6] Further progression leads to the appearance of clinical

This work was supported by the Social Renewal Operational Programme [TÁMOP-4.2.2.A-11/1/KONV-2012-0045], by a Hungarian Scientific Research Fund [OTKA K 109083], and by the European Union Project FP7-HEALTH-2010: "MEDIA-Metabolic Road to Diastolic Heart Failure" MEDIA-261409.
The authors have nothing to disclose.
Division of Clinical Physiology, Faculty of Medicine, Institute of Cardiology, University of Debrecen, Móricz Zs. krt. 22, Debrecen 4032, Hungary
* Corresponding author.
E-mail address: pappz@med.unideb.hu

Heart Failure Clin 10 (2014) 389–398
http://dx.doi.org/10.1016/j.hfc.2014.04.002
1551-7136/14/$ – see front matter

symptoms at rest: dyspnea, fatigue, coughing, and lung crepitation caused by pulmonary congestion, often accompanied by paroxysmal attacks of acute HF episodes with pulmonary edema.[7] In addition, patients with HFPEF are vulnerable to small changes in volume regulation, resulting in severe hypotension or hypertensive crisis.[8]

HFPEF: A SYNDROME OF DERANGED VENTRICULAR-ARTERIAL COUPLING
Interaction Between the Heart and Vasculature Is the Achilles Heel of the Cardiovascular System

HFPEF is increasingly recognized as a disease of abnormal ventricular-arterial coupling in association with decreased exercise tolerance.[9] To understand the main pathologic pathways leading to this exercise intolerance, basic issues of hemodynamic coupling between the heart and the vasculature should be reviewed under physiologic and pathologic conditions.

The term of ventricular-arterial coupling refers to an interaction between the heart and the vascular system, because the stroke volume (SV) from the LV is transferred toward the vascular tree.[10] Ideal coupling provides optimal working efficiency for the cardiovascular system in several ways. On the one hand, good ventricular-arterial coupling maintains continuous blood flow without exaggerated fluctuations in blood pressure (BP) and hence it protects peripheral organs. On the other hand, an optimal ventricular-arterial coupling allows the mobilization of cardiovascular reserve mechanisms during conditions of increased metabolic demands.[11]

To investigate the relationship between the heart and the vascular system, it is necessary to include indices characterizing ventricular and vascular properties within the same framework. One of the models allowing this type of analysis operates with LV end-systolic elastance (E_{es}) and arterial elastance (E_a), both derived from the LV pressure-volume (P-V) relationship of the cardiac cycle (**Fig. 1A**).[12] Ventricular function can be

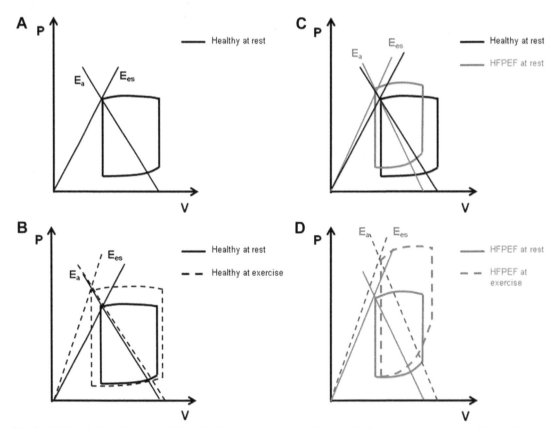

Fig. 1. LV P-V relationships in healthy individuals and patients with HFPEF. (*A*) Ventricular contractility, E_{es} (ie, the slope of the LV end-systolic P-V relationship) and the E_a (ie, the negative slope of the line through the end-systolic and end-diastolic P-V points of LV P-V relations) in healthy individuals at rest. Under normal conditions E_{es} is increased during exercise (*B*). HFPEF is associated with increased baseline E_{es} values at rest (caused by increased LV stiffness) and with increased LV end-diastolic pressure (LVEDP) (*C*). Dynamic exercise results in augmented increases in arterial BP caused by increased ventricular and arterial stiffness in patients with HFPEF (*D*).

characterized by its capacity to empty its SV into the vasculature: ie, LVEF reflects the systolic functions, but it also tightly depends on hemodynamic external forces (preload and afterload) modulating the cardiovascular performance.[13] An alternative measure of LV contractility (reflecting also the loading conditions) is E_{es}, which is the slope of the LV end-systolic P-V relationship.[14] E_a characterizes the vascular part of the coupling and it is shown as the negative slope of the line through the end-systolic and end-diastolic P-V points of the LV P-V relationship.[15] Ventricular-arterial coupling when expressed as the ratio of E_a and E_{es} (E_a/E_{es}) is considered to be optimal when it ranges between 0.6 and 1.2.[16] The reserve function of ventricular-arterial coupling can be shown during physical exercise, when E_a/E_{es} ratio typically decreases as a result of a greater enhancement in E_{es} exceeding that of E_a (**Fig. 1B**).[17] Baseline values for E_a/E_{es} ratio are maintained during aging as a result of similar trends in gradually increasing E_a and E_{es} parameters. Nevertheless, aging in women leads to higher increases in E_a and E_{es} than in those of age-matched men, resulting in distinctions between ventricular-arterial coupling in aged women and aged men, even at rest.[18] The exercise-induced decrease in E_a/E_{es} (representing cardiovascular reserve) is attenuated by aging, thereby contributing to exercise intolerance; moreover, this phenomenon is more pronounced in the presence of other precipitating factors of ventricular-arterial uncoupling, as detailed later.[19]

Ventricular-Arterial Stiffening in HFPEF Resulting in Abnormal Ventricular-Arterial Coupling

The basic mechanism leading to impaired ventricular-arterial coupling in HFPEF is increased stiffening in the cardiovascular system, resulting in cardiac and vascular dysfunctions. Patients with HFPEF were reported to have decreased E_a/E_{es} ratios when compared with those of age-matched controls, but not when compared with hypertensive controls without HF (**Fig. 1C**).[18,20]

Diastolic dysfunction in HFPEF

The main features of LV diastolic dysfunction are: slowed LV relaxation, enhanced LV stiffness,[21] reduced ventricular restoring forces,[10] impaired diastolic suction,[22] and ventricular dyssynchrony.[23] From the practical point of view, characterization of diastolic function is more difficult than that of systolic function, and this is also reflected by the many currently used quantitative indices of LV diastolic function obtained by invasive hemodynamic tests and noninvasive investigations.

Borlaug and colleagues[24] emphasized that impaired early diastolic filling is well shown by the time constant of early diastolic pressure decay (τ). This parameter was described to be increased at rest and it failed to decrease during exercise. However, not all hemodynamic studies of this kind confirmed this finding, and conversely, some showed preserved isovolumic relaxation properties in patients with HFPEF.[25]

Early diastolic lengthening velocity (E') measured by tissue Doppler imaging is increasingly considered as a marker sensitive enough for the characterization of LV diastolic function.[26] In addition, the ratio of early mitral valve flow velocity (E) and E' shows a tight correlation with LV filling pressures (FPs).[27] Patients with HFPEF tend to have decreased early diastolic velocities (characterized by lower E' measures at rest), in combination with their inadequate enhancements during exercise.[28,29]

Increased LV stiffness can also evoke inadequate LV filling during diastole; it was reported by Kitzman and colleagues[30] as a result of a hypothetical failure of the Frank-Starling mechanism. In their studies, these investigators found a blunted end-diastolic volume (EDV) increase in response to invasive cardiopulmonary exercise testing. However, most recent studies[31] have not confirmed such a depletion of EDV response during exercise. What seems to be universally characteristic for the LV function is increased LV end-diastolic pressure (LVEDP), resulting in an upward and leftward shift of the LV P-V relationship when compared with that of control (**Fig. 1C**).[24,32]

In addition, HFPEF is often associated with cardiac dyssynchrony, resulting in further impairment of exercise capacity. Mechanical dyssynchrony is referred as differences in the onsets or peaks of contractions/relaxations between the LV and right ventricle (interventricular dyssynchrony), or between different myocardial segments of the LV (intraventricular dyssynchrony). Mechanical dyssynchrony can be assessed by two-dimensional or three-dimensional speckle tracking imaging via determining systolic and diastolic abnormalities of ventricular torsion, untwist, and longitudinal motion during contraction and relaxation.[23]

Abnormalities in ventricular suction mechanism may also contribute to deranged diastolic functions in HFPEF. In normal conditions, during the early phase of isovolumic relaxation, LV pressure decreases lower than the pressure of the left atrium (LA), providing a drive for blood flow toward the LV.[22] In addition, there is a progressive intraventricular pressure difference (IVPD) as well, extending from the LA to the LV apex, increasing in response to adrenergic stimulation.[33] These physiologic mechanisms allow the heart to function as a dynamic suction pump. A deranged ventricular suction has been shown by significantly increased LV minimal diastolic pressure values during diastolic recoil in patients with HFPEF.[32] Moreover, HFPEF is also associated with a reduced adrenergic augmentation of the IVPD to the LV apex, indicating less apical suction.[33] In a study by Tan and colleagues,[23] early diastolic mitral flow propagation velocity served as an approximation for suction and was found to be comparable between patients with HFPEF and control at rest, but it was reported to be significantly attenuated during exercise, with the inability to augment ventricular suction in patients with HFPEF.

Systolic dysfunction in HFPEF

Systolic abnormalities can also be associated with increased ventricular stiffness. Although systolic function and its measures (eg, EF) are preserved or slightly reduced at rest, the contractile responses in LVEF, SV, or cardiac output are often blunted during exercise in patients with HFPEF, resulting in further impairments in exercise capacity.[21,34] Theoretically, increased E_{es} may reflect enhanced LV contractility. However, in HFPEF, the high basal E_{es} indicates increased LV stiffness rather than enhanced contractility.[35]

Moreover, an increased steepness of the end-systolic P-V relationship with high basal E_{es} evokes hemodynamic instabilities. Accordingly, for a given increase in preload (eg, dynamic exercise, see **Fig. 1**D), systolic BP increases in an exaggerated fashion, whereas a decrease in preload (eg, diuretic therapy) evokes greater decreases of systolic BP in patients with HFPEF than is seen in healthy individuals.[36] In addition, mechanical cardiac dyssynchrony also contributes to the impairment of systolic function, because systolic longitudinal and radial strain, apical rotation, and longitudinal motions are all considered to be low in patients with HFPEF at rest, and they fail to increase during exercise.[23] Taken together, decreased systolic reserve capacity may contribute to exercise intolerance in HFPEF with normal or mildly reduced systolic functions.

Chronotropic incompetence in HFPEF

Chronotropic incompetence, the inability to increase heart rate [HR] during exercise, is tightly coupled to impaired systolic function in patients with HFPEF and it is believed to contribute to exercise intolerance.[37] Plasma catecholamine levels seem to be comparable between control and HF groups, suggesting perturbations in adrenergic signaling at the myocardial level.[37] Diminished chronotropic reserve capacity was also confirmed by a study of Phan and colleagues,[38] in which an impaired HR recovery was also described at the end of metabolic exercise tests in patients with HFPEF.

Vascular stiffening in HFPEF

In addition to the enhanced ventricular stiffness, decreased vascular compliance is also associated with HFPEF. However, increased arterial stiffness can also be shown in patients without HFPEF, because Goto and colleagues[12] reported significantly increased E_a in old, but otherwise healthy women. Generally speaking, high vascular stiffness can affect both the proximal[39] and distal[40] part of the vascular system. Decreased arterial compliance can be the consequence of inadequate peripheral vasodilatation caused by endothelial dysfunction, and this feature has been correlated with poor clinical outcome.[41,42] As a hemodynamic consequence, augmented pulse pressure waves are ejected during systoles. Moreover, arterial pressure waves rebounding from arterial bifurcations may be amplified by stiff proximal vessels.[43] All of these hemodynamic perturbations reflecting backwards to the chambers can further impair systolic and diastolic LV functions.[44]

RISK FACTORS AND COMORBIDITIES AS TRIGGERS IN HFPEF

Comorbidities have major influence on the pathogenesis of HFPEF. In addition to the primary age-dependent derangements between the myocardium and the vascular system,[18] various comorbidities may evoke additional adverse effects on ventricular and vascular functions[45] (**Fig. 2**). Moreover, the prognosis of HFPEF with comorbidities is worse than can be expected with comorbidities alone.[46]

Because multiple comorbidities influence the prognosis of HFPEF, their targeted treatment takes priority and may be more beneficial in HFPEF than in HFREF.[47] Hence, it has been suggested that the greatest reductions in overall morbidity and mortality may result from treating comorbidities with currently available therapies,[48] in contrast to HFREF, in which final common pathways such as the renin-angiotensin-aldosterone system and the high sympathetic activity can be effectively influenced, even at a late stage of the disease, irrespective of the initial cause.[49]

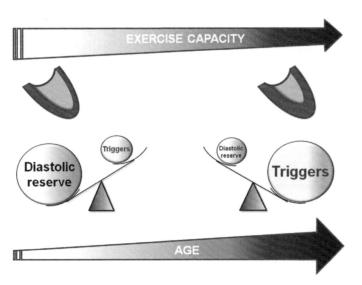

Fig. 2. HFPEF is a progressive disease developing in the context of cardiovascular aging, triggering comorbidities; it mostly associates with concentric hypertrophy. Aging of the cardiovascular system associates with reduced exercise capacity caused by limitations in diastolic reserve. Causes and comorbidities act like triggers and accelerate the development of HFPEF.

CELLULAR AND MOLECULAR MECHANISMS OF INCREASED STIFFNESS: TRANSLATION OF COMORBIDITIES TO PATHOPHYSIOLOGY

Myocardial remodeling in HFPEF differs from that in HFREF, in which myocardial remodeling is dominated by cardiomyocyte loss.[50] In contrast, in HFPEF, numerous comorbidities result in cellular and molecular changes that promote cardiac and vascular stiffening and contribute to LV diastolic dysfunction (**Fig. 3**).

Myofilament Determinants of Cellular Stiffness

With respect to myocardial stiffness, the contributions of myofilament proteins, especially titin, and of extracellular matrix (ECM) deserve attention. The giant titin molecule is known as one of the main determinants of Ca^{2+}-independent passive stiffness ($F_{passive}$) of isolated cardiomyocytes. Results of preclinical investigations by Linke and Kruger[51] have suggested that the biophysical properties of titin contribute more to $F_{passive}$ at lower sarcomere lengths (ie, between 1.9 μm and 2.2 μm), whereas the contribution of extracellular collagen to myocardial stiffness gains dominance around sarcomere lengths of 2.2 μm–2.3 μm. These observations suggest a more dominant role for collagen in the mechanical properties of dilated hearts than in hearts with normal LV dimensions.

Borbely and colleagues[52] reported increased $F_{passive}$ of isolated cardiomyocytes together with higher collagen volume fraction (CVF) as determinants of in vivo diastolic LV dysfunction in patients with HFPEF. Moreover, distinct changes of LV samples were recognized between HFPEF

and HFREF in myocardial structure (ie, characteristics of collagen deposition and cardiomyocyte hypertrophy) and function (ie, high LVEDP and $F_{passive}$).[53] Nevertheless, in both cases in vitro administration of protein kinase A (PKA) treatment in permeabilized cardiomyocyte preparations had the potential to normalize $F_{passive}$.

In addition to titin-dependent changes in increased cardiomyocyte $F_{passive}$, the phosphorylation status or other types of posttranslational modifications in myofilament proteins can also modulate cardiomyocyte relaxation through influencing the Ca^{2+} sensitivity of force production.[54]

In the mammalian heart, 2 isoforms of titin, a compliant N2BA (3.2–3.7 MDa) and a stiff N2B (~3.0 MDa) are coexpressed; however, their ratio can be shifted toward the stiffer N2B during certain pathologic conditions. Besides changes in isoform expression, the elastic properties of titin are also determined by complex phosphorylation mechanisms. PKA, protein kinase G (PKG), extracellular signal-regulated kinase 2, and Ca^{2+}/calmodulin-dependent protein kinase II phosphorylate the N2-B unique sequence (N2Bus) of titin, thereby decreasing its stiffness, whereas protein kinase C phosphorylates the PEVK domain of titin, thereby increasing its stiffness.[51] Multiple phosphorylations of titin at different phosphorylation sites fundamentally alter the flexibility of the molecule, and therefore ventricular stiffness.

HFPEF with its highly prevalent metabolic comorbidities such as obesity and DM has been associated with low intracellular cyclic guanosine monophosphate (cGMP) concentrations. In a study by van Heerebeek and colleagues,[55] low myocardial PKG activity led to increased cardiomyocyte $F_{passive}$, and this condition may be

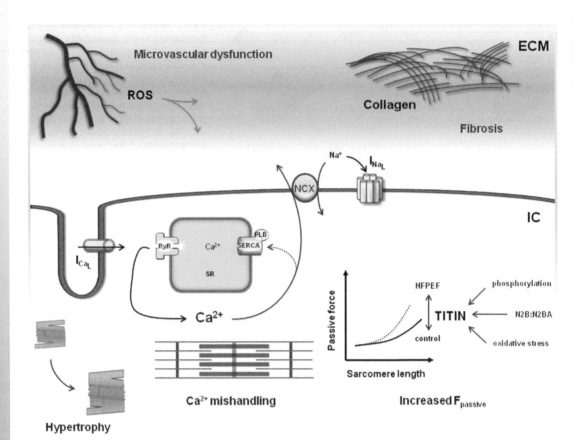

Fig. 3. Pathophysiologic mechanisms contributing to increased myocardial stiffness in HFPEF. Several pathogenic factors have been recognized in HFPEF, ranging from microvascular dysfunction to increased cardiomyocyte $F_{passive}$ (see text for details). (ECM, extracellular matrix; $F_{passive}$, cardiomyocyte passive stiffness; IC, intracellular space; I_{Ca_L}, ion current through L-type Ca^{2+}-channel; I_{Na_L}, ion current through late Na^+-channel; NCX, Na^+/Ca^{2+} exchanger; PLB, phospholamban; ROS, reactive oxygen species; RyR, ryanodine receptor; SERCA, sarcoplasmic reticulum Ca^{2+} ATPase; SR, sarcoplasmic reticulum).

caused by higher myocardial nitrosative/oxidative stress originating from comorbidities themselves. Titin can be modified by oxidative stress, which could be an additional contributor to the increased diastolic LV stiffness. By promoting the formation of disulfide bridges within the cardiac N2Bus domain, oxidative stress can stiffen the whole titin molecule, resulting in increased $F_{passive}$.[51]

Aortic stenosis (AS) as a frequent pathology in old patients increases LV afterload. When AS was complicated with DM, LV end-diastolic distensibility was reduced more than without DM. This more severe diastolic LV dysfunction in patients with AS and DM predisposing to HF was associated with high CVF, increased intramyocardial vascular advanced glycation end product (AGE) deposition, and high cardiomyocyte $F_{passive}$ caused by hypophosphorylation of the N2B titin isoform.[56] These findings support a role for disease modifier comorbidities in the pathophysiology of HFPEF.

Titin Versus Collagen

Basic mechanisms leading to increased diastolic stiffness seem to be different in diabetic patients with HFREF or with HFPEF. Deposition of AGEs and fibrosis are more important for the increased LV stiffness in diabetic patients with HFREF, whereas high cardiomyocyte $F_{passive}$ seems to be the main determinant of increased LV stiffness in diabetic patients with HFPEF.[57] In hypertensive patients with or without HF, the amount of collagen tissue, the extent of collagen type I deposition, and the coronary or peripheral PICP (carboxy-terminal propeptide of procollagen type I, as an index of collagen type I synthesis) were higher than those in normotensives.[58] Moreover, in hypertensive patients with HFPEF, LV FPs were increased and showed an apparent correlation with the pattern of collagen metabolism. In the study of Gonzalez and colleagues,[59] in patients with increased FPs, increased collagen synthesis was accompanied by unchanged collagen degradation because of a relative excess of TIMP-1, the tissue inhibitor of matrix metalloproteinase 1 (MMP-1), as well as a decrease in the major collagenase system (MMP-1) in the heart. Moreover, increased expression of profibrotic growth factor (transforming growth factor β) produced by a subgroup of inflammatory cells has also been documented in patients with HFPEF. The apparent relationship among cardiac collagen, the amount of inflammatory cells, and diastolic dysfunction suggests a direct influence of inflammation on myocardial fibrosis, triggering diastolic dysfunction.[60]

When analyzing early pathophysiologic events in HFPEF, studies with congenital heart disease may have particular significance. For example, in hypertrophic cardiomyopathy (HCM), besides pathologic alterations in Ca^{2+}-regulated ventricular relaxation, accumulation of interstitial collagen was also documented.[61] Increased levels of serum PICP showed increased myocardial collagen synthesis in sarcomere-mutation carriers of patients with HCM without overt disease, suggesting that the stimulus for myocardial fibrosis is a fundamental, early manifestation of sarcomere-gene mutations.[62] Observations[63] carried out on endomyocardial ventricular biopsies obtained at open heart surgery showed that systolic pressure overload resulted both in increased cardiomyocyte stiffness and ECM reorganization.

Coronary Microvascular Oxidative Stress

A new concept from Paulus and Tschope[50] about cellular and molecular processes in HFPEF is based on a systemic proinflammatory state induced by multiple comorbidities such as obesity, HT, DM, chronic obstructive pulmonary disease, and anemia. These conditions are accompanied by oxidative stress in the coronary microvascular endothelium, reducing nitric oxide (NO) bioavailability, cGMP content, and PKG activity in the adjacent cardiomyocytes. Low PKG activity promotes hypertrophy and (through PKG-mediated hypophosphorylation of titin) it increases passive stiffness of cardiomyocytes. Both stiff cardiomyocytes and interstitial fibrosis contribute to high diastolic LV stiffness and HF development. Although peripheral endothelial dysfunction correlates with future cardiovascular events in patients with HFPEF,[42] cardiac oxidation by itself can lead to uncoupled cardiac NO synthase and thereby diastolic dysfunction, even in the absence of significant changes in the vasculature.[64]

Disturbances in Ca^{2+}-Related Relaxation

Diastolic properties of the LV are determined not only by its passive mechanical characteristics, but also the active processes of myocardial relaxation. The latter refers mostly to the intracellular Ca^{2+} handling mechanisms; the abnormalities of these mechanisms may contribute to impaired ventricular relaxation during diastole. Collectively, all those pathologic processes, in which Ca^{2+} mishandling leads to increased resting Ca^{2+} concentrations, can result in increased ventricular tension during diastole.[65] Under normal conditions, cytosolic Ca^{2+} is either transferred either into the sarcoplasmic reticulum (SR) via SERCA, the phospholamban-regulated SR Ca^{2+} adenosine triphosphatase (ATPase), or pumped out from the cytosol toward the extracellular space by the Na^+/Ca^{2+} exchanger (NCX).

Oxidative posttranslational modifications (eg, carbonylation) and decreased expression of SERCA proteins can diminish SR Ca^{2+} uptake.[66,67] Rats with LV diastolic dysfunction showed derangements in the expression both of SERCA and of its regulatory molecule phospholamban.[66] In addition to potential disturbances in SERCA function, NCX may also contribute to increased intracellular Ca^{2+} loading during Na^+ accumulation (eg, because of reduced Na^+-K^+-ATPase activity).[68] In addition, ryanodine receptor Ca^{2+} leakage may also promote such perturbations in Ca^{2+} handling.[65,69] It is debated whether late sodium current (I_{Na_L}) is an important contributor to diastolic dysfunction in HFPEF. Previous experimental studies[70] showed positive results for I_{Na_L} inhibitor ranolazine improving diastolic functions. However, clinical trials were performed mostly in patient populations with systolic ventricular dysfunction and ischemic cardiomyopathy. Hence, future studies should make further efforts to avoid such overlaps between HFPEF and HFREF to elucidate the role of I_{Na_L} in HFPEF.[71]

SUMMARY

The pathophysiology of HFPEF is driven by interactions among age-dependent and gender-dependent characteristics of ventricular-arterial coupling and various predisposing comorbidities and risk factors. Ventricular diastolic dysfunction is central in the pathogenesis of HFPEF as a result of increased ventricular stiffness and it is responsible for limited exercise tolerance. At tissue, cellular, and molecular levels, concentric myocardial hypertrophy, alterations in ECM and fibrosis, expressional changes, and posttranslational modifications of titin (leading to increased cardiomyocyte $F_{passive}$) as well as perturbations of intracellular Ca^{2+} handling have been implicated. All these molecular mechanisms have the potential to contribute to LV stiffness; nevertheless, their contribution may depend on the given combination of predisposing pathogenic factors. Hence, further phenotyping of patients with HFPEF and preclinical studies in animal models of HFPEF may bring further insights into the pathogenesis of the complex syndrome of HFPEF. These efforts may help to pinpoint the central molecular mechanisms in the pathophysiology of HFPEF, with the hope of finding more effective future therapeutic approaches than currently available.

REFERENCES

1. Owan TE, Hodge DO, Herges RM, et al. Trends in prevalence and outcome of heart failure with preserved ejection fraction. N Engl J Med 2006;355: 251–9.
2. Zile MR, Gottdiener JS, Hetzel SJ, et al. Prevalence and significance of alterations in cardiac structure and function in patients with heart failure and a preserved ejection fraction. Circulation 2011;124: 2491–501.
3. Velagaleti RS, Gona P, Pencina MJ, et al. Left ventricular hypertrophy patterns and incidence of heart failure with preserved versus reduced ejection fraction. Am J Cardiol 2014;113:117–22.
4. Shah AM. Ventricular remodeling in heart failure with preserved ejection fraction. Curr Heart Fail Rep 2013;10:341–9.
5. Borbely A, Papp Z, Edes I, et al. Molecular determinants of heart failure with normal left ventricular ejection fraction. Pharmacol Rep 2009;61:139–45.
6. Borlaug BA, Nishimura RA, Sorajja P, et al. Exercise hemodynamics enhance diagnosis of early heart failure with preserved ejection fraction. Circ Heart Fail 2010;3:588–95.
7. Banerjee P, Clark AL, Nikitin N, et al. Diastolic heart failure. Paroxysmal or chronic? Eur J Heart Fail 2004;6:427–31.
8. Schwartzenberg S, Redfield MM, From AM, et al. Effects of vasodilation in heart failure with preserved or reduced ejection fraction implications of distinct pathophysiologies on response to therapy. J Am Coll Cardiol 2012;59:442–51.
9. Antonini-Canterin F, Carerj S, Di Bello V, et al. Arterial stiffness and ventricular stiffness: a couple of diseases or a coupling disease? A review from the cardiologist's point of view. Eur J Echocardiogr 2009;10(1):36–43.
10. Frenneaux M, Williams L. Ventricular-arterial and ventricular-ventricular interactions and their relevance to diastolic filling. Prog Cardiovasc Dis 2007;49:252–62.
11. O'Rourke MF, Yaginuma T, Avolio AP. Physiological and pathophysiological implications of ventricular/vascular coupling. Ann Biomed Eng 1984;12: 119–34.
12. Goto T, Ohte N, Fukuta H, et al. Relationship between effective arterial elastance, total vascular resistance, and augmentation index at the ascending aorta and left ventricular diastolic function in older women. Circ J 2013;77:123–9.
13. Dong SJ, Hees PS, Huang WM, et al. Independent effects of preload, afterload, and contractility on left ventricular torsion. Am J Physiol 1999;277(3 Pt 2): H1053–60.
14. Starling MR. Left ventricular-arterial coupling relations in the normal human heart. Am Heart J 1993;125:1659–66.
15. Sunagawa K, Maughan WL, Sagawa K. Optimal arterial resistance for the maximal stroke work studied in isolated canine left ventricle. Circ Res 1985;56:586–95.
16. Chantler PD, Lakatta EG, Najjar SS. Arterial-ventricular coupling: mechanistic insights into cardiovascular performance at rest and during exercise. J Appl Physiol (1985) 2008;105:1342–51.
17. De Tombe PP, Jones S, Burkhoff D, et al. Ventricular stroke work and efficiency both remain nearly optimal despite altered vascular loading. Am J Physiol 1993;264:H1817–24.
18. Redfield MM, Jacobsen SJ, Borlaug BA, et al. Age- and gender-related ventricular-vascular stiffening: a community-based study. Circulation 2005;112: 2254–62.
19. Chantler PD, Lakatta EG. Arterial-ventricular coupling with aging and disease. Front Physiol 2012;3:90.
20. Lam CS, Roger VL, Rodeheffer RJ, et al. Cardiac structure and ventricular-vascular function in persons with heart failure and preserved ejection fraction from Olmsted County, Minnesota. Circulation 2007;115(15):1982–90.
21. Phan TT, Abozguia K, Nallur Shivu G, et al. Heart failure with preserved ejection fraction is characterized by dynamic impairment of active relaxation and contraction of the left ventricle on exercise and associated with myocardial energy deficiency. J Am Coll Cardiol 2009;54:402–9.
22. Gillebert TC, De Buyzere ML. HFpEF, diastolic suction, and exercise. JACC Cardiovasc Imaging 2012;5:871–3.
23. Tan YT, Wenzelburger F, Lee E, et al. The pathophysiology of heart failure with normal ejection fraction: exercise echocardiography reveals complex abnormalities of both systolic and diastolic ventricular function involving torsion, untwist, and longitudinal motion. J Am Coll Cardiol 2009;54:36–46.
24. Borlaug BA, Jaber WA, Ommen SR, et al. Diastolic relaxation and compliance reserve during dynamic exercise in heart failure with preserved ejection fraction. Heart 2011;97:964–9.
25. Kawaguchi M, Hay I, Fetics B, et al. Combined ventricular systolic and arterial stiffening in patients

with heart failure and preserved ejection fraction: implications for systolic and diastolic reserve limitations. Circulation 2003;107:714–20.

26. Sohn DW, Chai IH, Lee DJ, et al. Assessment of mitral annulus velocity by Doppler tissue imaging in the evaluation of left ventricular diastolic function. J Am Coll Cardiol 1997;30:474–80.

27. Park JH, Marwick TH. Use and limitations of E/e' to assess left ventricular filling pressure by echocardiography. J Cardiovasc Ultrasound 2011;19:169–73.

28. Ha JW, Oh JK, Pellikka PA, et al. Diastolic stress echocardiography: a novel noninvasive diagnostic test for diastolic dysfunction using supine bicycle exercise Doppler echocardiography. J Am Soc Echocardiogr 2005;18:63–8.

29. Paulus WJ, Tschope C, Sanderson JE, et al. How to diagnose diastolic heart failure: a consensus statement on the diagnosis of heart failure with normal left ventricular ejection fraction by the Heart Failure and Echocardiography Associations of the European Society of Cardiology. Eur Heart J 2007; 28(20):2539–50.

30. Kitzman DW, Higginbotham MB, Cobb FR, et al. Exercise intolerance in patients with heart failure and preserved left ventricular systolic function: failure of the Frank-Starling mechanism. J Am Coll Cardiol 1991;17:1065–72.

31. Zile MR, Kjellstrom B, Bennett T, et al. Effects of exercise on left ventricular systolic and diastolic properties in patients with heart failure and a preserved ejection fraction versus heart failure and a reduced ejection fraction. Circ Heart Fail 2013;6:508–16.

32. Zile MR, Baicu CF, Gaasch WH. Diastolic heart failure–abnormalities in active relaxation and passive stiffness of the left ventricle. N Engl J Med 2004; 350:1953–9.

33. Ohara T, Niebel CL, Stewart KC, et al. Loss of adrenergic augmentation of diastolic intra-LV pressure difference in patients with diastolic dysfunction: evaluation by color M-mode echocardiography. JACC Cardiovasc Imaging 2012;5:861–70.

34. Abudiab MM, Redfield MM, Melenovsky V, et al. Cardiac output response to exercise in relation to metabolic demand in heart failure with preserved ejection fraction. Eur J Heart Fail 2013;15:776–85.

35. Borlaug BA, Lam CS, Roger VL, et al. Contractility and ventricular systolic stiffening in hypertensive heart disease insights into the pathogenesis of heart failure with preserved ejection fraction. J Am Coll Cardiol 2009;54:410–8.

36. Borlaug BA, Kass DA. Ventricular-vascular interaction in heart failure. Heart Fail Clin 2008;4:23–36.

37. Borlaug BA, Melenovsky V, Russell SD, et al. Impaired chronotropic and vasodilator reserves limit exercise capacity in patients with heart failure and a preserved ejection fraction. Circulation 2006; 114:2138–47.

38. Phan TT, Shivu GN, Abozguia K, et al. Impaired heart rate recovery and chronotropic incompetence in patients with heart failure with preserved ejection fraction. Circ Heart Fail 2010;3:29–34.

39. Tartiere-Kesri L, Tartiere JM, Logeart D, et al. Increased proximal arterial stiffness and cardiac response with moderate exercise in patients with heart failure and preserved ejection fraction. J Am Coll Cardiol 2012;59:455–61.

40. Haykowsky MJ, Liang Y, Pechter D, et al. A meta-analysis of the effect of exercise training on left ventricular remodeling in heart failure patients: the benefit depends on the type of training performed. J Am Coll Cardiol 2007;49:2329–36.

41. Matsue Y, Suzuki M, Nagahori W, et al. Endothelial dysfunction measured by peripheral arterial tonometry predicts prognosis in patients with heart failure with preserved ejection fraction. Int J Cardiol 2013; 168:36–40.

42. Akiyama E, Sugiyama S, Matsuzawa Y, et al. Incremental prognostic significance of peripheral endothelial dysfunction in patients with heart failure with normal left ventricular ejection fraction. J Am Coll Cardiol 2012;60:1778–86.

43. Nichols WW, Edwards DG. Arterial elastance and wave reflection augmentation of systolic blood pressure: deleterious effects and implications for therapy. J Cardiovasc Pharmacol Ther 2001;6:5–21.

44. Weber T, O'Rourke MF, Ammer M, et al. Arterial stiffness and arterial wave reflections are associated with systolic and diastolic function in patients with normal ejection fraction. Am J Hypertens 2008;21:1194–202.

45. Abramov D, He KL, Wang J, et al. The impact of extra cardiac comorbidities on pressure volume relations in heart failure and preserved ejection fraction. J Card Fail 2011;17:547–55.

46. Mohammed SF, Borlaug BA, Roger VL, et al. Comorbidity and ventricular and vascular structure and function in heart failure with preserved ejection fraction: a community-based study. Circ Heart Fail 2012;5:710–9.

47. Edelmann F, Stahrenberg R, Gelbrich G, et al. Contribution of comorbidities to functional impairment is higher in heart failure with preserved than with reduced ejection fraction. Clin Res Cardiol 2011;100:755–64.

48. Shah SJ, Gheorghiade M. Heart failure with preserved ejection fraction: treat now by treating comorbidities. JAMA 2008;300:431–3.

49. Pieske B. Heart failure with preserved ejection fraction–a growing epidemic or 'The Emperor's New Clothes?'. Eur J Heart Fail 2011;13:11–3.

50. Paulus WJ, Tschope C. A novel paradigm for heart failure with preserved ejection fraction: comorbidities drive myocardial dysfunction and remodeling

through coronary microvascular endothelial inflammation. J Am Coll Cardiol 2013;62:263–71.

51. Linke WA, Kruger M. The giant protein titin as an integrator of myocyte signaling pathways. Physiology (Bethesda) 2010;25:186–98.

52. Borbely A, van der Velden J, Papp Z, et al. Cardiomyocyte stiffness in diastolic heart failure. Circulation 2005;111:774–81.

53. van Heerebeek L, Borbely A, Niessen HW, et al. Myocardial structure and function differ in systolic and diastolic heart failure. Circulation 2006;113:1966–73.

54. Hamdani N, Bishu KG, von Frieling-Salewsky M, et al. Deranged myofilament phosphorylation and function in experimental heart failure with preserved ejection fraction. Cardiovasc Res 2013;97:464–71.

55. van Heerebeek L, Hamdani N, Falcao-Pires I, et al. Low myocardial protein kinase G activity in heart failure with preserved ejection fraction. Circulation 2012;126:830–9.

56. Falcao-Pires I, Hamdani N, Borbely A, et al. Diabetes mellitus worsens diastolic left ventricular dysfunction in aortic stenosis through altered myocardial structure and cardiomyocyte stiffness. Circulation 2011;124:1151–9.

57. van Heerebeek L, Hamdani N, Handoko ML, et al. Diastolic stiffness of the failing diabetic heart: importance of fibrosis, advanced glycation end products, and myocyte resting tension. Circulation 2008;117:43–51.

58. Querejeta R, Lopez B, Gonzalez A, et al. Increased collagen type I synthesis in patients with heart failure of hypertensive origin: relation to myocardial fibrosis. Circulation 2004;110:1263–8.

59. Gonzalez A, Lopez B, Querejeta R, et al. Filling pressures and collagen metabolism in hypertensive patients with heart failure and normal ejection fraction. Hypertension 2010;55:1418–24.

60. Westermann D, Lindner D, Kasner M, et al. Cardiac inflammation contributes to changes in the extracellular matrix in patients with heart failure and normal ejection fraction. Circ Heart Fail 2011;4:44–52.

61. Carrier L, Schlossarek S, Willis MS, et al. The ubiquitin-proteasome system and nonsense-mediated mRNA decay in hypertrophic cardiomyopathy. Cardiovasc Res 2010;85:330–8.

62. Ho CY, Lopez B, Coelho-Filho OR, et al. Myocardial fibrosis as an early manifestation of hypertrophic cardiomyopathy. N Engl J Med 2010;363:552–63.

63. Chaturvedi RR, Herron T, Simmons R, et al. Passive stiffness of myocardium from congenital heart disease and implications for diastole. Circulation 2010;121:979–88.

64. Silberman GA, Fan TH, Liu H, et al. Uncoupled cardiac nitric oxide synthase mediates diastolic dysfunction. Circulation 2010;121:519–28.

65. Periasamy M, Janssen PM. Molecular basis of diastolic dysfunction. Heart Fail Clin 2008;4:13–21.

66. Dupont S, Maizel J, Mentaverri R, et al. The onset of left ventricular diastolic dysfunction in SHR rats is not related to hypertrophy or hypertension. Am J Physiol Heart Circ Physiol 2012;302:H1524–32.

67. Shao CH, Capek HL, Patel KP, et al. Carbonylation contributes to SERCA2a activity loss and diastolic dysfunction in a rat model of type 1 diabetes. Diabetes 2011;60:947–59.

68. Louch WE, Hougen K, Mork HK, et al. Sodium accumulation promotes diastolic dysfunction in end-stage heart failure following Serca2 knockout. J Physiol 2010;588:465–78.

69. Fischer TH, Maier LS, Sossalla S. The ryanodine receptor leak: how a tattered receptor plunges the failing heart into crisis. Heart Fail Rev 2013;18:475–83.

70. Sossalla S, Wagner S, Rasenack EC, et al. Ranolazine improves diastolic dysfunction in isolated myocardium from failing human hearts–role of late sodium current and intracellular ion accumulation. J Mol Cell Cardiol 2008;45:32–43.

71. Papp Z, Borbely A, Paulus WJ. CrossTalk opposing view: the late sodium current is not an important player in the development of diastolic heart failure (heart failure with a preserved ejection fraction). J Physiol 2014;592(Pt 3):415–7.

Diagnosis of Heart Failure with Preserved Ejection Fraction

Rolf Wachter, MD*, Frank Edelmann, MD

KEYWORDS

- Heart failure with preserved ejection fraction • Diastolic heart failure • Diagnosis • Biomarkers
- Echocardiographic • Diastolic dysfunction

KEY POINTS

- Heart failure with preserved ejection fraction (HFpEF) is characterized by typical signs and symptoms of heart failure, a preserved left ventricular ejection fraction, and functional and/or structural alterations of left ventricular function.
- Comorbidities (eg, chronic obstructive pulmonary disease, renal insufficiency) are frequent and may cause similar symptoms as HFpEF, and therefore must be addressed in the differential diagnosis.
- Different clinical settings for HFpEF are discussed.

INTRODUCTION

Nature of the Problem

Heart failure is the leading cause of hospitalization in the Western world, and heart failure with preserved ejection fraction (HFpEF) is now considered the major phenotype of heart failure within an aging population.[1]

Heart failure with preserved ejection fraction is often also referred to as *diastolic heart failure*, because abnormalities of diastolic dysfunction are common. However, diastolic dysfunction is also highly prevalent in patients with cardiovascular risk factors but without heart failure symptoms, and in patients with heart failure and reduced ejection fraction. Hence, the more descriptive phrase *heart failure with preserved ejection fraction* is now the commonly accepted term used in scientific literature.

Heart failure with preserved ejection fraction was probably first described as early as 1985 by Topol and colleagues.[2] These investigators described 21 cases of elderly, predominantly female, and predominantly black patients with hypertrophied left ventricles and heart failure symptoms in the absence of severe coronary artery disease and with a very high left ventricular ejection fraction, but abnormal diastolic function.

These findings have fostered research at a basic science level, in patient-oriented research, and in population-based cohorts. Most of the early findings by Topol and colleagues[2] have been confirmed, and this review focuses on the current understanding of modalities to diagnose HFpEF and to distinguish the impact of comorbidities, which play an important role in the disease.

Diagnosing HFpEF: What Do the Guidelines Say?

Diagnosing HFpEF is often more challenging than diagnosing heart failure with reduced ejection fraction (HFrEF) (ie, systolic heart failure). With HFrEF, the presence of systolic dysfunction (especially

Conflict of Interest: None.

Clinic for Cardiology and Pneumology, DZHK (German Center for Cardiovascular Research), University of Göttingen, Göttingen, Germany

* Corresponding author. Clinic for Cardiology and Pneumology, Universitätsmedizin Göttingen, Robert-Koch-Str.40, 37075 Göttingen, Germany.

E-mail address: wachter@med.uni-goettingen.de

Heart Failure Clin 10 (2014) 399–406

http://dx.doi.org/10.1016/j.hfc.2014.04.010

through assessing the left ventricular ejection fraction) has been widely accepted as the key objective diagnostic criterion. In the former, recent European and American guidelines address the diagnostic challenges, and various algorithms for the diagnosis of HFpEF have been proposed.[3] To date there is still no uniformly accepted consensus on a diagnostic approach or specific cutoffs for diagnostic criteria, and adequately powered trials to validate different diagnostic approaches are lacking. Moreover, different pathophysiologies may underlie different diseases that all manifest as heart failure, and hence HFpEF may be the end of the line of different diseases but with a similar clinical picture that makes the (differential) diagnosis even more difficult.

The definitions of heart failure used in the 2012 European Society of Cardiology (ESC) Guidelines for the diagnosis and treatment of acute and chronic heart failure[4] and the 2013 American College of Cardiology Foundation/American Heart Association (ACCF/AHA)[5] Guideline for the management of heart failure are summarized in **Table 1**.[6] A consensus document by the Heart Failure and Echocardiography Associations of the European Society of Cardiology[3] also exists, which differs slightly from the ESC guidelines in that it includes specific definitions for invasively measured alterations in relaxation and filling pressures (eg, elevated left ventricular end diastolic pressure, left ventricular stiffness) and different cutoffs for natriuretic peptides. Specific clinical

factors that increase the likelihood of diagnosis of HFpEF should also be taken into consideration, such as the presence of atrial fibrillation and female sex, whereas coronary artery disease, ST elevation, and left bundle branch block favor HFrEF.[7]

Symptom Criteria

In the European Guideline, the diagnosis of heart failure requires the presence of signs and symptoms of heart failure.[4] Typical signs and symptoms are displayed in **Table 2**. The specificity of different clinical signs for heart failure may be difficult, and possible other causal diagnoses must be considered. Typical symptoms of heart failure include breathlessness, orthopnea, paroxysmal nocturnal dyspnea, reduced exercise tolerance, and fatigue.

CLINICAL FINDINGS
Physical Examination

Clinical findings in HFpEF do not substantially differ from those in HFrEF. Specific findings during physical examination are elevated jugular venous pressure, hepatojugular reflux, third heart sound, laterally displaced apical impulse, and cardiac murmur. Peripheral edema, especially at the ankles, is common and pulmonary crepitations are often heard, especially if the onset of symptoms is acute. Physical examination should also focus on common comorbidities (eg, anemia, chronic

---

Table 1
Comparison of recent European and American Guidelines regarding the definition and classification of heart failure

	2012 ESC Guidelines for the Diagnosis and Treatment of Acute and Chronic Heart Failure	2013 ACCF/AHA Guideline for the Management of Heart Failure
HF definition	Abnormality of cardiac structure or function leading to failure of the heart to deliver oxygen at a rate commensurate with the requirement of the metabolizing tissues, despite normal filling pressure (or only at the expense of increased filling pressures)	Complex clinical syndrome that results from any structural or functional impairment of ventricular filling or ejection of blood
HF-PEF diagnosis	Requires 4 conditions to be satisfied • Typical symptoms of HF • Typical signs of HF • Preserved ejection fraction (EF ≥45%) and left ventricle not dilated • Relevant structural heart disease and/or diastolic dysfunction	Stage C heart failure • Known structural heart disease • Typical signs and symptoms • Preserved ejection fraction (EF ≥50% → HF-PEF, EF 41%–50% → borderline HF-PEF)

Abbreviations: EF, ejection fraction; HF, heart failure; PEF, preserved ejection fraction.
Adapted from Rigolli M, Whalley GA. Heart failure with preserved ejection fraction. J Geriatr Cardiol 2013;10:369–76.

Table 2	
Signs and symptoms of heart failure	
Symptoms	Signs
Typical	**More specific**
Breathlessness	Elevated jugular venous pressure
Orthopnea	Hepatojugular reflux
Paroxysmal nocturnal dyspnea	Third heart sound (gallop rhythm)
Reduced exercise tolerance	Laterally displaced apical impulse
Fatigue, tiredness, increased time to recover after exercise	Cardiac murmur
Ankle swelling	
Less typical	**Less specific**
Nocturnal cough	Peripheral edema (ankle, sacral, scrotal)
Wheezing	Pulmonary crepitations
Weight gain (>2 kg/wk)	Reduced air entry and dullness to percussion at lung bases (pleural effusion)
Weight loss (in advanced heart failure)	Tachycardia
Bloated feeling	Irregular pulse
Loss of appetite	Tachypnea (>16 breaths/min)
Confusion (especially in the elderly)	Hepatomegaly
Depression	Ascites

Adapted from McMurray JJ, Adamopoulos S, Anker SD, et al. ESC guidelines for the diagnosis and treatment of acute and chronic heart failure 2012: The Task Force for the Diagnosis and Treatment of Acute and Chronic Heart Failure 2012 of the European Society of Cardiology. Developed in collaboration with the Heart Failure Association (HFA) of the ESC. Eur J Heart Fail 2012;14:1795; with permission.

kidney disease, muscle wasting, fluid overload, chronic pulmonary disease).

Diagnostic Modalities

Diagnostics in patients with suspected HFpEF should comply with usual diagnostics in every patient with heart failure. Essential diagnostic tools include electrocardiography, echocardiography, and laboratory tests. A chest radiograph should be considered in patients with a more chronic history of the disease, but should be performed immediately in patient with an acute onset of symptoms.

Routine laboratory testing should include sodium, potassium, creatinine, estimated glomerular filtration rate (eGFR), and hematology testing (hemoglobin, hematocrit, leukocytes, ferritin, and platelets). Additionally, measuring thyroid-stimulating hormone, liver enzymes (aspartate amino transferase, alanine amino transferase), and glucose levels should be considered.[4] Testing for B-type natriuretic peptide (BNP) and N-terminal pro-BNP (NT-proBNP) is strongly recommended. Upcoming new biomarkers, such as growth differentiation factor 15,[8] are summarized elsewhere.[9]

Echocardiography is the cornerstone of HFpEF diagnostics. Despite the evaluation of left ventricular ejection fraction and the assessment of valvular function, left atrial size and relaxation/stiffness should be analyzed. E/é (pulsed-wave Doppler E wave velocity divided by tissue Doppler E wave velocity) is the most commonly used continuous marker of left ventricular end-diastolic pressure (LVEDP) and left ventricular stiffness. E/é greater than 15 is usually considered to prove an elevation of LVEDP and establish the diagnosis of HFpEF in symptomatic patients. In patients with E/é between 8 and 15, NT-proBNP greater than 220 pg/mL or BNP greater than 200 pg/mL establishes the diagnosis of HFpEF. Alternatively to natriuretic peptide levels, the diagnosis can be established using other echocardiographic measurements.[3] The gold standard remains the invasive determination of left ventricular relaxation, pressures, and stiffness using pressure-volume-loop diagnostics,[10,11] but this modality is mostly neither necessary nor performed.

In patients with pulmonary hypertension, right heart catheterization, ideally with fluid challenge, should be performed (see also section on Pulmonary Hypertension and Saline Infusion).

The diagnostic workup should also rule out possible differential diagnoses. Therefore, pulmonary function test (eg, spirometry) for chronic pulmonary disease should always be performed. Depending on the results of the clinical examination and the patient's medical history, other tests may be added.

DIFFERENTIAL DIAGNOSIS AND DIAGNOSTIC DILEMMAS

Patients complaining of dyspnea are not necessarily considered to have heart failure. Differential diagnoses are numerous and are listed in **Box 1**.

Dyspnea on exertion is the major complaint in patients being evaluated in cardiac outpatient clinics. However, these patients may also be seen initially by pneumologists, and therefore

Box 1
Possible differential diagnoses in patients with symptoms suggestive of HFpEF preserved ejection fraction

Pulmonary

- Chronic obstructive pulmonary disease
- Emphysema
- Pneumonia
- Tuberculosis of the lung
- Pulmonary fibrosis
- Lung cancer
- Asthma
- Pulmonary embolism
- Pneumothorax
- Pleural effusions

Cardiovascular

- HFrEF
- Pulmonary hypertension for reasons other than HFpEF (eg, arterial pulmonary hypertension)
- Valvular heart disease
- Arrhythmia (eg, paroxysmal atrial fibrillation)
- Constrictive pericarditis
- Hypertension and hypertensive crisis

Head-nose-throat diseases

- Tracheal stenosis
- Diseases of the vocal cord (eg, vocal cord dysfunction)

Neuromuscular diseases

Anemia

Medication

Adipositas

Lack of training, muscle wasting

need to be referred for further cardiologic workup. The consensus document of the ESC working groups provides reasonable algorithms for ruling in and out HFpEF.[3] The algorithm to rule in HFpEF is shown in **Fig. 1**. Different pathways for cardiac and noncardiac evaluation may also be used. For instance, every patient with echocardiographic signs of pulmonary hypertension should be carefully evaluated for having HFpEF, especially if right heart catheterization shows signs of elevated filling pressures and left ventricular systolic dysfunction, and significant valvular diseases have been ruled out.

Process of Elimination

The ESC consensus document describes a pathway to exclude HFpEF as a cause of symptoms.[3] Diagnostic procedures should be chosen according to possible differential diagnoses based on medical history, physical examination, and initial diagnostic findings.

Comorbidities

Comorbidities in HFpEF are frequent and may dissimilate signs and symptoms of heart failure; this confers to chronic kidney disease, chronic pulmonary disease, and deconditioning. Numerous comorbidities (eg, anemia, chronic kidney disease, diabetes, obesity) are associated with unique clinical, structural, functional, and prognostic profiles in HFpEF.[12] Researchers have postulated that comorbidities drive myocardial dysfunction and remodeling through coronary microvascular endothelial inflammation.[13] Frequent comorbidities are described in the following section.

CASE STUDIES

In general, in the authors' experience, HFpEF has 2 distinct clinical presentations (**Table 3**). Past HFpEF trials have reported on both of these entities.

Currently, whether these are actually 2 different entities or the same disease at different stages is unclear. Ongoing prospective observational trials (eg, Diast-CHF) and epidemiologic trials are currently investigating the incidence and clinical predictors of progression from the early to the late presentation.

Patients Hospitalized for Heart Failure and HFpEF

More than half of patients hospitalized with heart failure have preserved ejection fraction, and mortality rates are similarly grim as for those with heart failure with reduced ejection fraction.[1,14] The proportion of patients with heart failure and preserved ejection fraction has been increasing in recent years, which may be attributed to a higher awareness of physicians and/or an aging population.

Dyspnea on Exertion and HFpEF

In 359 patients with dyspnea on exertion and preserved ejection fraction (>50%) who were scheduled for cardiac catheterization, 71 (20%) were diagnosed to have definite and 223 (62%) to have possible HFpEF, based on NT-proBNP levels and right heart catheterization results.[15] The authors' group diagnosed HFpEF as defined by the ESC consensus criteria[3] in 66% of ambulatory

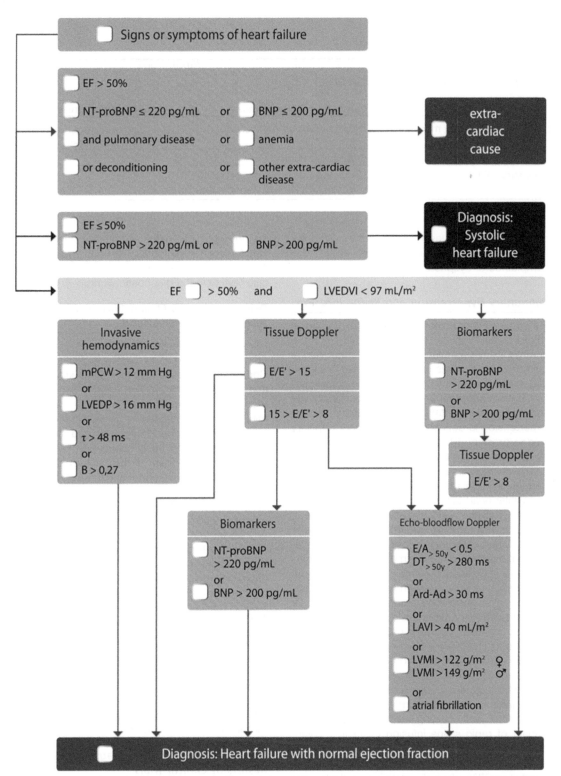

Fig. 1. Diagnostic algorithm for the diagnosis of heart failure with normal ejection fraction. Ad, duration of mitral valve atrial wave flow; Ard, duration of reverse pulmonary vein atrial systole flow; b, constant of left ventricular chamber stiffness; BNP, brain natriuretic peptide; DT, deceleration time; E, early mitral valve flow velocity; E', early TD lengthening velocity; E/A, ratio of early (E) to late (A) mitral valve flow velocity; LAVi, left atrial volume indexed; LVEDDi, left ventricular end diastolic diameter indexed; LVEDVi, left ventricular end diastolic volume indexed; LVEDP, left ventricular end-diastolic pressure; LVEF, left ventricular ejection fraction; LVMi, left ventricular mass indexed; mPCW, mean pulmonary capillary wedge pressure; NT-proBNP, N-terminal-pro brain natriuretic peptide; τ, time constant of left ventricular relaxation. (*Adapted from* Paulus WJ, Tschöpe C, Sanderson JE, et al. How to diagnose diastolic heart failure: a consensus statement on the diagnosis of heart failure with normal left ventricular ejection fraction by the Heart Failure and Echocardiography Associations of the European Society of Cardiology. Eur Heart J 2007;28(20):2544; with permission.)

Table 3
Early and late clinical presentation of HFpEF

	Early Clinical Presentation	Late Clinical Presentation
Reason for seeking medical attention	Dyspnea/fatigue on exertion	Cardiac decompensation, fluid overload
Typical clinical setting	Outpatient clinic	Hospital
5-y survival rate	Unknown but probably better than in the late clinical presentation	≈40%

patients with cardiovascular risk factors (Wachter and colleagues, unpublished data, 2014) who complained of dyspnea.

Pulmonary Hypertension and Saline Infusion

Pulmonary hypertension is a frequent finding in HFpEF, and 83% of participants in the community-based Olmsted County study had a pulmonary artery pressure of 45 mm Hg or higher and a strong mortality predictor.[16] The differentiation between arterial and venous pulmonary hypertension is important, and pulmonary venous hypertension is defined as a pulmonary capillary wedge pressure (PCWP) greater than 15 mm Hg in addition to an elevated mean pulmonary pressure of at least 25 mm Hg.[17] Pulmonary venous hypertension results from left ventricular myocardial or valvular heart disease, and, if systolic dysfunction and valvular heart disease can be ruled out, HFpEF is the most likely differential diagnosis.[18] Robbins and colleagues[19] investigated the prevalence of overt and occult pulmonary venous hypertension in patients undergoing right heart catheterization for evaluation of pulmonary hypertension. The population studied was typical for arterial pulmonary hypertension, with female predominance and a mean age of 55 years. However, 32 patients (13%) were diagnosed with overt pulmonary venous hypertension and an additional 46 (18%) with occult pulmonary venous hypertension, which appeared after a challenge of 0.5 L of saline infused rapidly (5–10 minutes).

Fujimoto and colleagues[20] investigated the impact of rapid saline infusion in healthy volunteers and in women with HFpEF. Two liters of rapid saline infusion increased PCWP to 15 mm Hg or greater in 92% of study participants (both men and women), most of them without HFpEF. These results challenge the 15 mm Hg cutoff for PCWP to establish the diagnosis of HFpEF, which was proposed previously.[21] However, the increase in PCWP was significantly higher in women with HFpEF than in healthy volunteers. In summary, these data support the use of fluid challenge

during right heart catheterization in patients with risk factors for pulmonary venous hypertension. An (even better) alternative may be to include exercise testing in the diagnostic workup.[22]

Patients with HFpEF and Chronic Kidney Disease or Fluid Overload

Chronic kidney disease has an enormous impact on the prognosis of patients with HFpEF. Compared with patients with normal kidney function, an eGFR of 15 to 29 mL/min/1.73 m² doubles the risk of death and an eGFR of less than 15 mL/min/1.73 m² increases it 7-fold.[23] In patients treated with peritoneal dialysis for end-stage renal disease, 39% had heart failure and HFpEF was more prominent than HFrEF, but patients with HFpEF had a lower mortality risk than those with HFrEF.[24] Many biomarkers (eg, BNP, galectin-3)[25] strongly correlate with kidney function, which hampers their diagnostic value in concomitant kidney disease. Alterations in cardiac structure and function detected on echocardiography should be thoroughly weighed against the degree of renal impairment in the diagnosis of HFpEF in this patient population.

Patients with HFpEF and Chronic Pulmonary Disease

Spirometry can be used to evaluate pulmonary function. B-type natriuretic peptide has repeatedly been shown to be of great clinical value in distinguishing pulmonary and cardiac causes of dyspnea. Spiroergometry allows further evaluation for the cause of symptoms.

Criteria for Heart Failure Diagnostics and Results of Clinical Trials

The aforementioned differentiation of early and late clinical presentation may also explain different results in clinical trials. For instance, in the large TOPCAT trial (spironolactone vs placebo in HFpEF), patients with wither presentation could be included.[26] Of 22 prespecified strata for the primary end point, a significant interaction ($P = .013$)

was seen in the primary outcome (hospitalization for heart failure, cardiovascular death, or aborted cardiac arrest) only for patients included for high natriuretic peptide level (BNP $\geq$100 pg/mL or NT-proBNP $\geq$360 pg/mL; ie, early manifestation of HFpEF) and those included for hospitalization for heart failure (ie, late manifestation of HFpEF). Patients with early-stage HFpEF showed benefit, and patients included for late-stage HFpEF showed neutral results.[27] In addition, in the Aldo-DHF trial (spironolactone vs placebo in patients with symptomatic diastolic dysfunction [early HFpEF]), similarly positive effects on left ventricular form (left ventricular hypertrophy), biomarkers (NT-proBNP), and function (E/é reduced) could be seen, whereas HFpEF symptoms remained unchanged.[28] Future trials in HFpEF should more precisely refer to only one of these entities. Patients with late manifestation of HFpEF mostly die from noncardiovascular causes,[29] and any intervention to change cardiac structure or function may just come too late. Therefore, in the authors' opinion, future HFpEF trials should focus on the early manifestation of HFpEF. Because of the possibly slow progression of the disease, longer follow-ups than in current heart failure trials may be necessary for positive results.

SUMMARY

Diagnosing HFpEF is challenging. Patients may present with different clinical pictures; they may be hospitalized for heart failure, complaining of dyspnea on exertion, or scheduled for right cardiac catheterization with echocardiographic signs of pulmonary hypertension.

In addition to a thorough evaluation of signs and symptoms, minimal diagnostics should include electrocardiography, echocardiography, and laboratory testing. In many cases, right heart catheterization or exercise testing should be added. Left heart catheterization with conductance technique–based analysis of left ventricular pressure-volume loop, ideally with preload and/or postload change (eg, exercise, handgrip, fluid), is considered the diagnostic gold standard but is rarely necessary and performed. Relevant and frequent comorbidities (eg, chronic pulmonary obstructive lung disease) should be ruled out based on past medical history, physical examination, and adequate testing.

REFERENCES

1. Owan TE, Hodge DO, Herges RM, et al. Trends in prevalence and outcome of heart failure with preserved ejection fraction. N Engl J Med 2006; 355:251–9.
2. Topol EJ, Traill TA, Fortuin NJ. Hypertensive hypertrophic cardiomyopathy of the elderly. N Engl J Med 1985;312:277–83.
3. Paulus WJ, Tschöpe C, Sanderson JE, et al. How to diagnose diastolic heart failure: a consensus statement on the diagnosis of heart failure with normal left ventricular ejection fraction by the Heart Failure and Echocardiography Associations of the European Society of Cardiology. Eur Heart J 2007;28: 2539–50.
4. McMurray JJ, Adamopoulos S, Anker SD, et al. ESC guidelines for the diagnosis and treatment of acute and chronic heart failure 2012: the Task Force for the Diagnosis and Treatment of Acute and Chronic Heart Failure 2012 of the European Society of Cardiology. Developed in collaboration with the Heart Failure Association (HFA) of the ESC. Eur J Heart Fail 2012;14:803–69.
5. Yancy CW, Jessup M, Bozkurt B, et al. 2013 ACCF/AHA Guideline for the Management of Heart Failure: a report of the American College of Cardiology Foundation/American Heart Association Task Force on Practice Guidelines. J Am Coll Cardiol 2013;62: e147–239.
6. Rigolli M, Whalley GA. Heart failure with preserved ejection fraction. J Geriatr Cardiol 2013;10:369–76.
7. Ho JE, Gona P, Pencina MJ, et al. Discriminating clinical features of heart failure with preserved vs. reduced ejection fraction in the community. Eur Heart J 2012;33:1734–41.
8. Stahrenberg R, Edelmann F, Mende M, et al. The novel biomarker growth differentiation factor 15 in heart failure with normal ejection fraction. Eur J Heart Fail 2010;12:1309–16.
9. Becher PM, Lindner D, Fluschnik N, et al. Diagnosing heart failure with preserved ejection fraction. Expert Opin Med Diagn 2013;7:463–74.
10. Westermann D, Kasner M, Steendijk P, et al. Role of left ventricular stiffness in heart failure with normal ejection fraction. Circulation 2008;117:2051–60.
11. Wachter R, Schmidt-Schweda S, Westermann D, et al. Blunted frequency-dependent upregulation of cardiac output is related to impaired relaxation in diastolic heart failure. Eur Heart J 2009;30: 3027–36.
12. Mohammed SF, Borlaug BA, Roger VL, et al. Comorbidity and ventricular and vascular structure and function in heart failure with preserved ejection fraction: a community-based study. Circ Heart Fail 2012; 5:710–9.
13. Paulus WJ, Tschöpe C. A novel paradigm for heart failure with preserved ejection fraction: comorbidities drive myocardial dysfunction and remodeling through coronary microvascular endothelial inflammation. J Am Coll Cardiol 2013;62:263–71.

14. Quiroz R, Doros G, Shaw P, et al. Comparison of characteristics and outcomes of patients with heart failure preserved ejection fraction reduced left ventricular ejection fraction in an urban cohort. Am J Cardiol 2014;113:691–6.

15. Weber T, Wassertheurer S, ÓRourke MF, et al. Pulsatile hemodynamics in patients with exertional dyspnea. Potentially of value in the diagnostic evaluation of suspected heart failure with preserved ejection fraction. J Am Coll Cardiol 2013;61: 1874–83.

16. Lam CS, Roger VL, Rodeheffer RJ, et al. Pulmonary hypertension in heart failure with preserved ejection fraction: a community-based study. J Am Coll Cardiol 2009;53:1119–26.

17. Galiè N, Hoeper MM, Humbert M, et al, ESC Committee for Practice Guidelines (CPG). Guidelines for the diagnosis and treatment of pulmonary hypertension: the Task Force for the Diagnosis and Treatment of Pulmonary Hypertension of the European Society of Cardiology (ESC) and the European Respiratory Society (ERS), endorsed by the International Society of Heart and Lung Transplantation (ISHLT). Eur Heart J 2009;30:2493–537.

18. Simonneau G, Gatzoulis MA, Adatia I, et al. Updated clinical classification of pulmonary hypertension. J Am Coll Cardiol 2013;62(Suppl 25):D34–41.

19. Robbins IM, Hemnes AR, Pugh ME, et al. High prevalence of occult pulmonary venous hypertension revealed by fluid challenge in pulmonary hypertension. Circ Heart Fail 2014;7:116–22.

20. Fujimoto N, Borlaug BA, Lewis GD, et al. Hemodynamic responses to rapid saline loading: the impact of age, sex, and heart failure. Circulation 2013;127: 55–62.

21. Hoeper M, Barberà JA, Channick RN, et al. Diagnosis, assessment, and treatment of non-pulmonary arterial hypertension pulmonary hypertension. J Am Coll Cardiol 2009;54:S85–96.

22. Van Empel VP, Kaye DM. Integration of exercise evaluation into the algorithm for evaluation of patients with suspected heart failure with preserved ejection fraction. Int J Cardiol 2013;168:716–22.

23. Smith DH, Thorp ML, Gurwitz JH, et al. Chronic kidney disease and outcomes in heart failure with preserved versus reduced ejection fraction: the Cardiovascular Research Network PRESERVE Study. Circ Cardiovasc Qual Outcomes 2013;6:333–42.

24. Wang AY, Wang M, Lam CW, et al. Heart failure with preserved or reduced ejection fraction in patients treated with peritoneal dialysis. Am J Kidney Dis 2013;61:975–83.

25. Gopal DM, Kommineni M, Ayalon N, et al. Relationship of plasma galectin-3 to renal function in patients with heart failure: effects of clinical status, pathophysiology of heart failure, and presence or absence of heart failure. J Am Heart Assoc 2012;1:e000760.

26. Desai AS, Lewis EF, Li R, et al. Rationale and design of the treatment of preserved cardiac function heart failure with an aldosterone antagonist trial: a randomized, controlled study of spironolactone in patients with symptomatic heart failure and preserved ejection fraction. Am Heart J 2011;162:966–72.

27. Pitt B, Pfeffer MA, Assmann SF, et al. Spironolactone for Heart Failure with Preserved Ejection Fraction. N Engl J Med 2014;370:1383–92.

28. Edelmann F, Wachter R, Schmidt AG, et al. Effect of spironolactone on diastolic function and exercise capacity in patients with heart failure with preserved ejection fraction: the Aldo-DHF randomized controlled trial. JAMA 2013;309:781–91.

29. Henkel DM, Redfield MM, Weston SA, et al. Death in heart failure: a community perspective. Circ Heart Fail 2008;1:91–7.

Phenotypic Spectrum of Heart Failure with Preserved Ejection Fraction

Sanjiv J. Shah, MD[a],*, Daniel H. Katz, BA[b], Rahul C. Deo, MD, PhD[c]

KEYWORDS

- Heart failure with preserved ejection fraction • Phenotype • Phenomics • Etiology
- Pathophysiology • Classification • Clinical trials

KEY POINTS

- Patients with heart failure and preserved ejection fraction (HFpEF) are united by the presence of (1) increased left ventricular (LV) filling pressures and/or reduced cardiac output at rest or with exertion and (2) a preserved left ventricular ejection fraction (LVEF), typically defined as LVEF greater than 45% to 50%; however, the etiology and pathophysiology underlying the HFpEF syndrome—the phenotypic spectrum—vary widely among patients with the syndrome.
- The heterogeneity of the HFpEF syndrome may be a key reason why clinical trials have largely failed to show improved outcomes in these patients.
- Improved classification of the HFpEF syndrome, whether by etiology, pathophysiology, and/or type of clinical presentation, should lead to better matching of appropriate therapies to patients, thereby leading to improved outcomes for these patients.
- Phenomapping is a novel technique that uses machine learning to define clusters of patients based on dense phenotypic data, thereby providing an unbiased way to classify hetereogeneous clinical syndromes such as HFpEF.
- Future clinical trials of HFpEF should account for the heterogeneity of HFpEF when considering inclusion/exclusion criteria, study design, phenotyping tools, and outcome measures, and should a priori consider subgroup analyses to highlight specific HFpEF subtypes that may derive greater benefit from a particular HFpEF drug.

INTRODUCTION

Heart failure (HF) is a common clinical syndrome with high morbidity and mortality and one that is increasing in prevalence with the aging population.[1–4] Regardless of underlying ejection fraction (EF), HF is a heterogeneous syndrome.[5–7] HF is the result of 1 or more risk factors that lead to abnormal cardiac structure and function, which ultimately cause reduced cardiac output and/or elevated cardiac filling pressures at rest or with exertion.[1] Although HF with reduced EF (HFrEF) can be heterogeneous in etiology, chronic HFrEF

Disclosures: None.
Grant Support: National Institutes of Health R01 HL107577 and American Heart Association 0835488N to S.J. Shah; and NIH K08 HL098361 to R.C. Deo.
a Heart Failure with Preserved Ejection Fraction Program, Division of Cardiology, Department of Medicine, Feinberg Cardiovascular Research Institute, Northwestern University Feinberg School of Medicine, Chicago, IL, USA; b Division of Cardiology, Department of Medicine, Feinberg Cardiovascular Research Institute, Northwestern University Feinberg School of Medicine, Chicago, IL, USA; c Division of Cardiology, Department of Medicine, Cardiovascular Research Institute, University of California, San Francisco, San Francisco, CA, USA
* Corresponding author.
E-mail address: sanjiv.shah@northwestern.edu

in particular has proved to respond to a one-size-fits-all approach; several drugs and devices have improved outcomes in randomized clinical trials of patients with HFrEF.[1]

Unlike HFrEF, however, clinical trials of pharmacologic agents in HFpEF, previously termed diastolic HF, have not shown significant benefits, and no treatments have been found effective in this group of patients.[8,9] In HFpEF, the underlying phenotypic heterogeneity is most likely much greater than HFrEF[5,6] and may be a key reason for the poor track record of HFpEF clinical trials. Therefore, understanding the phenotypic spectrum of HFpEF, which includes the etiologic and pathophysiologic heterogeneity of the syndrome, may allow for more targeted clinical diagnosis and management of HFpEF patients and more successful clinical trials.

HETEROGENEITY OF HFpEF: EPIDEMIOLOGIC STUDIES VERSUS PATHOPHYSIOLOGIC STUDIES

Prior observational registries and epidemiologic studies that have included patients with HFpEF, such as the Acute Decompensated Heart Failure National Registry and the Rochester Epidemiology Project, have enrolled a broad array of patients with a wide variety of HF etiologies and pathophysiologies.[10,11] Detailed mechanistic studies of HFpEF, however, often only enroll very specific subsets of HFpEF patients, thereby limiting generalizability to the overall population of HFpEF patients. For example, in a detailed pathophysiologic study of HFpEF,[12] Prasad and colleagues[12] began with 1119 patients hospitalized for HF with EF greater than 50% but ended up with only 23 (2%) patients who were eligible for their study after applying a lengthy list of exclusion criteria, including atrial fibrillation, chronic kidney disease, myocardial infarction, cognitive impairment, and other common HFpEF comorbidities.

Several studies have now shown that HFpEF is heterogeneous from both an etiologic and pathophysiologic standpoint,[6,13–15] and previous pathophysiologic studies that have concluded that HFpEF is mainly a disease of diastolic dysfunction have been challenged.[16] The complexity and heterogeneity of HFpEF is readily apparent when caring for patients suffering from this syndrome. Consider an 86-year-old woman with systemic hypertension, diabetes, chronic kidney disease, signs and symptoms of HF (New York Heart Association functional class III), a preserved LVEF of 65%, mild concentric LV hypertrophy with mild superimposed basal septal hypertrophy, severe left atrial enlargement, and moderate (grade II) diastolic dysfunction. This description is typical for a HFpEF patient; however, consider her color Doppler echocardiographic findings (**Fig. 1**), which

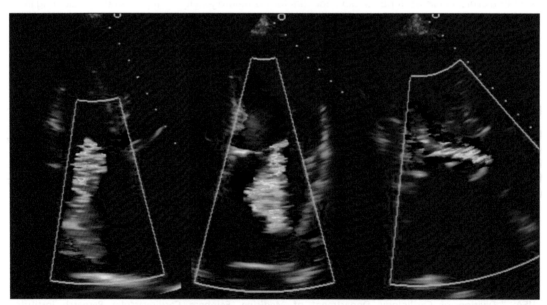

Fig. 1. Color Doppler echocardiography from a patient with HFpEF showing multiple moderate valvular lesions. (*Left panel*) Apical 4-chamber view of the right heart showing moderate tricuspid regurgitation. (*Middle panel*) Apical 4-chamber view of the left heart showing moderate mitral regurgitation. (*Right panel*) Apical 3-chamber view showing moderate aortic regurgitation. (*From* Oktay AA, Shah SJ. Heart failure with preserved ejection fraction. In: Levine G, editor. Color atlas of clinical cardiology. New Delhi (India): Jaypee Medical Publishers; 2014; with permission.)

show moderate aortic regurgitation, moderate mitral regurgitation, and moderate tricuspid regurgitation. Although none of these valvular lesions meets criteria for surgical treatment, they nevertheless combine with the intrinsic myocardial abnormalities to exacerbate the HF syndrome, and treatment of diastolic dysfunction and fluid overload alone may not improve symptoms in this type of patient.

It is now well known that comorbidities are important in both the development of HFpEF and in driving outcomes in these patients.[17–21] Accumulation of comorbidities predisposes to stage B HF and ultimately leads to stage C (symptomatic) HF, including HFpEF. Many different combinations of comorbidities can occur, however, and these combinations of risk factors, along with genetic and environmental factors, lead to different varieties of HF that are more complex than simply systolic versus diastolic HF (**Fig. 2**). A critical unmet need is the determination of which combinations of risk factors lead to which specific phenotypes of HFpEF. Such information would allow for targeted screening and diagnostic strategies for the prevention of the spectrum of HFpEF.

PHENOTYPIC CLASSIFICATION OF HFpEF

An appropriate analogy to help understand the pitfalls of the current diagnosis and treatment strategy in HFpEF is cancer. Imagine a world where all patients with cancer were viewed similarly; the

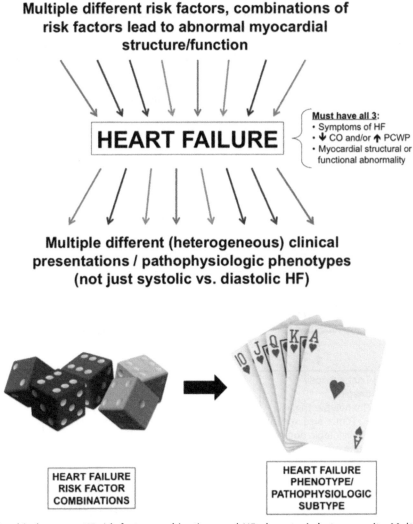

Multiple different risk factors, combinations of risk factors lead to abnormal myocardial structure/function

HEART FAILURE

Must have all 3:
- Symptoms of HF
- ↓ CO and/or ↑ PCWP
- Myocardial structural or functional abnormality

Multiple different (heterogeneous) clinical presentations / pathophysiologic phenotypes (not just systolic vs. diastolic HF)

HEART FAILURE RISK FACTOR COMBINATIONS

HEART FAILURE PHENOTYPE/ PATHOPHYSIOLOGIC SUBTYPE

Fig. 2. Relationship between HF risk factor combinations and HF phenotypic heterogeneity. Multiple different risk factors can lead to different patterns and types of the HF syndrome. Particular combinations of risk factors (ie, a roll of dice) may lead to different types of HF phenotypes (ie, a particular hand of cards). CO, cardiac output; PCWP, pulmonary capillary wedge pressure.

diagnosis of cancer was based only on symptoms and the presence of a tumor; clinical trials were designed to treat the general disease of cancer; and physicians did not further categorize cancer before or after entering patients in clinical trials—and we wonder in amazement that all treatments for cancer have failed.

This description of cancer—the concept of cancer as one single disease—sounds foreign and even laughable. If the word "cancer" were replaced with the word "HFpEF" and the word "tumor" with "normal EF" in the preceding paragraph, that would describe the current state of affairs for the diagnosis and management of HFpEF. Although the field of oncology has benefited greatly from improved phenotypic classification of cancer (eg, type of cancer, size of tumor, histologic subtype, extent of growth, presence of metastases, biomarker levels, and even genetic testing and gene expression of tumor cells), comparably little has been done in HF and even less for HFpEF (**Fig. 3**). Thus, new ways to classify and categorize the HFpEF syndrome are sorely needed.

This article describes the rationale, benefits, and pitfalls of 4 types of classification schemas for HFpEF: (1) pathophysiologic classification, (2) clinical/etiologic classification, (3) classification based on type of clinical presentation, and (4) phenomics (phenomapping) of HFpEF.

Pathophysiologic Classification of HFpEF

From a pathophysiologic standpoint, the primary abnormality underlying HFpEF was initially thought to be diastolic dysfunction—both impaired LV relaxation and decreased LV compliance, hence the term, *diastolic heart failure*.[22] Although diastolic dysfunction is a prominent part of the HFpEF syndrome, it is now well known that the pathophysiology of HFpEF is heterogeneous (**Fig. 4**).[6,8,23] Pathophysiologic abnormalities known to be present in HFpEF include (1) diastolic dysfunction (impaired relaxation and/or reduced compliance)[24]; (2) longitudinal systolic dysfunction (eg, decreased longitudinal systolic tissue velocities and decreased global longitudinal strain)[25,26]; (3) endothelial dysfunction[20]; (4) abnormal ventricular-arterial coupling[27]; (5) impaired systemic vasodilator reserve[28]; (6) pulmonary hypertension and pulmonary vascular disease with right HF in the setting of left heart disease[29,30]; (7) chronotropic incompetence[28,31]; and (8) extracardiac causes of volume overload in the susceptible heart (examples include obesity, chronic kidney disease, and anemia, each of which can cause diastolic dysfunction along with extracardiac fluid retention, thereby combining to contribute to the HFpEF syndrome).[15] Adding to the complexity of HFpEF is that these patients often have more than one pathophysiology of HFpEF that contribute to their clinical syndrome.

Clinical/Etiologic Classification of HFpEF

Clinically, several patterns are evident when caring for HFpEF patients, even when those with severe valvular disease, prior history of HFrEF (ie, recovered LVEF), and constrictive pericarditis are

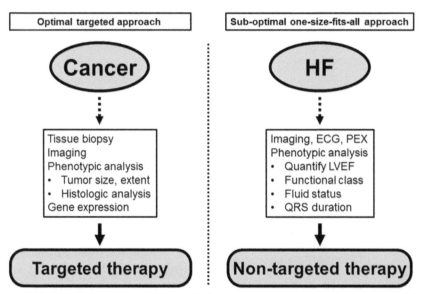

Fig. 3. Illustration of a targeted diagnostic approach (eg, cancer) versus a one-size-fits-all approach (eg, HF). Treatment of cancer has benefited from an increasingly targeted approach whereas current HF treatment is more generalized with few exceptions (eg, cardiac resynchronization therapy). PEX, physical examination.

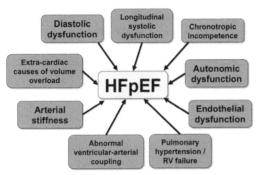

Fig. 4. Multiple pathophysiologic contributors to the HFpEF syndrome. (*From* Oktay AA, Shah SJ. Heart failure with preserved ejection fraction. In: Levine G, editor. Color atlas of clinical cardiology. New Delhi (India): Jaypee Medical Publishers; 2014; with permission.)

excluded. Clinical phenotypes of HFpEF include (1) garden-variety HFpEF, which is associated with hypertension, obesity, diabetes/metabolic syndrome, and/or chronic kidney disease; (2) coronary artery disease (CAD)-associated HFpEF[25] (these patients typically have multivessel CAD, and the CAD seems to be driving the HFpEF syndrome)[25]; (3) atrial fibrillation–predominant HFpEF (these patients frequently have uncontrolled atrial fibrillation, which seems to drive the HFpEF syndrome); (4) right HF–predominant HFpEF (these patients have pulmonary venous hypertension [occasionally with superimposed pulmonary arterial hypertension] and right ventricular [RV] dysfunction in the setting of significant diastolic dysfunction; however, the right HF drives their clinical course)[29,32]; (5) hypertrophic cardiomyopathy–induced or hypertrophic cardiomyopathy–like HFpEF (these patients typically have small LV cavities with thick walls and respond best to negative inotropes); (6) multivalvular HFpEF (these patients typically have 2 or more moderate valvular lesions that do not meet operative criteria but nevertheless contribute to HFpEF, usually in the setting of other risk factors and causes of HFpEF); and (7) restrictive cardiomyopathies, such as cardiac amyloidosis.[2]

Although useful from a clinical standpoint, clinical classification of HFpEF can be problematic because these categories are not mutually exclusive; therefore, it is sometimes difficult to place patients into a single category to guide treatment. Nevertheless, when diagnosing and managing patients with HFpEF, the clinical/etiologic classification system can be helpful in guiding initial treatment (**Table 1**). The clinical/etiologic classification of HFpEF remains, however, empiric and anecdotal for the most part; clinical trials are

necessary to prove the utility of the classification and management strategies outlined in **Table 1**.

Classification of HFpEF Based on Clinical Presentation

The underlying pathophysiology and etiology of HFpEF is not the only basis for heterogeneity of the HFpEF syndrome. Clinical presentation of HFpEF varies considerably as well. Patients tend to present in 1 of 3 types of categories that correlate with the clinical severity of the HFpEF syndrome,[7] as shown in **Fig. 5**.

The first category, representing the lowest-risk type of patient but also the most difficult to diagnose, is exercise-induced increases in LV filling pressures, also known as exercise-induced diastolic dysfunction.[33,34] Exertional dyspnea is the predominant symptom in these patients. They typically do not have overt signs of volume overload, such as lower extremity edema, and are rarely hospitalized for HF. Therefore, clinical diagnosis rests on a combination of abnormalities in cardiac structure (LV hypertrophy and/or left atrial enlargement) and evidence of exercise-induced elevations in LV filling pressure, either invasively (ie, pulmonary capillary wedge pressure >25 mm Hg at peak exercise during invasive hemodynamic testing in the cardiac catheterization laboratory)[33] or noninvasively (ie, diastolic stress echocardiography—increased [>13] septal ratio of early mitral inflow to early mitral annular diastolic tissue velocity [E/e'] at peak exercise).[35–37] Cardiopulmonary exercise testing can also be helpful to exclude poor effort (reduced peak respiratory exchange ratio <1.0); obesity (normal peak absolute oxygen consumption [$\dot{V}o_2$] with reduced relative $\dot{V}o_2$ when indexed to weight); or pulmonary abnormalities as causes of exercise intolerance. HFpEF patients who fit into the category of exercise-induced elevation in LV filling pressure typically have normal or only mildly elevated B-type natriuretic peptide (BNP) levels, and the risk of major morbidity or mortality at this stage of the HFpEF syndrome is low.[33,34,38]

The second type of clinical presentation of HFpEF is the common one that clinicians often easily recognize: overt volume overload. Besides dyspnea, exercise intolerance, and abnormalities in cardiac structure (LV hypertrophy and/or left atrial enlargement), these HFpEF patients have lower extremity edema, elevated jugular venous pressure, and even bibasilar crackles when severe. In addition, these patients typically (but not always) have elevated BNP or N-terminal–proBNP levels and typically have a history of HF hospitalization, after which morbidity and mortality are

Table 1
Management of heart failure with preserved ejection fraction by phenotypic classification

Phenotypic Classification	Management Strategies
Garden-variety HFpEF	• Treat comorbidities • Enroll in HFpEF clinical trial
CAD-HFpEF	• Consider revascularization • Aggressive medical management of CAD
Right HF–predominant HFpEF	• Diuresis/ultrafiltration • Digoxin (dose qMWF if elderly and/or if CKD is present) • Midodrine to support systemic blood pressure if systemically hypotensive • PDE5 inhibition if superimposed pulmonary arterial hypertension is present (ie, if PA diastolic pressure – pulmonary capillary wedge pressure >5 mm Hg)
Atrial fibrillation–predominant HFpEF	• Typically require rate/rhythm control more than antihypertensive therapy • Trial of cardioversion or ablation, especially if very symptomatic loss of atrial contraction • Anticoagulation unless contraindicated
Hypertrophic cardiomyopathy–like HFpEF	• Verapamil, diltiazem, long-acting metoprolol; cautious use of diuretics and vasodilators (use only if absolutely necessary)
Valvular HFpEF	• Medical treatment of underlying valve disease if possible • Surgical treatment of valvular disease if indicated
High-output HFpEF	• Determine underlying cause of high output state (ie, anemia, liver disease, AV fistula, hyperthyroidism) • Treat underlying cause of high output state • Diuretics/ultrafiltration typically necessary
Rare causes of HFpEF (zebras)	• Determine underlying cause • Treat underlying cause • Enroll in clinical trial if possible

Abbreviations: AV, arteriovenous; GFR, glomerular filtration rate; LVEDP, LV end-diastolic pressure; PA, pulmonary artery; PDE5, phosphodiesterase-5 inhibitor; qMWF, every Monday, Wednesday, and Friday.
From Oktay AA, Shah SJ. Diagnosis and management of heart failure with preserved ejection fraction: 10 key lessons. Curr Cardiol Rev 2013. [Epub ahead of print]; with permission.

high. These are also the patients who are frequently enrolled in HFpEF clinical trials that require high BNP levels or previous HF hospitalization.[39] Although diagnosis is often straightforward in these patients, sometimes the diagnosis is missed, especially in those with concomitant obesity (difficult to visualize jugular venous pressure and lower BNP levels) or lung disease. In these patients, confirmation of the HFpEF diagnosis with right heart catheterization for evaluation of invasive hemodynamics can be useful.

The third type of HFpEF clinical presentation is that of pulmonary hypertension with right HF.[29,30,32] This is the highest-risk clinical subset of HFpEF, with high morbidity and mortality. These patients often have the highest BNP levels, but this is not true in all cases. Furthermore, some of these patients have superimposed pulmonary arterial hypertension on top of pulmonary venous hypertension,[40] which adds to the propensity for right HF. In HFpEF, the presence of RV hypertrophy and/or RV dysfunction is associated with worse outcomes, even after controlling for other HFpEF risk markers.[23]

Although some patients can transition from one type of HFpEF clinical presentation to the other, there are patients who first present with one predominant type of HFpEF and do not progress. Whether this phenomenon has to do with duration of the HF syndrome, dietary factors, severity of underlying abnormalities in cardiac structure/function, or other factors is unknown.

Phenomics (Phenomapping) of HFpEF

Several sophisticated phenotyping tools, ranging from a multitude of biomarkers to comprehensive cardiovascular imaging modalities to environmental characterization using tools such as geocoding are now available in the era of deep

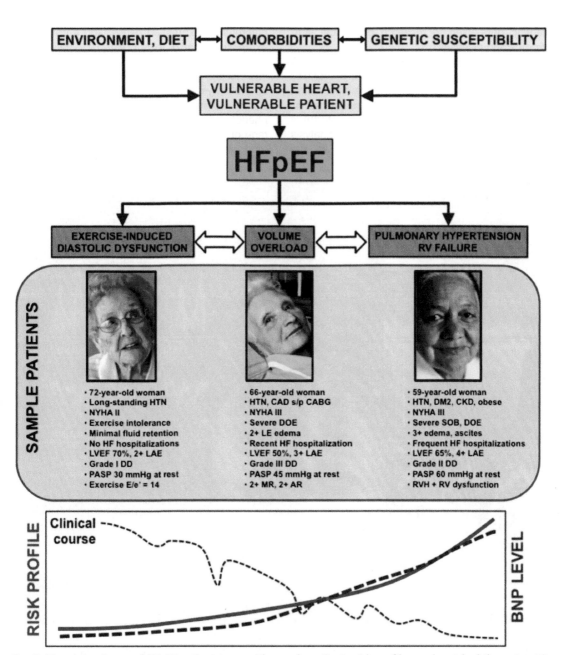

Fig. 5. Theoretic schema of HFpEF patient types with sample patients, risk profiles, and matched therapies. AR, aortic regurgitation; ARNI, angiotensin receptor/neprilysin inhibitor; CABG, coronary artery bypass grafting; CKD, chronic kidney disease; DD, diastolic dysfunction; DM2, type 2 diabetes mellitus; DOE, dyspnea on exertion; HTN, hypertension; If, inward funny channel; LAE, left atrial enlargement; LE, lower extremity; MR, mitral regurgitation; MRA, mineralocorticoid receptor antagonist; NYHA, New York Heart Association; PASP, pulmonary artery systolic pressure; PDE5, phosphodiesterase-5; RVH, RV hypertrophy; s/p, status post; SOB, shortness of breath. (*From* Shah SJ. Matchmaking for the optimization of clinical trials of heart failure with preserved ejection fraction: no laughing matter. J Am Coll Cardiol 2013;62(15):33; with permission.)

phenotyping.[41] These comprehensive phenotyping tools, along with genomics and systems biology, can improve characterization of heterogeneous syndromes like HFpEF. Combined with "big data" machine learning algorithms to find patterns in dense, multidimensional data, novel phenotypic characterization of HFpEF should be possible in the near future. Although machine learning analyses are not new, they have been popularized in recent years with the advent of large quantities of genetic data used in research of clinical syndromes and diseases.

For example, in gene expression analyses, RNA is isolated from a specific tissue, and microarray analyses are used to quantify gene expression with interrogation of several pathways (inflammation, fibrosis, cell cycle mediators, and so forth).[42] Next, unbiased hierarchical clustering analysis is performed to determine patterns in the differentially expressed genes, and a visual gene expression heat map is created.[43] The resultant gene expression signatures can provide insight into disease pathogenesis and potential therapeutic pathways. A similar type of analysis, unsupervised cluster analysis, can be performed using phenotypic data. In HFpEF, we can take advantage of the large quantity of available phenotypic data, such as a wide variety of quantitative data

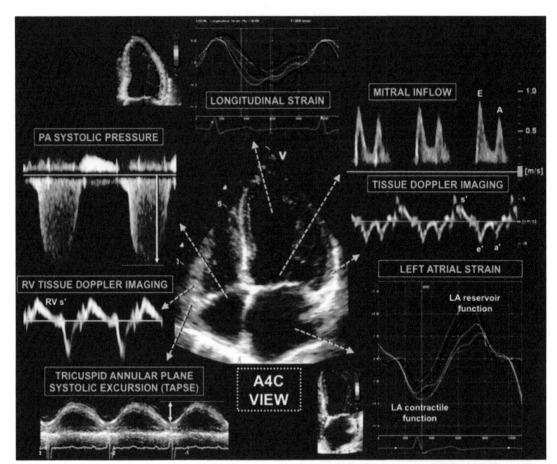

Fig. 6. Comprehensive echocardiographic phenotypic analysis of HFpEF. Comprehensive echocardiography, including 2-D, Doppler, tissue Doppler, and speckle tracking, allows for detailed phenotypic analysis of cardiac structure, function, and mechanics in patients with HFpEF. The figure shows examples of information that can be obtained from the apical 4-chamber view. Clockwise from the top: speckle-tracking echocardiography for assessment of LV regional and global longitudinal strain (early diastolic strain rate can also be obtained in this view). Mitral inflow and tissue Doppler imaging of the septal and lateral mitral annulus provide information on LV diastolic function grade and estimated LV filling pressure (E/e' ratio), along with assessment of longitudinal systolic (s') and atrial (a') function. Speckle-tracking analysis of LA function provides peak LA contractile function (peak negative longitudinal LA strain) and LA reservoir function (peak positive longitudinal LA strain). Tricuspid annular plane systolic function (TAPSE) and basal RV free wall peak longitudinal tissue Doppler velocity (RV s') provide information on longitudinal RV function, as does speckle tracking echocardiography of the RV (not shown). Finally, analysis of the tricuspid regurgitant jet Doppler profile, when added to the estimated RA pressure, provides an estimate of the PA systolic pressure. Additional data available from the apical 4-chamber view include assessment of LV volumes and EF, LA volume, and RV size and global systolic function (eg, RV fractional area change). A4C, apical 4-chamber; LA, left atrial; PA, pulmonary artery; RA, right atrial. (*From* Butler J, Fonarow G, Zile MR, et al. Developing therapies for heart failure with preserved ejection fraction: current state and future directions. JACC Heart Fail 2014;2(2):97–112; with permission.)

available from comprehensive echocardiography (including Doppler, tissue Doppler, and speckle-tracking analysis), as shown in **Fig. 6**. Phenotypic heat maps can be created that are akin to gene expression heat maps, thereby allowing for novel categorization of patients (**Fig. 7**). In addition, dense, multidimensional phenotypic data from HFpEF clinical trials could be distilled down to a few dimensions using principal components analysis (**Fig. 8**).

Table 2 summarizes the phenomapping approach to the categorization of clinical syndromes, including HFpEF. These types of analyses have several advantages: (1) they take into consideration immense quantitative phenotypic data; (2) it is possible to visualize the heterogeneity of the clinical syndrome; (3) they provide mutually exclusive classification of a clinical syndrome; and (4) the clustering of patients into categories is unsupervised and thus does not rely on knowledge of a specific outcome, which is required for more traditional clustering analyses and supervised statistical analyses, such as classification and regression tree (CART) analysis.[44]

Once performed for HFpEF, phenomapping analyses can be applied to clinical trials to determine whether certain subgroups of patients with a particular phenotype signature are more responsive to the investigational drug or device compared with other types of patients, thereby leading to theranostics, a combined diagnostic and therapeutic strategy.[45]

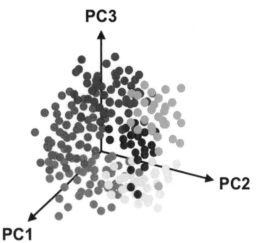

Fig. 8. 3-D principal components analysis plot. In this theoretic example, patients are grouped based on 3 principal components (PC1, PC2, and PC3) in 3 dimensions. Each color represents a group of patients that corresponds to a particular cluster based on phenotypic similarities.

THE VALUE OF ENHANCED CLASSIFICATION OF HFpEF IN FUTURE CLINICAL TRIALS

Future clinical trials can harness these advances in phenotypic categorization in 2 key ways. First, phase II clinical trials of HFpEF may benefit greatly from advanced phenotyping of potential subjects by matching the mechanism of a particular drug with a specific HFpEF phenotype. For

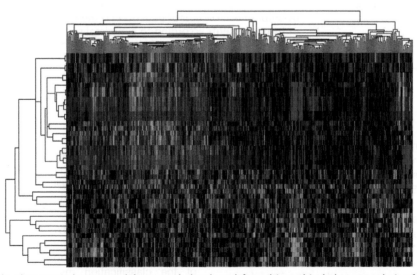

Fig. 7. Sample phenotypic heat map (phenomap) developed from hierarchical cluster analysis of quantitative echocardiographic data. The rows in the heat map correspond to the various quantitative echocardiographic phenotypes (eg, septal wall thickness, EF, and early diastolic [e'] tissue velocity), whereas the columns represent individual patients. Red, increased values; green, decreased values. The dendrogram across the top of the heat map is a tree diagram that demonstrates the clustering of patients; the dendrogram on the left side of the heat map illustrates clustering of phenotypes.

Table 2
Analytic methods for phenomapping analyses

Methodology	Description
Preparation of quantitative phenotypic variables	• Collect a large amount of phenotypic data in the patients being studied. • Standardize each quantitative variable to a mean of 0 and standard deviation of 1 (ie, mean $\pm$ SD of 0 $\pm$ 1). • Remove any variables with large amounts of missing information and, for all other variables with missing data, perform multiple imputation to fill in missing values.
Explore redundancy among phenotypic variables	• Generate a correlation matrix of phenotypic variables by assigning correlation coefficients to each bivariate comparison. • Visualize correlations among phenotypic variables through the use of hierarchical clustering to create a heat map of bivariate correlations (with the color intensity of each cell in the matrix corresponding to the strength of the correlation between any 2 quantitative phenotypes). • Use the heat map to highlight similarities among phenotypic variables and visualize and unanticipated correlations across phenotypes.
Principal components analysis	• Perform principal components analysis as an alternate method to find orthogonal axes of phenotypic variation within the data set. • Interpret top principal components according to combinations of conventional phenotypic features. • Classify patients according to contribution of individual components.
Model-based clustering with bayesian information criterion analysis	• Use model-based clustering, which achieves parameter fitting and assigns patients to clusters by minimizing a penalized likelihood, to determine phenotypic signatures of patients.[46,47] • Incorporate bayesian information criterion analysis to penalize increases in model complexity (eg, greater number of clusters) to create the most parsimonious solution (this approach is termed, *regularization*, in machine learning, and allows increased generalizability to other data sets[44]).
Multinomial logistic regression with lasso penalty	• Build a generalizable logistic regression model (using multinomial logistic regression with L1 norm [lasso] technique)[48] to define membership for each cluster of patients in order to (1) permit classification of future patients according to a minimal set of quantitative phenotypes and (2) identify those features most informative for categorization of patients.

example, a drug that ameliorates ischemia and improves myocyte relaxation would benefit most from enrolling patients with a history of CAD and reduced tissue Doppler e' velocities on echocardiography. Second, in phase II and III clinical trials, deep phenotyping of study participants using banked blood and cardiac imaging (such as comprehensive echocardiography), along with other tools (quality of life, exercise tests, and so forth) as needed, will allow for the development of phenomaps, as described previously. Investigators can then use the resultant phenotypic signatures to determine groups of patients most likely to benefit from a particular drug or device.

SUMMARY

HFpEF is a heterogeneous syndrome, a key reason that may explain why (1) diagnosing and treating HFpEF is so challenging and (2) clinical trials in HFpEF have failed thus far. Here we have reviewed 4 ways of categorizing HFpEF patients based on pathophysiology, clinical/etiologic subtype, type of clinical presentation, and quantitative phenomics (phenomapping analysis). Regardless of the classification method used, improved phenotypic characterization of HFpEF patients in both clinics and in clinical trials, and matching of targeted therapies with specific patient subtypes, will be critical if outcomes are to be improved in this increasingly prevalent patient population.

REFERENCES

1. Yancy CW, Jessup M, Bozkurt B, et al. 2013 ACCF/AHA guideline for the management of heart failure: a report of the American College of Cardiology Foundation/American Heart Association Task Force on Practice Guidelines. J Am Coll Cardiol 2013; 62(16):e147–239.

2. Oktay AA, Shah SJ. Diagnosis and management of heart failure with preserved ejection fraction: 10 key lessons. Curr Cardiol Rev 2013. [Epub ahead of print].

3. Oktay AA, Rich JD, Shah SJ. The emerging epidemic of heart failure with preserved ejection fraction. Curr Heart Fail Rep 2013;10(4):401–10.

4. Go AS, Mozaffarian D, Roger VL, et al. Heart disease and stroke statistics–2013 update: a report from the American Heart Association. Circulation 2013;127(1):e6–245.

5. Shah AM, Pfeffer MA. The many faces of heart failure with preserved ejection fraction. Nat Rev Cardiol 2012;9(10):555–6.

6. Shah AM, Solomon SD. Phenotypic and pathophysiological heterogeneity in heart failure with preserved ejection fraction. Eur Heart J 2012;33(14):1716–7.

7. Shah SJ. Matchmaking for the optimization of clinical trials of heart failure with preserved ejection fraction: no laughing matter. J Am Coll Cardiol 2013; 62(15):1339–42.

8. Borlaug BA, Paulus WJ. Heart failure with preserved ejection fraction: pathophysiology, diagnosis, and treatment. Eur Heart J 2011;32(6):670–9.

9. Borlaug BA, Redfield MM. Diastolic and systolic heart failure are distinct phenotypes within the heart failure spectrum. Circulation 2011;123(18):2006–13 [discussion: 2014].

10. Yancy CW, Lopatin M, Stevenson LW, et al. Clinical presentation, management, and in-hospital outcomes of patients admitted with acute decompensated heart failure with preserved systolic function: a report from the Acute Decompensated Heart Failure National Registry (ADHERE) Database. J Am Coll Cardiol 2006;47(1):76–84.

11. Bursi F, Weston SA, Redfield MM, et al. Systolic and diastolic heart failure in the community. JAMA 2006; 296(18):2209–16.

12. Prasad A, Hastings JL, Shibata S, et al. Characterization of static and dynamic left ventricular diastolic function in patients with heart failure with a preserved ejection fraction. Circ Heart Fail 2010;3(5): 617–26.

13. Maurer MS, King DL, El-Khoury Rumbarger L, et al. Left heart failure with a normal ejection fraction: identification of different pathophysiologic mechanisms. J Card Fail 2005;11(3):177–87.

14. Kliger C, King DL, Maurer MS. A clinical algorithm to differentiate heart failure with a normal ejection fraction by pathophysiologic mechanism. Am J Geriatr Cardiol 2006;15(1):50–7.

15. Bench T, Burkhoff D, O'Connell JB, et al. Heart failure with normal ejection fraction: consideration of mechanisms other than diastolic dysfunction. Curr Heart Fail Rep 2009;6(1):57–64.

16. Burkhoff D, Maurer MS, Packer M. Heart failure with a normal ejection fraction: is it really a disorder of diastolic function? Circulation 2003;107(5):656–8.

17. Ather S, Chan W, Bozkurt B, et al. Impact of noncardiac comorbidities on morbidity and mortality in a predominantly male population with heart failure and preserved versus reduced ejection fraction. J Am Coll Cardiol 2012;59(11):998–1005.

18. Edelmann F, Stahrenberg R, Gelbrich G, et al. Contribution of comorbidities to functional impairment is higher in heart failure with preserved than with reduced ejection fraction. Clin Res Cardiol 2011;100(9):755–64.

19. Mohammed SF, Borlaug BA, Roger VL, et al. Comorbidity and ventricular and vascular structure and function in heart failure with preserved ejection fraction: a community-based study. Circ Heart Fail 2012; 5(6):710–9.

20. Paulus WJ, Tschope C. A novel paradigm for heart failure with preserved ejection fraction: comorbidities drive myocardial dysfunction and remodeling through coronary microvascular endothelial inflammation. J Am Coll Cardiol 2013;62(4):263–71.

21. Shah SJ, Gheorghiade M. Heart failure with preserved ejection fraction: treat now by treating comorbidities. JAMA 2008;300(4):431–3.

22. Aurigemma GP, Gaasch WH. Clinical practice. Diastolic heart failure. N Engl J Med 2004;351(11): 1097–105.

23. Burke MA, Katz DH, Beussink L, et al. Prognostic importance of pathophysiologic markers in patients with heart failure and preserved ejection fraction. Circ Heart Fail 2014;7(2):288–99.

24. Zile MR, Baicu CF, Gaasch WH. Diastolic heart failure–abnormalities in active relaxation and passive stiffness of the left ventricle. N Engl J Med 2004; 350(19):1953–9.

25. Shah SJ. Evolving approaches to the management of heart failure with preserved ejection fraction in patients with coronary artery disease. Curr Treat Options Cardiovasc Med 2010;12(1):58–75.

26. Liu YW, Tsai WC, Su CT, et al. Evidence of left ventricular systolic dysfunction detected by automated function imaging in patients with heart failure and preserved left ventricular ejection fraction. J Card Fail 2009;15(9):782–9.

27. Kawaguchi M, Hay I, Fetics B, et al. Combined ventricular systolic and arterial stiffening in patients with heart failure and preserved ejection fraction: implications for systolic and diastolic reserve limitations. Circulation 2003;107(5):714–20.

28. Borlaug BA, Melenovsky V, Russell SD, et al. Impaired chronotropic and vasodilator reserves limit exercise capacity in patients with heart failure and a preserved ejection fraction. Circulation 2006; 114(20):2138–47.

29. Thenappan T, Shah SJ, Gomberg-Maitland M, et al. Clinical characteristics of pulmonary hypertension in patients with heart failure and preserved ejection fraction. Circ Heart Fail 2011;4(3):257–65.

30. Lam CS, Roger VL, Rodeheffer RJ, et al. Pulmonary hypertension in heart failure with preserved ejection fraction: a community-based study. J Am Coll Cardiol 2009;53(13):1119–26.

31. Phan TT, Shivu GN, Abozguia K, et al. Impaired heart rate recovery and chronotropic incompetence in patients with heart failure with preserved ejection fraction. Circ Heart Fail 2010;3(1):29–34.

32. Shah SJ. Pulmonary hypertension. JAMA 2012; 308(13):1366–74.

33. Borlaug BA, Nishimura RA, Sorajja P, et al. Exercise hemodynamics enhance diagnosis of early heart failure with preserved ejection fraction. Circ Heart Fail 2010;3(5):588–95.

34. Maeder MT, Thompson BR, Htun N, et al. Hemodynamic determinants of the abnormal cardiopulmonary exercise response in heart failure with preserved left ventricular ejection fraction. J Card Fail 2012;18(9):702–10.

35. Burgess MI, Jenkins C, Sharman JE, et al. Diastolic stress echocardiography: hemodynamic validation and clinical significance of estimation of ventricular filling pressure with exercise. J Am Coll Cardiol 2006;47(9):1891–900.

36. Ha JW, Oh JK, Pellikka PA, et al. Diastolic stress echocardiography: a novel noninvasive diagnostic test for diastolic dysfunction using supine bicycle exercise Doppler echocardiography. J Am Soc Echocardiogr 2005;18(1):63–8.

37. Kane GC, Oh JK. Diastolic stress test for the evaluation of exertional dyspnea. Curr Cardiol Rep 2012; 14(3):359–65.

38. Anjan VY, Loftus TM, Burke MA, et al. Prevalence, clinical phenotype, and outcomes associated with normal B-type natriuretic Peptide levels in heart failure with preserved ejection fraction. Am J Cardiol 2012;110(6):870–6.

39. Shah SJ, Heitner JF, Sweitzer NK, et al. Baseline characteristics of patients in the treatment of preserved cardiac function heart failure with an aldosterone antagonist (TOPCAT) trial. Circ Heart Fail 2013; 6(2):184–92.

40. Gerges C, Gerges M, Lang MB, et al. Diastolic pulmonary vascular pressure gradient: a predictor of prognosis in "out-of-proportion" pulmonary hypertension. Chest 2013;143(3):758–66.

41. Tracy RP. 'Deep phenotyping': characterizing populations in the era of genomics and systems biology. Curr Opin Lipidol 2008;19(2):151–7.

42. Ballman KV. Genetics and genomics: gene expression microarrays. Circulation 2008;118(15):1593–7.

43. Eisen MB, Spellman PT, Brown PO, et al. Cluster analysis and display of genome-wide expression patterns. Proc Natl Acad Sci U S A 1998;95(25):14863–8.

44. Lemon SC, Roy J, Clark MA, et al. Classification and regression tree analysis in public health: methodological review and comparison with logistic regression. Ann Behav Med 2003;26(3):172–81.

45. Shah SJ, Wasserstrom JA. SERCA2a gene therapy for the prevention of sudden cardiac death: a future theranostic for heart failure? Circulation 2012; 126(17):2047–50.

46. Fraley C, Raftery AE. Model-based clustering, discriminant analysis, and density estimation. J Am Stat Assoc 2002;97:611–31.

47. Hastie T, Tibshirani R, Friedman J. Unsupervised learning: hierarchical clustering. In: Hastie T, Tibshirani R, Friedman J, editors. The elements of statistical learning. 2nd edition. New York: Springer; 2009. p. 520–8.

48. Friedman J, Hastie T, Tibshirani R. Regularization paths for generalized linear models via coordinate descent. J Stat Softw 2010;33(1):1–22.

Imaging in Heart Failure with Preserved Ejection Fraction

Deepak K. Gupta, MD[a], Scott D. Solomon, MD[b],*

KEYWORDS

- Left ventricular ejection fraction • Echocardiography • Diastolic dysfunction
- Myocardial deformation • Stress testing

KEY POINTS

- Cardiac imaging is needed to define left ventricular ejection fraction (LVEF), but the cut point for defining preserved versus reduced LVEF remains controversial.
- Identifying cardiac dysfunction in heart failure (HF) with preserved EF (HFpEF) can be challenging and requires an integrated assessment of cardiac structure and function.
- Transthoracic echocardiography is the first-line noninvasive imaging test for evaluating cardiac structure and function in patients with HF.
- HFpEF is characterized by heterogeneity in phenotype and includes not only diastolic dysfunction but also systolic abnormalities not identifiable by LVEF alone.
- Abnormalities of cardiac function may not be present at rest in HFpEF but may be unmasked with exercise or pharmacologic testing.

INTRODUCTION

The objective demonstration of cardiac dysfunction through imaging supports the diagnosis of heart failure (HF). Cardiac dysfunction is readily apparent when the left ventricular ejection fraction (LVEF) is reduced; but when the LVEF is preserved, identifying cardiac dysfunction is more challenging. As HF with preserved EF (HFpEF) is becoming the predominant form of HF, understanding cardiac structure and function in this syndrome is highly relevant for diagnosis, prognosis, pathophysiology, and management.

HFpEF was initially recognized when patients with clinical HF were found to have preserved LVEF by nuclear and echocardiographic techniques; consequently, HFpEF was attributed to diastolic dysfunction.[1,2] However, with advances in cardiac imaging, systolic abnormalities not captured by LVEF have been identified in HFpEF, thereby challenging the prevailing concept of isolated diastolic HF.[3–6] Furthermore, characterization of cardiac structure in HFpEF populations has revealed significant heterogeneity rather than a uniform finding of the classic description of a small LV cavity with thick walls and an enlarged left atrium (LA).[7–11] It is also becoming apparent that patients with HFpEF frequently have symptoms only with exertion and that imaging tests performed at rest may be insensitive for identifying cardiac dysfunction, such that stress testing for the detection of cardiac dysfunction in HFpEF may play an increasing role.[12–14] The expanding literature on HFpEF reveals it to be a challenging syndrome with significant heterogeneity, both clinically and with regard to cardiac structure and

Disclosures: None.
[a] Vanderbilt Heart and Vascular Institute, Department of Medicine, Vanderbilt University Medical Center, 2525 West End Ave, Suite 300, Nashville, TN 37203, USA; [b] Division of Cardiology, Department of Medicine, Brigham and Women's Hospital, Harvard Medical School, 75 Francis Street, Boston, MA 02115, USA
* Corresponding author.
E-mail address: ssolomon@rics.bwh.harvard.edu

Heart Failure Clin 10 (2014) 419–434
http://dx.doi.org/10.1016/j.hfc.2014.04.004
1551-7136/14/$ – see front matter © 2014 Elsevier Inc. All rights reserved.

function. In this article, cardiac imaging in HFpEF is reviewed with attention to the choice of imaging modality, technique, and interpretation.

PLANNING CARDIAC IMAGING

Any patient presenting with new-onset HF or prevalent HF with a change in clinical status should undergo cardiac imaging to quantify LVEF and assess for underlying causes.[15] Cardiac imaging provides essential information for diagnosis, prognosis, and management, especially if a reversible cause or specific cause for HF, such as coronary artery, valvular, pericardial, hypertrophic, infiltrative, or congenital heart disease, is identified.

Selection of Imaging Modality

Several noninvasive cardiac imaging modalities, including echocardiography (echo), magnetic resonance (MR), nuclear, and computed tomography (CT), are available (**Fig. 1**). The history, physical, and laboratory data, with attention to such factors as weight, pulmonary disease, chest wall deformities, renal dysfunction, metal objects or devices, ability to lay flat and follow commands, respiratory status, and/or claustrophobia may help inform the decision regarding which imaging test to obtain. However, transthoracic echo is the recommended first-line noninvasive imaging test for evaluating patients with HF because of its safety, availability, relatively low cost, and ability to provide detailed information regarding cardiac structure, systolic and diastolic function, and hemodynamics.[15]

MR, nuclear, and CT imaging are complementary to echo in the evaluation of patients with HFpEF (**Table 1**).[2,16–18] MR overcomes poor imaging windows that may limit some echocardiographic examinations, has excellent spatial resolution, has a high signal-to-noise ratio yielding clear delineation of the blood-endocardial interface, can provide tissue characterization with regard to myocardial edema and fibrosis, can quantify diastolic function through phase contrast sequences, and is able to assess myocardial mechanics through tagging or feature tracking. In addition, myocardial perfusion imaging with MR can be used to evaluate for coronary artery disease.[16] Nuclear techniques, such as single-photon emission computed tomography (SPECT), positron emission tomography (PET), and radionuclide ventriculography, are well established for quantifying ventricular volumes and EF and provided some of the early literature regarding diastolic dysfunction in the setting of HFpEF.[2,17] SPECT and PET imaging are also robust techniques for evaluating coronary artery disease, cardiac metabolism, and sympathetic innervation.[19,20] CT is a rapidly developing cardiac imaging technology that is becoming more widely available. It has high spatial resolution allowing imaging of the coronary and pulmonary vasculature, chamber sizes, volumes, and EF. However, temporal resolution is often low in CT; patients are

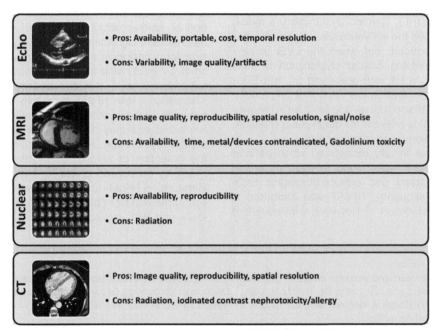

Fig. 1. Noninvasive cardiac imaging modalities. Echo, MR imaging (MRI), nuclear, and CT are the most commonly used cardiac imaging modalities. Each modality has their advantages and disadvantages.

Table 1
Strengths and weaknesses of different cardiac imaging modalities

Parameters	Echo	MRI	Nuclear	CT
Chamber size, wall thickness, volumes	+++	++++	++	+++
LVEF	+++	++++	+++	+++
LV diastolic function	++++	++	+	?
Hemodynamics	++++	++	−	?
Right ventricular size and function	+++	++++	++	+++
Coronary artery disease & vasculature	++	+++	++	+++
Valves: aortic, mitral, tricuspid, pulmonic	++++	++	−	+
Myocardial deformation/mechanics	++++	++++	+	+
Pericardial disease	++	++++	−	+++
Tissue characterization (fibrosis)	+	++++	++	++

Abbreviation: MRI, MR imaging.

exposed to radiation and nephrotoxic contrast agents; therefore, cardiac CT is rarely used in the initial evaluation of patients with HFpEF.[16] MR, nuclear, and CT are individually robust cardiac imaging techniques that may offer complementary information to that obtained by echo; however, these modalities have not been validated against outcomes to the same extent as echo with regard to HFpEF.[10,21–23] Therefore, the remainder of the article focuses on the echo evaluation of patients with HFpEF.

ECHO IMAGING TECHNIQUE

The characterization of cardiac structure and function in HFpEF depends on *quantitative* echo; therefore, meticulous attention to optimization of images is essential for accurate measurement and interpretation. In order to obtain the best quality data, appropriate patient preparation, positioning, and careful imaging technique are required. Common pitfalls that reduce the quality of data include a lack of comprehensive examination, foreshortening particularly of apical views, poor alignment of the Doppler beam, and low frame rates.

Standard transthoracic echo is performed with patients comfortably situated in the left lateral decubitus or supine position. Electrocardiogram leads should be positioned to produce a signal that clearly displays the cardiac cycle. Heart rate, rhythm, blood pressure, height, and weight should be recorded. Comprehensive 2-dimensional (2D), M-mode, and Doppler examination should be performed from the parasternal, apical, subcostal, and suprasternal windows, with careful attention paid to the optimization of each image (**Table 2**).[24] At least 3 and 5 full cardiac cycles should be captured for each image for patients in sinus rhythm and atrial fibrillation, respectively.

In the parasternal long-axis view, it is important that the imaging plane be parallel to the true long axis of the LV and aorta, with visualization of the mid to basal LV, both leaflets of the mitral valve, the aortic valve, LA, and right ventricle (RV). In this orientation, the LV minor axis diameter is at its greatest and where LV wall thicknesses and cavity dimensions should be measured for quantification of LV mass and geometry, which are of prognostic importance in HFpEF.

In the apical views, care should be taken to obtain images demonstrating the full length of the LV without foreshortening. The apical 4- and 2-chamber views are of particular importance for the calculation of LVEF using Simpson's biplane method; therefore, accurate classification of a patient as having HFpEF depends on high-quality apical views. If 2 or more endocardial segments cannot be visualized, then intravenous echocardiographic contrast should be used to improve image quality.[25,26]

From the apical 4-chamber view, several Doppler indices important for characterizing systolic and diastolic function, as well as hemodynamics, should be obtained as these are of particular relevance in describing the cardiac phenotype of patients with HFpEF. These indices include mitral and tricuspid annular tissue Doppler systolic (S') and diastolic (e' and a') velocities, transmitral spectral Doppler LV inflow, pulmonary venous flow, and mitral and tricuspid regurgitation. A focused 2D view of the RV should also be obtained along with M-mode interrogation of the lateral tricuspid annulus planar systolic excursion. Nonforeshortened images focused and zoomed on the LA should also be obtained in the apical 4- and 2-chamber views for quantification of LA volumes.

Table 2
Protocol for comprehensive 2D, M-mode, and Doppler transthoracic echo as it relates to the evaluation of patients with HFpEF

Window	2D View	M-mode	Doppler	Additional/Advanced
Parasternal	Long axis	RV, LV, MV, AV, LA	MV & AV (color)	—
	RV inflow	—	RV inflow (spectral) TV (color & spectral)	—
	Short axis (base, MV, mid LV, apex)	AV	AV, TV, & PV (color) TV & PV (spectral) RVOT (spectral)	Circumferential & radial S & SR Twist/torsion/untwist
Apical	4 Chamber	—	MV annulus (TDI) Transmitral LV inflow (spectral) Pulmonary vein (spectral) MV (color & spectral)	Zoomed LA Color M-mode of LV inflow Longitudinal S & SR
	RV focused	TAPSE	TV (spectral) TV annulus (TDI)	—
	2 Chamber	—	MV (color & spectral)	Zoomed LA Longitudinal strain & strain rate
	Long axis	—	AV (color & spectral)	—
	5 Chamber	—	AV, IVRT	—
Subcostal	4 Chamber	—	TV (color & spectral) IAS (color)	—
	IVC & hepatic veins	—	Hepatic veins (color & spectral)	Sniff
Suprasternal	Aorta	—	Ascending (spectral) Descending (spectral)	—

Abbreviations: AV, aortic valve; IAS, interatrial septum; IVC, inferior vena cava; IVRT, isovolumic relaxation time; MV, mitral valve; PV, pulmonic valve; RVOT, right ventricular outflow tract; S, strain; SR, strain rate; TAPSE, tricuspid annular planar systolic excursion; TDI, tissue Doppler imaging; TV, tricuspid valve.

INTERPRETATION/ASSESSMENT OF CLINICAL IMAGES
LVEF

Accurately quantifying LVEF is centrally important to the care of patients with HF. When categorizing a patient as HFpEF or heart failure with reduced ejection fraction attention must be paid to the method for determining LVEF as well as the quality and reliability of LVEF assessment. There is a variety of methods for estimating LVEF with echo,[27,28] including visual estimation, Teichcholz' method, Simpson's biplane, and more recently 3-dimensional (3D) imaging,[29] with Simpson's biplane method currently recommended.[27] The LVEF value for defining HFpEF remains controversial, with cut points ranging from more than 40% to more than 55% in various clinical trials and observational registries (**Table 3**).[7] The rationale for each of these LVEF values can be justified; however, the controversy regarding the LVEF for defining HFpEF will likely remain until a therapy is demonstrated to reduce mortality, which to date is lacking. Although guidelines from the American Heart Association, American College of Cardiology, and European Society of Cardiology recommend an LVEF of 50% or more,[15,30] most clinical trials in HFpEF have or are using an LVEF of 45% more as an inclusion criterion; therefore, this value may become the benchmark in the future.

Cardiac Structure

Although the classic description of cardiac structure in HFpEF is one with thick LV walls and a small LV cavity, this pattern is not universally present.[31] Findings from epidemiologic cohorts and clinical trials consistently demonstrate diverse cardiac phenotypes in HFpEF, with pooled estimates suggesting that approximately 70% of patients with HFpEF have abnormal LV geometry (28% concentric remodeling, 35% concentric hypertrophy, and 7% eccentric hypertrophy), whereas 30% have normal LV geometry (see **Table 3**).[7] Although some of the heterogeneity may be attributable to differences in study populations, these findings have diagnostic implications, namely, the presence of normal LV wall thickness and cavity size does not exclude the syndrome of HFpEF and that the presence of cardiac remodeling or hypertrophy, although supportive, is not required in HFpEF. Importantly, patterns of LV geometry in HFpEF are of prognostic importance as the presence of hypertrophy seems to confer an increased risk of death or cardiovascular hospitalization, as compared to normal geometry or concentric remodeling.[8,10]

The different patterns of cardiac structure in HFpEF may also inform underlying pathophysiologic mechanisms. For example, in the Cardiovascular Health Study, participants with HFpEF were characterized as having larger LV size and stroke volume as compared with hypertensive and healthy controls, suggesting volume overload in those with HFpEF.[32] In contrast, findings from Olmsted County, MN indicated that patients with HFpEF, as compared with hypertensive controls, had lower stroke volume, smaller LV size, and more impaired diastolic function despite similar resting vascular and LV stiffening, suggesting primary diastolic abnormalities of cardiomyocytes and/or the extracellular matrix.[11] Together these data highlight the need to better understand the pathophysiologic mechanisms underlying the variations in structural phenotypes that may inform future preventive and therapeutic strategies in HFpEF.

Diastolic Function

HF is present when the heart is unable to produce sufficient cardiac output to meet the body's physiologic demands or is only able to do so at the expense of elevated filling pressures.[33] HFpEF is classically attributed to elevated LV filling pressures as a consequence of diastolic dysfunction; therefore, the assessment of LV filling pressures and diastolic function are essential components in the evaluation of patients with HFpEF.

Diastole begins with aortic valve closure and includes isovolumic relaxation, rapid filling, diastasis, and atrial contraction.[34] LV relaxation is an energy-dependent process largely driven by the active reuptake of cytoplasmic calcium into the sarcoplasmic reticulum and occurs during isovolumic relaxation and rapid filling phases. During this time, cardiac myofilaments lengthen (relax), leading to an expansion of the LV cavity with a resultant decline in LV pressure to less than that of the LA. When LV pressure decreases to less than LA pressure, the mitral valve opens with rapid filling of the LV as blood is sucked from the LA into the expanding LV. As blood moves between the LA and LV, the pressure gradient between these chambers decreases to zero, representing diastasis. Finally, in late diastole, atrial contraction increases LA pressure more than that of the LV and a compliant LV accepts the additional volume of blood pumped in by atrial systole.[34]

Echocardiographic parameters of diastolic function have been validated against invasive cardiac catheterization[35–37] and have prognostic significance with regard to the risk of developing HF, HF hospitalizations, and mortality.[10,21–23] In particular, 2D and Doppler indices can be integrated to define whether diastolic dysfunction is present (**Fig. 2**)[21] and whether LV filling pressure is elevated (**Fig. 3**).[36] These indices include mitral annular tissue Doppler velocities, LA volume, transmitral spectral Doppler inflow, isovolumic relaxation time, as well as the patterns and duration of pulmonary venous flow and pulmonary artery systolic pressure.[21,36] In the setting of preserved LVEF, transmitral spectral Doppler flow velocities and patterns have weaker correlations with LV filling pressures, whereas mitral annular tissue Doppler velocities better characterize diastolic function. The ratio of the early transmitral spectral Doppler velocity (E) to the early tissue Doppler mitral annular velocity (e') is highly correlated with the pulmonary capillary wedge pressure, LA pressure, and LV end diastolic pressure in the setting of preserved LVEF.[38]

In community studies and clinical trials of HFpEF, up to one-third of subjects have normal patterns of diastolic function as assessed by resting echo (see **Table 3**).[7,10,39] This finding may be in part related to differences in study populations, variability in methodology for defining the presence and/or severity of diastolic dysfunction by echo, as well as the limitations of echo with regard to the sensitivity to detect diastolic dysfunction. However, the data regarding the prevalence of diastolic dysfunction by echo in HFpEF also highlight the heterogeneity of this syndrome and emphasize that normal diastolic function does not exclude the syndrome of HFpEF. Moreover, metrics of diastolic function change with age; given that HFpEF most commonly occurs in the elderly, caution should be exercised in the interpretation of diastolic function in older age groups, as impaired relaxation can be a normal age-related finding.[22] Similarly, left atrial size or volume, which is considered to be an integrated barometer of diastolic function, can be enlarged in atrial fibrillation; therefore, left atrial enlargement may not be specific for diastolic dysfunction in the setting of atrial fibrillation. Altogether, these data support the concepts that (1) diastolic dysfunction is present in most patients with HFpEF, (2) HFpEF is not synonymous with diastolic HF, and (3) HFpEF may not be caused by diastolic dysfunction alone.

Table 3
Cardiac structure and function in selected HFpEF trials, epidemiologic cohorts, and registries

	TOPCAT[7]	I-PRESERVE[10]	Aldo-DHF[80]	PARAMOUNT[48]	Northwestern Registry[8]	Olmsted County[11]	Cardiovascular Health Study[32]
n	935	745	422	292	402	244	167
Key inclusion criteria	LVEF ≥45%, HF hosp, or BNP ≥100 or NTproBNP ≥360 pg/mL	LVEF ≥45%, NSR at echo	LVEF ≥50%, NSR at echo, DD on echo or AF, pVO2 ≤25	LVEF ≥45%, NTproBNP >400 pg/mL	LVEF >50%	LVEF ≥50%	LVEF ≥55%
Age (y)	69.9 ± 9.7	72 ± 7	67 ± 8	70.6 ± 9.1	65 ± 13	76 (22–99)	76 ± 7
Women (%)	49	62	52	56	62	55	57
LVEF (%)	59.6 ± 8.0	64 ± 9	67 ± 8	57.7 ± 7.9	61 ± 6	62 ± 6	72 ± 7
LVEDD (cm)	4.80 ± 0.58	4.8 ± 0.6	4.65 ± 0.62	4.64 ± 0.48	4.63 ± 0.63	n/a	5.1 ± 0.8
LVESD (cm)	3.37 ± 0.51	3.2 ± 0.7	2.55 ± 0.64	2.99 ± 0.70	2.94 ± 0.65	n/a	3.0 ± 0.7
LVEDVI (mL/m²)	49.9 ± 15.5	49 ± 14	n/a	61.4 ± 15.4	40.6 ± 11.0	56.4 ± 14.4	69 ± 22
LVESVI (mL/m²)	20.7 ± 9.8	18 ± 9	n/a	26.5 ± 10.4	16.2 ± 6.3	n/a	20 ± 10
LV mass (g)	223 ± 71	164 ± 48	n/a	148 ± 43	210 ± 79	200.4 ± 67.1	176 ± 64
LVMI (g/m²)	111 ± 31	n/a	109 ± 28	79.1 ± 22.2	103 ± 38	102.1 ± 29.0	98 ± 34
Normal geometry (%)	14	46	n/a	72	12	31	n/a

Conc remodeling (%)	34	25	n/a	14	28	27	n/a
Conc hypertrophy (%)	43	29	n/a	7	48	26	n/a
Ecc hypertrophy (%)	9	0	n/a	7	12	16	n/a
Diastolic dysfxn (any) (%)	66	69	100	92	91	n/a	n/a
None (%)	34	31	0	8	n/a	n/a	n/a
Grade I (%)	22	29	77	31	n/a	n/a	n/a
Grade II (%)	34	36	21	43	n/a	n/a	n/a
Grade III (%)	10	4	2	18	n/a	n/a	n/a
LAVI (mL/m^2)	29.8 ± 12.5	n/a	28.0 ± 8.4	35.9 ± 13.5	34 ± 14	n/a	n/a
E/A	1.2 ± 0.7	1.05 ± 0.74	0.91 ± 0.33	1.1 ± 0.62	1.4 ± 0.7	1.21 ± 0.69	1.3 ± 1.2
TDI E' lat	8.2 ± 3.2	9.1 ± 3.4	n/a	7.5 ± 2.8	9.3 ± 3.9	n/a	n/a
TDI E' sept	6.1 ± 2.2	7.2 ± 2.9	5.9 ± 1.3	5.8 ± 2.0	7.0 ± 2.7	6.0 ± 2.1	n/a
E/e' lat	11.8 ± 5.9	10.0 ± 4.5	n/a	12.7 ± 7.4	n/a	n/a	n/a
E/e' sept	15.6 ± 6.8	n/a	12.8 ± 4.0	15.9 ± 7.3	17 ± 9	18.4 ± 9.7	n/a
TR velocity (m/s)	2.8 ± 0.5	n/a	n/a	2.5 ± 0.4	3.0 ± 0.6	n/a	n/a
RVSP (mm Hg)	n/a	37 ± 13	n/a	n/a	n/a	n/a	n/a

Abbreviations: AF, atrial fibrillation; BNP, b-type natriuretic peptide; Conc, concentric; DD, diastolic dysfunction; DHF, diastolic heart failure; e', mitral annular early relaxation velocity; E/A, transmitral spectral Doppler E wave velocity/A wave velocity; E/e', transmitral spectral Doppler E wave velocity/mitral annular relaxation velocity; Ecc, eccentric; EDD, end diastolic diameter; EDVI, end diastolic volume index; ESD, end systolic diameter; ESVI, end systolic volume index; hosp, hospitalization; I-PRESERVE, Irbesartan in Heart Failure with Preserved Ejection Fraction Study; lat, lateral; LAVI, left atrial volume index; MI, mass index; n/a, not applicable; NSR, normal sinus rhythm; NTproBNP, N-terminal pro–B-type natriuretic peptide; PARAMOUNT, Prospective comparison of ARNI with ARB on Management Of heart failUre with preserved ejectioN fracTion; pVO2, peak oxygen consumption; RVSP, right ventricular systolic pressure; sept, septal; TDI, tissue Doppler imaging; TOPCAT, Treatment of Preserved Cardiac Function Heart Failure with an Aldosterone Antagonist; TR, tricuspid regurgitation.
Data from Refs.[7,8,10,11,32,48,80]

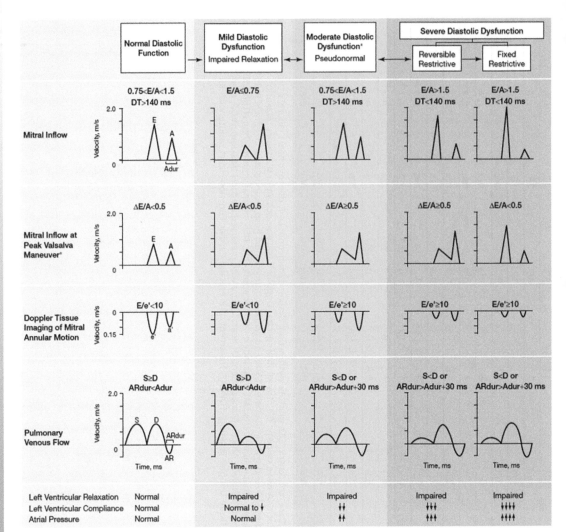

Fig. 2. Echocardiographic criteria and algorithm for identifying diastolic dysfunction. a', velocity of mitral annulus motion with atrial systole; A, velocity at atrial contraction; Adur, A duration; AR, pulmonary venous atrial reversal flow; ARdur, AR duration; D, diastolic forward flow; DT, mitral E velocity deceleration time; e', velocity of mitral annulus early diastolic motion; E, peak early filling velocity; S, systolic forward flow. * Corrected for E/A fusion. (*From* Redfield MM, Jacobsen SJ, Burnett JC Jr, et al. Burden of systolic and diastolic ventricular dysfunction in the community: appreciating the scope of the heart failure epidemic. JAMA 2003;289(2):196; with permission.)

Myocardial Mechanics

Characterizing myocardial mechanical events has provided fundamental insights into cardiac dysfunction in HFpEF by demonstrating abnormalities of systolic function[40] and highlighting that LVEF is not a sensitive measure of contractile dysfunction.[41] The heart is composed of a helical band of myocardial fibers that are oriented longitudinally in the endocardium and epicardium and radially in the midmyocardium, such that when myocytes contract and relax, cardiac mechanical events occur in the longitudinal, circumferential, and radial directions (**Fig. 4**).[42] Noninvasive cardiac

imaging techniques, such as tissue Doppler and speckle tracking echo,[43] as well as tagging and feature tracking MR,[44] can be used to quantify myocardial deformation (**Fig. 5**).

Systolic abnormalities have been described in patients defined as diastolic HF challenging the concept that HFpEF is caused by pure or isolated diastolic dysfunction.[3–6,40,45–48] A recent speckle tracking echo analysis demonstrated that abnormal global longitudinal (GLS) and circumferential systolic strains (GCS) were common in HFpEF, present in 67% and 40% of patients, respectively.[48] This study also compared

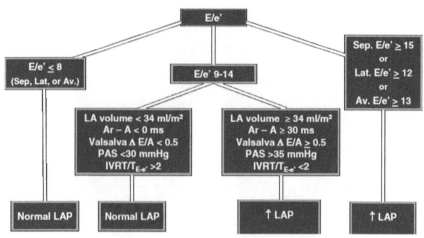

Fig. 3. Estimation of filling pressures in patients with preserved EF. A, transmitral spectral Doppler A wave duration; Ar, pulmonary venous atrial reversal duration; Av, average; e', mitral annular tissue Doppler e' velocity; E, transmitral spectral Doppler E velocity; IVRT, isovolumic relaxation time; LAP, left atrial pressure; Lat, lateral; PAS, pulmonary artery systolic pressure; Sep, septal; $T_{E-e'}$, time from R wave to E wave, time from R wave to e'. (*From* Nagueh SF, Appleton CP, Gillebert TC, et al. Recommendations for the evaluation of left ventricular diastolic function by echocardiography. J Am Soc Echocardiogr 2009;22(2):127; with permission.)

GLS and GCS in HFpEF to patients with hypertension without HF and healthy controls (**Fig. 6**).[48] GLS was impaired in a graded fashion from healthy to hypertensive to HFpEF, consistent with prior studies that suggested that the subendocardial fibers responsible for longitudinal contraction may be most susceptible to the adverse effects of hypertension, diabetes mellitus and ischemia.[48,49] GCS was also impaired in HFpEF when compared with healthy subjects and patients with hypertension, suggesting that

deterioration of GCS may contribute to the transition from compensated hypertension to HFpEF in some patients.[48]

Noninvasive imaging of myocardial deformation has also led to insights into diastolic function. Given the helical fiber orientation of cardiomyocytes in the LV, myocardial contraction has been described as analogous to the wringing of a rag, with clockwise rotation at the base and counterclockwise rotation at the apex.[50] This twisting and shortening motion during systole stores

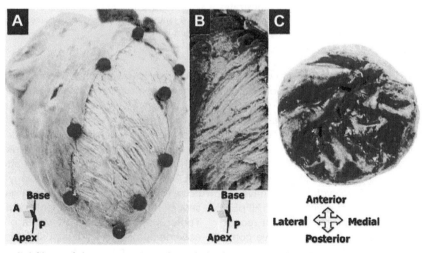

Fig. 4. Myocardial fibers of the LV are oriented in a helical pattern in this adult porcine heart. The muscle fibers are directed in a left-handed helix in the subepicardium (*A*) to right-handed helix in the subendocardium (*B*). The subendocardial helix is also seen in the apical trabeculae (*C*). (*From* Sengupta PP, Korinek J, Belohlavek M, et al. Left ventricular structure and function: basic science for cardiac imaging. J Am Coll Cardiol 2006;48(10):1991; with permission.)

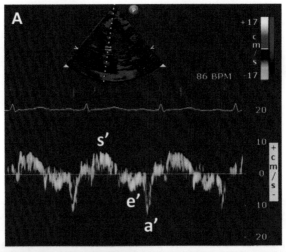

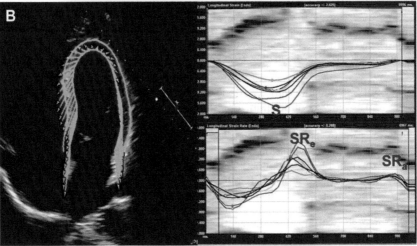

Fig. 5. Systolic and diastolic myocardial mechanics in the longitudinal direction assessed by echo. (*A*) Tissue Doppler imaging of the mitral annulus demonstrates a systolic wave (s′), early diastolic wave (e′), and atrial contraction wave (a′). (*B*) Speckle tracking echo in the apical 4-chamber view (*left*) with corresponding longitudinal strain (S) (*top right*) and strain rate (SR$_e$ and SR$_a$) (*bottom right*) curves.

potential energy that is released in early diastole when untwisting occurs, producing suction that draws blood from the LA toward the LV apex.[50,51] Abnormal twist mechanics have been identified in HFpEF and are thought to contribute to impaired LV filling.[52,53]

Myocardial deformational imaging has also informed understanding of other abnormalities of cardiac function in HFpEF. Several groups have reported the presence of LV dyssynchrony in HFpEF despite narrow QRS complexes.[54–59] In a recent substudy of the PARAMOUNT (Prospective comparison of ARNI with ARB on Management Of heart failUre with preserved ejectioN fracTion) trial, LV dyssynchrony was present among patients with HFpEF when compared with age- and gender-matched healthy controls; LV systolic dyssynchrony was most strongly correlated with tissue Doppler mitral annular relaxation velocities and LV mass, which may indicate disrupted coordination of systolic and diastolic events.[59] Whether LV dyssynchrony is a marker of HFpEF or a modifiable contributor in HFpEF remains to be determined.

There has also been increasing attention given to LA function on the pathophysiology of and prognosis in HFpEF.[60–62] Left atrial enlargement is present in most (50%–66%) patients with HFpEF (see **Table 3**) and is associated with a greater risk of adverse outcomes.[7,10] It is postulated that the LA dilates in response to chronically elevated filling pressures; however, a substantial percentage of patients with HFpEF have normal LA size. Abnormalities of LA function, which can be measured by emptying fraction, tissue Doppler imaging, or

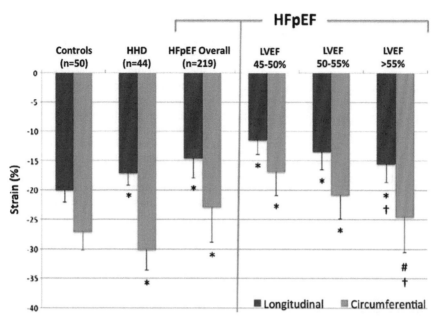

Fig. 6. Systolic dysfunction is present in HFpEF from speckle tracking echo. GLS (longitudinal) and GCS (circumferential) were compared in HFpEF with patients with hypertensive heart disease (HHD) without HF and healthy controls. * P<.0001 compared with controls and between HHD and HFpEF overall for GLS and GCS; # P = .0002 compared with controls; † LVEF adjusted P value <.001 compared with controls. (*From* Kraigher-Krainer E, Shah AM, Gupta DK, et al. Impaired systolic function by strain imaging in heart failure with preserved ejection fraction. J Am Coll Cardiol 2014;63:451; with permission.)

LA strain and strain rate from speckle tracking echo, have been demonstrated in HFpEF independent of LA size.[63] The findings of LA dysfunction also seem to be independent of LV function; therefore, a noncompliant and dysfunctional LA may be the primary contributor to the pathophysiology of HFpEF in some patients.[64] It has also been suggested that LA dysfunction may be more accurate than LA enlargement for identifying diastolic dysfunction and HFpEF.[63] Additionally, impairments of LA function may be exacerbated in the setting of exercise, which may contribute to exercise intolerance, which is a common symptom in HFpEF.[65]

Although not currently performed in routine clinical practice, quantification of myocardial mechanics with noninvasive imaging has potential for improving the understanding of cardiac dysfunction in HFpEF.[41] However, at this time, further studies are needed to validate indices of myocardial deformation against outcomes, assess their incremental prognostic significance beyond current conventional measures of cardiac function, and determine the feasibility and reproducibility of these measures in the clinical setting.[41]

RV Dysfunction and Pulmonary Hypertension

RV dysfunction and pulmonary hypertension are increasingly being recognized in HFpEF.[66–70]

Studies from the Mayo Clinic demonstrated that RV dysfunction was present in 33% to 50% of patients with HFpEF,[68] whereas pulmonary hypertension, defined as a pulmonary artery systolic pressure more than 35 mm Hg, was present in 83%, correlated with LV filling pressures (E/e'), and was highly accurate (area under the curve = 0.91) for distinguishing patients with HFpEF from those with hypertension alone.[69] Importantly, patients with HFpEF with and without pulmonary hypertension seem to be a distinct group with differing clinical and echocardiographic features as well as prognosis as patients with HFpEF with RV hypertrophy/dysfunction and/or pulmonary hypertension seem to be at an increased risk for death or cardiovascular hospitalization.[66,69,70]

Vascular Imaging

Comorbidities that affect the vasculature are common in HFpEF; therefore, attention has been given to understanding vascular dysfunction and its relationship to ventricular performance.[9] Vascular function can be characterized noninvasively by evaluating endothelial function and arterial stiffness. Endothelial function can be assessed through flow-mediated dilation (ultrasound imaging of the brachial or radial artery) or peripheral artery tonometry. Arterial stiffness can be estimated from pulse-wave velocity, which tracks the timing and waveforms of pulse waves at different segments of the arterial tree (eg, carotid and femoral) over the cardiac cycle, and is measured by Doppler ultrasound or MR imaging. A detailed discussion of these techniques is beyond the scope of this article, but vascular imaging techniques in HF have been reviewed elsewhere.[71] Vascular imaging in HFpEF populations have demonstrated the presence of endothelial dysfunction and arterial stiffening in HFpEF, which may contribute to systolic and diastolic dysfunction in these patients.[45,72,73] Furthermore, arterial stiffening may be worsened with exercise, which may contribute to exercise intolerance, which is a common symptom in HFpEF; peripheral endothelial dysfunction in HFpEF has been associated with adverse prognosis.[13,72]

Exercise/Stress Testing

Most echocardiographic algorithms for cardiac structure, function, and hemodynamics use information obtained at rest. However, symptoms and signs of HF that are present only with exertion are common in HFpEF; these patients have objectively reduced exercise performance.[12] Consequently, there has been increased attention given to identifying cardiac dysfunction during exercise or under pharmacologic stress conditions.[74] Compared with healthy controls, patients with HFpEF demonstrate blunted augmentation of LVEF, stroke volume, and cardiac output with exercise.[13,75] Reduced longitudinal LV function, as measured by mitral annular tissue Doppler S' velocities and speckle tracking GLS, and increases in filling pressures (E/e') have also been reported with exercise in patients with HFpEF.[14,76,77]

Despite the fact that many patients with HFpEF experience symptoms only with exertion, the current guidelines do not incorporate stress testing into algorithms for diagnosing HFpEF. This fact may, in part, be caused by the difficulty with obtaining diastolic parameters while at peak exercise or early into recovery because of tachypnea and tachycardia. In addition, threshold values for systolic and diastolic indices for defining an abnormal response to stress testing have not been established and validated in HFpEF. Nevertheless, stress testing, not only for the evaluation of coronary artery disease, which is present in 40% to 60% of patients with HFpEF,[78] but also for the identification of cardiac dysfunction that may not be readily apparent at rest, will likely become an important component in the evaluation of patients with HFpEF.[79]

SUMMARY

HFpEF is becoming the predominant form of HF; understanding cardiac structure and function in this syndrome is highly relevant for diagnosis, prognosis, pathophysiology, and management. However, identifying cardiac dysfunction in HFpEF can be challenging and requires an integrated assessment of cardiac structure, systolic and diastolic function, and hemodynamics. Comprehensive transthoracic echo is the noninvasive imaging test of choice for evaluating patients with HF, with the recognition that abnormalities of cardiac function may not be present at rest in HFpEF but may be unmasked with exercise or pharmacologic stress testing. Cardiac imaging is an integral component to understanding the pathophysiology and diagnosis of and prognosis in HFpEF, although many questions about cardiac structure and function in HFpEF remain; further research is needed to better understand this complex syndrome (**Box 1**).

Box 1
Ongoing and future research topics related to imaging in HFpEF

Complementary roles of multimodality imaging

Diagnostic and prognostic role of integrated measures of cardiac performance (eg, MPI)

Feasibility, reproducibility, diagnostic, and prognostic value of 3D echo

Role of mitral regurgitation and exercise-induced mitral regurgitation

Ethnic differences in cardiac structure and function

Impact of aging on cardiac structure and function

Contribution and impact of coronary artery disease (epicardial and microvascular)

Sympathetic innervation

Contribution and impact of atrial fibrillation on cardiac structure and function

Cardiac metabolism

Myocardial fibrosis

Ventricular-vascular coupling

Contribution and impact of comorbidities on cardiac structure and function

Changes in cardiac structure and function in response to therapies

Abbreviation: MPI, myocardial performance index.

REFERENCES

1. Dougherty AH, Naccarelli GV, Gray EL, et al. Congestive heart failure with normal systolic function. Am J Cardiol 1984;54:778–82.

2. Soufer R, Wohlgelernter D, Vita NA, et al. Intact systolic left ventricular function in clinical congestive heart failure. Am J Cardiol 1985;55:1032–6.

3. Yu CM, Lin H, Yang H, et al. Progression of systolic abnormalities in patients with "isolated" diastolic heart failure and diastolic dysfunction. Circulation 2002;105:1195–201.

4. Yip G, Wang M, Zhang Y, et al. Left ventricular long axis function in diastolic heart failure is reduced in both diastole and systole: time for a redefinition? Heart 2002;87:121–5.

5. Petrie MC, Caruana L, Berry C, et al. Diastolic heart failure or heart failure caused by subtle left ventricular systolic dysfunction? Heart 2002;87:29–31.

6. Nikitin NP, Witte KK, Clark AL, et al. Color tissue Doppler-derived long-axis left ventricular function in heart failure with preserved global systolic function. Am J Cardiol 2002;90:1174–7.

7. Shah AM, Shah SJ, Anand IS, et al. Cardiac structure and function in heart failure with preserved ejection fraction: baseline findings from the echocardiographic study of the treatment of preserved cardiac function heart failure with an aldosterone antagonist trial. Circ Heart Fail 2013;7:104–15.

8. Katz DH, Beussink L, Sauer AJ, et al. Prevalence, clinical characteristics, and outcomes associated with eccentric versus concentric left ventricular hypertrophy in heart failure with preserved ejection fraction. Am J Cardiol 2013;112:1158–64.

9. Mohammed SF, Borlaug BA, Roger VL, et al. Comorbidity and ventricular and vascular structure and function in heart failure with preserved ejection fraction: a community-based study. Circ Heart Fail 2012;5:710–9.

10. Zile MR, Gottdiener JS, Hetzel SJ, et al. Prevalence and significance of alterations in cardiac structure and function in patients with heart failure and a preserved ejection fraction. Circulation 2011;124:2491–501.

11. Lam CS, Roger VL, Rodeheffer RJ, et al. Cardiac structure and ventricular-vascular function in persons with heart failure and preserved ejection fraction from Olmsted County, Minnesota. Circulation 2007;115:1982–90.

12. Kitzman DW, Little WC, Brubaker PH, et al. Pathophysiological characterization of isolated diastolic heart failure in comparison to systolic heart failure. JAMA 2002;288:2144–50.

13. Borlaug BA, Olson TP, Lam CS, et al. Global cardiovascular reserve dysfunction in heart failure with preserved ejection fraction. J Am Coll Cardiol 2010;56:845–54.

14. Meluzin J, Sitar J, Kristek J, et al. The role of exercise echocardiography in the diagnostics of heart failure with normal left ventricular ejection fraction. Eur J Echocardiogr 2011;12:591–602.

15. Writing Committee Members, Yancy CW, Jessup M, et al. 2013 ACCF/AHA guideline for the management of heart failure: a report of the American College of Cardiology Foundation/American Heart Association task force on practice guidelines. Circulation 2013;128:e240–319.

16. Stacey RB, Hundley WG. The Role of cardiovascular magnetic resonance (CMR) and computed tomography (CCT) in facilitating heart failure management. Curr Treat Options Cardiovasc Med 2013;15:373–86.

17. Bonow RO. Radionuclide angiographic evaluation of left ventricular diastolic function. Circulation 1991;84:I208–15.

18. Salerno M. Multi-modality imaging of diastolic function. J Nucl Cardiol 2010;17:316–27.

19. Carrio I, Cowie MR, Yamazaki J, et al. Cardiac sympathetic imaging with mIBG in heart failure. JACC Cardiovasc Imaging 2010;3:92–100.

20. Peterson LR, Gropler RJ. Radionuclide imaging of myocardial metabolism. Circ Cardiovasc Imaging 2010;3:211–22.

21. Redfield MM, Jacobsen SJ, Burnett JC Jr, et al. Burden of systolic and diastolic ventricular dysfunction in the community: appreciating the scope of the heart failure epidemic. JAMA 2003;289:194–202.

22. Kane GC, Karon BL, Mahoney DW, et al. Progression of left ventricular diastolic dysfunction and risk of heart failure. JAMA 2011;306:856–63.

23. Aljaroudi W, Alraies MC, Halley C, et al. Impact of progression of diastolic dysfunction on mortality in patients with normal ejection fraction. Circulation 2012;125:782–8.

24. Armstrong WF, Ryan T, Feigenbaum H. Feigenbaum's echocardiography. 7th edition. Philadelphia: Wolters Kluwer Health/Lippincott Williams & Wilkins; 2010.

25. Mulvagh SL, Rakowski H, Vannan MA, et al. American Society of Echocardiography consensus statement on the clinical applications of ultrasonic contrast agents in echocardiography. J Am Soc Echocardiogr 2008;21:1179–201 [quiz: 1281].

26. Jenkins C, Moir S, Chan J, et al. Left ventricular volume measurement with echocardiography: a comparison of left ventricular opacification, three-dimensional echocardiography, or both with magnetic resonance imaging. Eur Heart J 2009;30:98–106.

27. Lang RM, Bierig M, Devereux RB, et al. Recommendations for chamber quantification: a report from the American Society of Echocardiography's guidelines and standards committee and the

chamber quantification writing group, developed in conjunction with the European Association of Echocardiography, a branch of the European Society of Cardiology. J Am Soc Echocardiogr 2005;18: 1440–63.

28. Nahar T, Croft L, Shapiro R, et al. Comparison of four echocardiographic techniques for measuring left ventricular ejection fraction. Am J Cardiol 2000;86:1358–62.

29. Pouleur AC, le Polain de Waroux JB, Pasquet A, et al. Assessment of left ventricular mass and volumes by three-dimensional echocardiography in patients with or without wall motion abnormalities: comparison against cine magnetic resonance imaging. Heart 2008;94:1050–7.

30. Paulus WJ, Tschope C, Sanderson JE, et al. How to diagnose diastolic heart failure: a consensus statement on the diagnosis of heart failure with normal left ventricular ejection fraction by the Heart Failure and Echocardiography Associations of the European Society of Cardiology. Eur Heart J 2007;28: 2539–50.

31. Shah AM, Pfeffer MA. The many faces of heart failure with preserved ejection fraction. Nat Rev Cardiol 2012;9:555–6.

32. Maurer MS, Burkhoff D, Fried LP, et al. Ventricular structure and function in hypertensive participants with heart failure and a normal ejection fraction: the cardiovascular health study. J Am Coll Cardiol 2007;49:972–81.

33. Borlaug BA, Redfield MM. Diastolic and systolic heart failure are distinct phenotypes within the heart failure spectrum. Circulation 2011;123: 2006–13 [discussion: 2014].

34. Braunwald E, Bonow RO. Braunwald's heart disease: a textbook of cardiovascular medicine. 9th edition. Philadelphia: Saunders; 2012.

35. Kasner M, Westermann D, Steendijk P, et al. Utility of Doppler echocardiography and tissue Doppler imaging in the estimation of diastolic function in heart failure with normal ejection fraction: a comparative Doppler-conductance catheterization study. Circulation 2007;116:637–47.

36. Nagueh SF, Appleton CP, Gillebert TC, et al. Recommendations for the evaluation of left ventricular diastolic function by echocardiography. J Am Soc Echocardiogr 2009;22:107–33.

37. Dokainish H, Nguyen J, Sengupta R, et al. New, simple echocardiographic indexes for the estimation of filling pressure in patients with cardiac disease and preserved left ventricular ejection fraction. Echocardiography 2010;27:946–53.

38. Nagueh SF, Middleton KJ, Kopelen HA, et al. Doppler tissue imaging: a noninvasive technique for evaluation of left ventricular relaxation and estimation of filling pressures. J Am Coll Cardiol 1997; 30:1527–33.

39. Persson H, Lonn E, Edner M, et al. Diastolic dysfunction in heart failure with preserved systolic function: need for objective evidence: results from the CHARM echocardiographic substudy-CHARMES. J Am Coll Cardiol 2007;49:687–94.

40. Nguyen JS, Lakkis NM, Bobek J, et al. Systolic and diastolic myocardial mechanics in patients with cardiac disease and preserved ejection fraction: impact of left ventricular filling pressure. J Am Soc Echocardiogr 2010;23:1273–80.

41. Shah AM, Solomon SD. Myocardial deformation imaging: current status and future directions. Circulation 2012;125:e244–8.

42. Torrent-Guasp F, Ballester M, Buckberg GD, et al. Spatial orientation of the ventricular muscle band: physiologic contribution and surgical implications. J Thorac Cardiovasc Surg 2001;122:389–92.

43. Mor-Avi V, Lang RM, Badano LP, et al. Current and evolving echocardiographic techniques for the quantitative evaluation of cardiac mechanics: ASE/EAE consensus statement on methodology and indications endorsed by the Japanese Society of Echocardiography. J Am Soc Echocardiogr 2011;24:277–313.

44. Ibrahim el SH, Miller AB, White RD. The relationship between aortic stiffness and E/A filling ratio and myocardial strain in the context of left ventricular diastolic dysfunction in heart failure with normal ejection fraction: insights from magnetic resonance imaging. Magn Reson Imaging 2011; 29:1222–34.

45. Borlaug BA, Lam CS, Roger VL, et al. Contractility and ventricular systolic stiffening in hypertensive heart disease insights into the pathogenesis of heart failure with preserved ejection fraction. J Am Coll Cardiol 2009;54:410–8.

46. Yip GW, Zhang Q, Xie JM, et al. Resting global and regional left ventricular contractility in patients with heart failure and normal ejection fraction: insights from speckle-tracking echocardiography. Heart 2011;97:287–94.

47. Cioffi G, Senni M, Tarantini L, et al. Analysis of circumferential and longitudinal left ventricular systolic function in patients with non-ischemic chronic heart failure and preserved ejection fraction (from the CARRY-IN-HFpEF study). Am J Cardiol 2012; 109:383–9.

48. Kraigher-Krainer E, Shah AM, Gupta DK, et al. Impaired systolic function by strain imaging in heart failure with preserved ejection fraction. J Am Coll Cardiol 2014;63:447–56.

49. Henein MY, Gibson DG. Long axis function in disease. Heart 1999;81:229–31.

50. Sengupta PP, Korinek J, Belohlavek M, et al. Left ventricular structure and function: basic science for cardiac imaging. J Am Coll Cardiol 2006;48: 1988–2001.

51. Ashikaga H, van der Spoel TI, Coppola BA, et al. Transmural myocardial mechanics during isovolumic contraction. JACC Cardiovasc Imaging 2009; 2:202–11.

52. Tan YT, Wenzelburger F, Lee E, et al. The pathophysiology of heart failure with normal ejection fraction: exercise echocardiography reveals complex abnormalities of both systolic and diastolic ventricular function involving torsion, untwist, and longitudinal motion. J Am Coll Cardiol 2009;54: 36–46.

53. Ohara T, Niebel CL, Stewart KC, et al. Loss of adrenergic augmentation of diastolic intra-LV pressure difference in patients with diastolic dysfunction: evaluation by color M-mode echocardiography. JACC Cardiovasc Imaging 2012;5:861–70.

54. De Sutter J, Van de Veire NR, Muyldermans L, et al. Prevalence of mechanical dyssynchrony in patients with heart failure and preserved left ventricular function (a report from the Belgian Multicenter Registry on dyssynchrony). Am J Cardiol 2005;96: 1543–8.

55. Wang J, Kurrelmeyer KM, Torre-Amione G, et al. Systolic and diastolic dyssynchrony in patients with diastolic heart failure and the effect of medical therapy. J Am Coll Cardiol 2007;49:88–96.

56. Lee AP, Song JK, Yip GW, et al. Importance of dynamic dyssynchrony in the occurrence of hypertensive heart failure with normal ejection fraction. Eur Heart J 2010;31:2642–9.

57. Phan TT, Abozguia K, Shivu GN, et al. Myocardial contractile inefficiency and dyssynchrony in heart failure with preserved ejection fraction and narrow QRS complex. J Am Soc Echocardiogr 2010;23: 201–6.

58. Morris DA, Vaz Perez A, Blaschke F, et al. Myocardial systolic and diastolic consequences of left ventricular mechanical dyssynchrony in heart failure with normal left ventricular ejection fraction. Eur Heart J Cardiovasc Imaging 2012;13:556–67.

59. Santos AB, Kraigher-Krainer E, Bello N, et al. Left ventricular dyssynchrony in patients with heart failure and preserved ejection fraction. Eur Heart J 2014;35:42–7.

60. Kurt M, Wang J, Torre-Amione G, et al. Left atrial function in diastolic heart failure. Circ Cardiovasc Imaging 2009;2:10–5.

61. Eicher JC, Laurent G, Mathe A, et al. Atrial dyssynchrony syndrome: an overlooked phenomenon and a potential cause of 'diastolic' heart failure. Eur J Heart Fail 2012;14:248–58.

62. Melenovsky V, Borlaug BA, Rosen B, et al. Cardiovascular features of heart failure with preserved ejection fraction versus nonfailing hypertensive left ventricular hypertrophy in the urban Baltimore community: the role of atrial remodeling/dysfunction. J Am Coll Cardiol 2007;49:198–207.

63. Khan UA, de Simone G, Hill J, et al. Depressed atrial function in diastolic dysfunction: a speckle tracking imaging study. Echocardiography 2013; 30:309–16.

64. Morris DA, Gailani M, Vaz Perez A, et al. Left atrial systolic and diastolic dysfunction in heart failure with normal left ventricular ejection fraction. J Am Soc Echocardiogr 2011;24:651–62.

65. Obokata M, Negishi K, Kurosawa K, et al. Incremental diagnostic value of la strain with leg lifts in heart failure with preserved ejection fraction. JACC Cardiovasc Imaging 2013;6:749–58.

66. Thenappan T, Shah SJ, Gomberg-Maitland M, et al. Clinical characteristics of pulmonary hypertension in patients with heart failure and preserved ejection fraction. Circ Heart Fail 2011;4:257–65.

67. Leung CC, Moondra V, Catherwood E, et al. Prevalence and risk factors of pulmonary hypertension in patients with elevated pulmonary venous pressure and preserved ejection fraction. Am J Cardiol 2010;106:284–6.

68. Puwanant S, Priester TC, Mookadam F, et al. Right ventricular function in patients with preserved and reduced ejection fraction heart failure. Eur J Echocardiogr 2009;10:733–7.

69. Lam CS, Roger VL, Rodeheffer RJ, et al. Pulmonary hypertension in heart failure with preserved ejection fraction: a community-based study. J Am Coll Cardiol 2009;53:1119–26.

70. Burke MA, Katz DH, Beussink L, et al. Prognostic importance of pathophysiologic markers in patients with heart failure and preserved ejection fraction. Circ Heart Fail 2014;7:288–99.

71. Marti CN, Gheorghiade M, Kalogeropoulos AP, et al. Endothelial dysfunction, arterial stiffness, and heart failure. J Am Coll Cardiol 2012;60: 1455–69.

72. Akiyama E, Sugiyama S, Matsuzawa Y, et al. Incremental prognostic significance of peripheral endothelial dysfunction in patients with heart failure with normal left ventricular ejection fraction. J Am Coll Cardiol 2012;60:1778–86.

73. Kitzman DW, Herrington DM, Brubaker PH, et al. Carotid arterial stiffness and its relationship to exercise intolerance in older patients with heart failure and preserved ejection fraction. Hypertension 2013;61:112–9.

74. van Empel VP, Kaye DM. Integration of exercise evaluation into the algorithm for evaluation of patients with suspected heart failure with preserved ejection fraction. Int J Cardiol 2013;168: 716–22.

75. Ennezat PV, Lefetz Y, Marechaux S, et al. Left ventricular abnormal response during dynamic exercise in patients with heart failure and preserved left ventricular ejection fraction at rest. J Card Fail 2008;14:475–80.

76. Donal E, Thebault C, Lund LH, et al. Heart failure with a preserved ejection fraction additive value of an exercise stress echocardiography. Eur Heart J Cardiovasc Imaging 2012;13:656–65.

77. Holland DJ, Prasad SB, Marwick TH. Contribution of exercise echocardiography to the diagnosis of heart failure with preserved ejection fraction (HFpEF). Heart 2010;96:1024–8.

78. Shah SJ. Evolving approaches to the management of heart failure with preserved ejection fraction in patients with coronary artery disease. Curr Treat Options Cardiovasc Med 2010;12:58–75.

79. Afsinoktay A, Shah SJ. Diagnosis and management of heart failure with preserved ejection fraction: 10 key lessons. Curr Cardiol Rev 2013. [Epub ahead of print].

80. Edelmann F, Wachter R, Schmidt AG, et al. Effect of spironolactone on diastolic function and exercise capacity in patients with heart failure with preserved ejection fraction: the Aldo-DHF randomized controlled trial. JAMA 2013;309:781–91.

Invasive Hemodynamic Characterization of Heart Failure with Preserved Ejection Fraction

Mads J. Andersen, MD, PhD[a,b], Barry A. Borlaug, MD[a,*]

KEYWORDS

- Invasive hemodynamic assessment • Heart failure with preserved ejection fraction • Dyspnea

KEY POINTS

- Invasive hemodynamic assessment in heart failure with preserved ejection fraction (HFpEF) was originally a primary research tool to advance the understanding of the pathophysiology of HFpEF.
- The role of invasive hemodynamic assessment in HFpEF is expanding to the diagnostic arena where invasive assessment offers a robust, sensitive, and specific way to diagnose or exclude HFpEF in patients with unexplained dyspnea and normal ejection fraction.
- In future years, invasive hemodynamic profiling may more rigorously phenotype patients to individualized therapy and, potentially, deliver novel device-based structural interventions.

INTRODUCTION

The circulatory system serves to deliver substrates to the body via the bloodstream while removing the byproducts of cellular metabolism. Hemodynamics broadly refers to the study of the forces involved in the circulation of blood, which are governed by to the physical properties of the heart and vasculature and their dynamic regulation by the autonomic nervous system. Before discussion of cardiac properties, the extrinsic forces modulating cardiac function must be defined.

Load and Cardiac Function

Afterload represents the forces opposing ventricular ejection and can be quantified by systolic left ventricular (LV) wall stress and aortic input impedance or its individual components (resistance, compliance, characteristic impedance).[1] Wall stress is inconvenient because it depends on heart size and geometry, whereas impedance is cumbersome because it is a frequency-domain parameter that cannot be easily coupled with time-domain measures of ventricular function. Effective arterial elastance (Ea), defined by the ratio of LV end-systolic pressure (ESP) to stroke volume, provides a robust measure of total arterial load. Ea is not a directly measured parameter but, instead, a net or lumped stiffness of the vasculature that incorporates both mean and oscillatory components of afterload (**Fig. 1**).[1]

Preload reflects the degree of myofiber stretch before the onset of contraction, which, in turn, dictates the force and velocity of contraction according to the Frank-Starling principle.[1] In everyday practice, preload is often conceptualized as equivalent to LV filling pressures. However, in fact, preload is most accurately reflected by the LV volume at end-diastole volume (EDV). Filling pressures are related to EDV by the LV diastolic chamber stiffness, which differs in healthy volunteers and subjects with HFpEF.

Conflicts: The authors have nothing to disclose.
[a] Division of Cardiovascular Diseases, Department of Medicine, Mayo Clinic, 200 First Street Southwest, Rochester, MN 55905, USA; [b] Department of Cardiology, Aarhus University Hospital, Brendstrupgårdsvej 100, DK-8200 Aarhus N, Aarhus, Denmark
* Corresponding author. Mayo Clinic College of Medicine, 200 First Street Southwest, Rochester, MN 55905.
E-mail address: borlaug.barry@mayo.edu

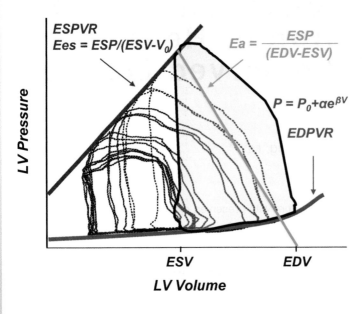

Fig. 1. Ventricular-arterial coupling in the pressure-volume plane. Pressure-volume loop at steady state is shown in dark black. The area subtended by the loop (*shaded*) represents the stroke work. Stroke volume is the difference between end-diastolic volume (EDV) and end-systolic volume (ESV). Ea is defined by the negative slope connecting the ESP and ESV coordinates with EDV and pressure = 0. With acute preload reduction (*dotted line loops*) there is progressive reduction in EDV, ESV, and ESP. The linear slope of the end-systolic pressure volume relationship (ESPVR) is LV end-systolic elastance (Ees). The curvilinear slope of the end-diastolic pressure–volume relationship (EDVPR) is derived by fitting pressure-volume coordinates measured during diastasis to the equation shown. The exponential power or stiffness constant (β) obtained is a measure of LV diastolic stiffness. (*Adapted from* Borlaug BA, Kass DA. Invasive hemodynamic assessment in heart failure. Heart Fail Clin 2009;5(2):217–28; with permission.)

Systolic Function

Ejection fraction (EF) is the most common clinical measure of LV systolic function, but EF is a poor measure of contractility because of its dependence on load and chamber size. For example, an acute decrease in afterload enhances EF in the absence of any change in contractility.[1] Isovolumic and ejection phase indices such as the maximal rate of pressure increase (dP/dt_{max}) and stroke work (SW) are independent of afterload but vary directly with preload (EDV).[2,3] More robust measures of contractility that are independent of preload and afterload include the slope of the relationship between SW and EDV (preload recruitable SW [PRSW]), stress-corrected fractional shortening (sc-FS), LV peak power index, and LV end-systolic elastance (Ees).[1,2,4,5] The latter, which describes the total stiffness attained by the LV at end-systole, is expressed graphically by the slope and intercept of the ESP–volume relationship (ESPVR). Ees is commonly examined in the context of Ea to assess ventricular-arterial coupling (see **Fig. 1**). In addition to inotropic state, Ees is sensitive to chamber remodeling and passive visco-elastic properties, meaning that it can be elevated even when systolic function is depressed.[5]

Diastolic Function

During early diastole there is rapid decay in LV pressure caused by active relaxation (thick-thin filament dissociation, ATP-dependent calcium

reuptake) and generation of negative intraventricular pressure gradients due to elastic recoil of constituents that were compressed in the preceding contraction.[6] This negative pressure gradient or suction effect enhances the atrioventricular pressure gradient leading to mitral valve opening.[7] This suction function is very important in the normal heart, which can fill even at zero pressure. Approximately 80% of filling is achieved during early diastole, with little increase in LV pressure. Invasively obtained parameters quantifying early-phase LV diastolic function include the time constant of pressure decay during isovolumic relaxation (τ), the maximal rate of pressure decay (dP/dt_{min}), and the minimal diastolic LV pressure achieved (LV_{min}).[8]

As chamber filling progresses, the atrioventricular pressure gradient dissipates and flow decelerates, leading to the period of diastasis in which mitral inflow is absent. Because flow is nil during this phase and relaxation is usually complete, diastasis represents the ideal period in which to assess passive LV stiffness. In research studies, passive chamber stiffness is assessed according to the slope and intercept of the diastolic pressure–volume relationship (DPVR; see **Fig. 1**).[8] Unlike the ESPVR, the DPVR is curvilinear, becoming more vertical (greater increase in pressure) at higher volumes. The DPVR can be assessed using single-beat and multibeat techniques. The single-beat technique simply plots LV pressure versus volume for a single heartbeat. Although the single-beat DPVR provides a useful measure of diastolic function, it is limited by the impact of external forces. Roughly 40% of the pressure component in the single-beat DPVR is accounted for by external forces (pericardial restraint and right heart compression).[1,8] To remove the impact of external pericardial constraint, the multibeat DPVR can be assessed wherein pressure-volume coordinates are obtained during diastasis at baseline and in each subsequent beat during acute preload reduction, usually achieved by transient caval occlusion (see **Fig. 1**). Atrial systole marks the final phase of diastole in which approximately 20%

of filling occurs in normal conditions owing to the booster function of the left atrium.

Ventricular-Arterial Interaction and Autonomic Influences

Ventricular-arterial interaction is assessed by relating Ees to Ea. In health, Ea and Ees are matched to provide optimal mechanical efficiency in the transfer of blood from the heart to the vascular system.[9] If the cardiac properties are held constant, an isolated decrease in afterload (Ea) will reduce blood pressure and increase stroke volume (**Fig. 2**A).[1] An increase in Ea will

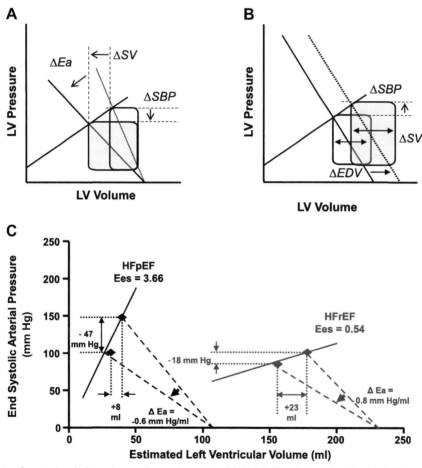

Fig. 2. Effects of acute load alteration on hemodynamics. (*A*) Isolated reduction in afterload (Ea) will increase in stroke volume (ΔSV) and reduce systolic blood pressure (ΔSBP), whereas (*B*) an isolated increase in preload (EDV) will increase in stroke volume and SBP. (*C*) The ESPVR in HFpEF (*black*) is steep (high Ees), particularly compared with HFrEF (*red*), meaning that, for any given reduction in Ea (as with a vasodilator), there is far greater drop in blood pressure and less enhancement in stroke volume in HFpEF compared with HFrEF. (*Adapted from* Borlaug BA, Kass DA. Ventricular-vascular interaction in heart failure. Heart Fail Clin 2008;4(1):27, with permission; and Schwartzenberg S, Redfield MM, From AM, et al. Effects of vasodilation in heart failure with preserved or reduced ejection fraction implications of distinct pathophysiologies on response to therapy. J Am Coll Cardiol 2012;59(5):448, with permission.)

have the opposite effect. Conversely, an isolated increase in preload will increase blood pressure and stroke volume by increasing EDV (see **Fig. 2**B), whereas an isolated decrease in preload will have the opposite effect. The absolute values of Ees and Ea dictate the magnitude of pressure change with these load alterations. Higher Ea (steeper ESPVR, higher Ees) leads to more dramatic shifts in arterial pressure for a given change in load (see **Fig. 2**C).

The interplay between the sympathetic and parasympathetic nervous systems plays a critical role in cardiovascular homeostasis. Baroreceptors located in the heart, aorta, and carotid bodies sense changes in deformation that lead to increased sympathetic outflow to increases arterial resistance and enhance venous return via venoconstriction.[10]

THE HEMODYNAMICS OF HFPEF

Heart failure (HF) is defined hemodynamically as an inability of the heart to pump blood to the body at a rate commensurate with its needs or to do so at the cost of elevated filling pressures.[11] This definition applies to both HFpEF and HF with reduced ejection fraction (HFrEF) and, indeed, invasive hemodynamics studies comparing the two have shown that both HF phenotypes share similar elevations in right atrial pressure (RAP) and left heart filling pressure (pulmonary capillary wedge pressure [PCWP]; LV end-diastolic pressure [LVEDP]) as well as similar degrees of pulmonary hypertension (PH) and pulmonary vascular disease.[12,13] Normal resting hemodynamics and typical values observed in early-stage and advanced HFpEF are indicated in **Table 1**.[14]

For years, left ventricular diastolic dysfunction was conceptualized as the pathophysiologic lynchpin of HFpEF because elevated filling pressures are observed in HFpEF at rest or during exercise and because high filling pressures plausibly explain symptoms. However, using the multibeat conductance catheter technique, Kawaguchi and colleagues[15] reported no difference in the shape of the DPVR and no differences in relaxation (τ) in subjects with HFpEF when compared with HF-free controls. In contrast, other groups have identified upward or leftward shifted DPVR (increased stiffness coefficient, β) and prolonged τ compared with control populations using modified single-beat[16] and multibeat techniques.[17,18] The reasons for these discrepant results are unclear but may relate to the increasingly appreciated mechanistic heterogeneity in HFpEF. Indeed, recent echocardiographic studies have reported that diastolic dysfunction (assessed noninvasively and at rest)

Table 1
Typical central hemodynamics in healthy adults and HFpEF

	Healthy Adults	Early HFpEF	Advanced HFpEF
Rest			
RAP (mm Hg)	0–6	0–8	$\geq$10
mPAP (mm Hg)	<20	<20	$\geq$25
PCWP (mm Hg)	6–15	6–18	$\geq$20
PVR (WU)	<2	<2	>2.5–3
CI (l/min*m²)	2.2–4.0	2.2–4.0	1.8–3.6
τ (ms)	<48	Variable	>48
β	0.21	Variable	>0.27
Exercise			
RAP (mm Hg)	<10	>12	>20
mPAP (mm Hg)	<25	$\geq$30	$\geq$40
PCWP (mm Hg)	<20	$\geq$25	$\geq$25
PVR (WU)	<1.5	<2	>2
ΔCO/ΔVO₂	$\geq$6	Variable	<6

Normative data for exercise cardiac index not provided because they vary with exercise intensity (Vo₂).

Abbreviations: CI, cardiac index; mPAP, mean pulmonary artery pressure; PVR, pulmonary vascular resistance; WU, Wood unit; ΔCO/ΔVo₂, change in cardiac output relative to change in oxygen consumption; β, monoexponential stiffness coefficient from the fitted LV DPVR.

is present in only approximately two-thirds of subjects with HFpEF.[19,20] In early-stage HFpEF, the elevation in PCWP is not present at rest but limited to exercise.[21] This increase in PCWP develops in response to increases in chamber stiffness (elevated DPVR), impaired diastolic suction (inability to lower LV$_{min}$ with stress), and inadequate relaxation (shortening of τ, enhancement in dP/dt$_{min}$) relative to the shortening in diastolic filling period with exercise-associated tachycardia[22] or rapid pacing (**Fig. 3**).[23] Although diastolic reserve impairments in HFpEF clearly increase filling pressures, recent studies have found that the increase in EDV achieved during exercise stress is similar in HFpEF and healthy controls.[11,24–26]

Abnormalities in longitudinal systolic function are well-described in HFpEF[27,28] and, although one study reported preserved chamber systolic function and contractility,[4] a larger, population-based study observed that LV contractility (PRSW, SW or EDV, sc-FS) is subtly but significantly impaired in subjects with HFpEF,[5] even though Ees is elevated. Notably, the degree of contractile dysfunction was predictive of worse outcome in HFpEF.[5] Mild systolic dysfunction has since been confirmed using strain-based

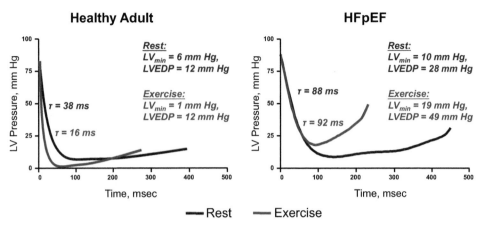

Fig. 3. Left ventricular diastolic reserve in HFpEF. In the normal healthy adult, the rate of LV pressure decay during isovolumic contraction (τ) is rapid and increases markedly during exercise in association with a reduction in LV_{min}, allowing for suction of blood into the LV, with no increase in left atrial pressure or LV end-diastolic pressure (LVEDP) despite an increase in LV end-diastolic volume and marked shortening of the cycle length. In HFpEF, relaxation is prolonged at baseline (increased τ) with inadequate hastening (shortening of τ) during exercise, contributing to an inability to reduce LV_{min} and, consequently, a complete lack of suction effects. LV filling then completely depends on left atrial hypertension, which develops in tandem with marked elevation in LVEDP. (*Data from* Borlaug BA, Jaber WA, Ommen SR, et al. Diastolic relaxation and compliance reserve during dynamic exercise in heart failure with preserved ejection fraction. Heart 2011;97(12):964–9.)

measures of systolic deformation.[29] Subtle abnormalities in resting contractility in HFpEF become dramatic during stress because of the inability to enhance systolic function that attenuates the increase in SV during exercise to limit cardiac output (CO) reserve.[26,30] Although resting EF, SV, and CO are generally normal in HFpEF, the ability to enhance EF, SV, and CO with exercise relative to metabolic needs is impaired.[11]

With chronic elevations in PCWP, there may be structural vascular remodeling and changes in pulmonary arterial (PA) tone leading to increases in pulmonary vascular resistance (PVR) and reductions in PA compliance (PAC, see **Table 1**). Lam and colleagues[31] demonstrated that echo-estimated PH was very common in HFpEF, present in greater than 80% of stable outpatients. For each 10 mm Hg increase in estimated PA pressures, there was a 30% increased risk of death. In an invasive hemodynamics study, Schwartzenberg and colleagues[12] found that the degree of PH was similar in subjects with HFpEF and HFrEF, and was largely reversible with acute infusion of sodium nitroprusside, suggesting that there is a substantial reactive component. Recently, in another invasive hemodynamics study, Melenovsky and colleagues[32] showed that, even after accounting for the extent of PH in HFpEF, there is primary right ventricular (RV) contractile dysfunction that is independently associated with

mortality. RV systolic dysfunction in HFpEF was associated with PA pressures as well as LVEF, male sex, coronary disease, and atrial fibrillation.

Invasive studies have shown that, on average, Ees is elevated in HFpEF, just as diastolic elastance is increased.[15] Lam and colleagues[33] showed similar findings in a large population-based noninvasive study. Increased ventricular-systolic stiffening in HFpEF is typically coupled to increased arterial stiffness (Ea),[1] which leads to a high-gain system wherein pressure fluctuations with load alteration are more dramatic. Schwartzenberg and colleagues[12] recently showed that nitroprusside infusion produced a much greater hypotensive response in HFpEF subjects compared with HFrEF subjects, owing to the steeper ESPVR in this population (see **Fig. 2**B). In addition, more than one-third of subjects with HFpEF in this study experienced a drop in stroke volume with nitroprusside (**Fig. 4**A). Because arterial afterload was reduced, this drop could only be explained by a reduction in preload (EDV), which is striking considering that the average PCWP in these subjects was 20 to 25 mm Hg. This reinforces the point that filling pressures do not really measure preload and that these data serve as important reminders that elevated filling pressures are often required in patients with HFpEF due to marked increases in LV diastolic chamber stiffness (see **Fig. 4**B).[12]

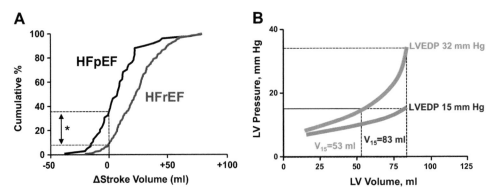

Fig. 4. Preload and filling pressures in HFpEF. (*A*) Cumulative distribution plot shows that acute changes in stroke volume with nitroprusside infusion are lower in HFpEF (*black*) compared with HFrEF (*red*). Because afterload (Ea) is lowered, any acute reduction in SV must be related to reduction in preload volume (EDV) and nearly 40% of HFpEF patients experienced stroke volume reduction with nitroprusside, despite high filling pressures (PCWP 20–25 mm Hg), indicating increased reliance on high pressures to achieve adequate EDV. *p<0.0001 compared with HFrEF. (*B*) LVEDP in a healthy adult (*blue*) and in a HFpEF patient with increased LV diastolic stiffness (*green*). At the same preload (EDV), pressure is more than twofold higher in HFpEF. In contrast, at the same LV diastolic pressure (15 mm Hg), LV volume is much lower in HFpEF, indicating decreased LV diastolic capacitance. V_{15}, volume at end-diastolic pressure = 15 mm Hg; LVEDP. (*Adapted from* Schwartzenberg S, Redfield MM, From AM, et al. Effects of vasodilation in heart failure with preserved or reduced ejection fraction implications of distinct pathophysiologies on response to therapy. J Am Coll Cardiol 2012;59(5):442–51; with permission.)

DIAGNOSIS OF HFPEF

HFpEF is defined at the bedside by clinical symptoms (dyspnea, fatigue), preserved LVEF (≥50%), and evidence of cardiac dysfunction that plausibly explains the symptoms.[34] Fulfilling the first two criteria is usually straightforward but the third component is often more challenging to prove. In HFrEF, the clinician needs only obtain an echocardiogram and demonstrate the presence of cardiac dysfunction (low EF). In HFpEF, LV size and EF are normal. There may be diastolic dysfunction but diastolic dysfunction is also part of normal aging and not specific to HFpEF, particularly when mild.[35,36] Congestive findings, such as jugular distention, rales, gallop sounds, and radiographic edema, provide convincing evidence of HF but are often absent, particularly among ambulatory patients. Echocardiography may allow for estimation of PCWP but lacks sensitivity.[30,37,38] Natriuretic peptide levels are helpful when elevated but normal levels do not exclude HFpEF.[21,39]

In the absence of clear-cut clinical, radiographic, or echocardiographic evidence of HFpEF, securing the diagnosis relies on the demonstration of elevated filling pressures, which are the ultimate downstream expression of LV diastolic dysfunction. Cardiac catheterization remains the gold standard for making this assessment. Demonstration of an elevation in PCWP or LVEDP (>15 mm Hg) in a patient with typical symptoms provides sufficient positive evidence of HFpEF.[34,40] Right heart catheterization can further allow for assessment of PA pressures, PVR, RAP, and CO. These parameters are frequently impaired in patients with more advanced HFpEF (see **Table 1**). They provide both prognostic insight and potential therapeutic targets for novel new treatments in the future. Left heart catheterization allows for direct measurement of LV_{min} and LVEDP, as well as the kinetics of relaxation (τ) and passive chamber stiffness (DPVR) but these assessments require high-fidelity micromanometer and conductance catheter systems that are not widely available clinically. The authors find that a high-quality PCWP tracing, with typical waveforms, verified by oximetry (saturation ≥94%), is just as robust as directly measured LVEDP is to make the diagnosis of HF.

Patients with early HFpEF experience dyspnea only during exercise and, accordingly, may not display an elevated PCWP at rest.[21] Invasive hemodynamic assessment during provocative maneuvers in these patients allows for greater sensitivity to positively diagnose or exclude HFpEF. Exercise provides the most robust and physiologically relevant stressor and can be performed safely in the supine or upright positions in virtually all patients. An increase in PCWP (or LVEDP) to greater than or equal to 25 mm Hg (≥20 mm Hg upright) is sufficient evidence to make the diagnosis of HFpEF (**Fig. 5**).[21,41] Measurements should be performed at end-expiration because the increased work of breathing during supine

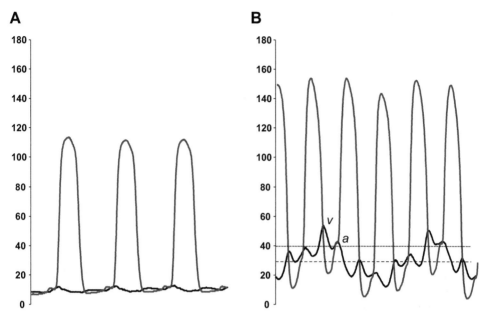

Fig. 5. Exercise hemodynamics in early stage HFpEF. (*A*) LV pressure (*red*) and PCWP (*black*) are normal at rest in a patient with HFpEF but (*B*) increase dramatically during 20-watt exercise, in which LVEDP and PCWP at end-expiration (measured at mid-a wave) are 40 mm Hg (*dotted line*). The average PCWP during the respiratory cycle (reported automatically by most recording systems) is substantially lower (30 mm Hg, *dashed line*) owing to the negative intrathoracic pressures generated during deep inspiration during exercise.

exercise frequently leads to large decreases in intrathoracic pressure, which tethers down all intracardiac pressures during stress (see **Fig. 5B**). This is particularly problematic in obese patients. Use of a micromanometer-tipped catheter provides greater accuracy and precision but is limited by cost and the need for additional monitoring equipment.

Invasive exercise testing also allows for assessment of CO responses to exercise, pulmonary vasodilator reserve, and estimation of the amount of pericardial restraint that may limit ventricular filling. At the Mayo Clinic, the practice is to directly measure oxygen consumption per unit time (Vo_2) to gauge the adequacy of CO reserve during exercise. In healthy humans, each 1 mL absolute increase in Vo_2 is matched with a 6 mL increase in CO.[11] Thus, if Vo_2 increases from 250 mL per minute at rest to 1250 mL per minute at peak exercise (+1000 mL/min), a 6 L per minute increase in CO is expected. If the observed increase in CO is less than 80% of the predicted value, this constitutes a CO reserve limitation and, as indicated above, this is common but not universal in HFpEF.[11]

It is also useful to measure RAP concomitantly with PCWP. An increased LVEDP is often equated with high diastolic stiffness (steep EDPVR) but this really represents the sum of intracavitary pressure and pericardial pressures.[42] Pericardial pressure

can be estimated by RAP.[43] Patients with tightly coupled increases in RAP and PCWP with exercise probably experience more pericardial restraint,[44] which may represent a different hemodynamic subtype of HFpEF compared with patients in whom PCWP greatly exceeds RAP, which suggests more isolated left heart impairment.

In normal adults and patients with early stage HFpEF, there is pulmonary vasodilation and reduction in PVR during exercise.[14,21] In more advanced HFpEF, there is loss of PVR reduction or even an apparent increase in PVR, with drop in PAC.[45] It may be that these patients will benefit from pulmonary vasodilating therapies, although this hypothesis remains untested. Finally, exercise testing also allows for direct measurement of PA pressure-flow relationships, which are believed to provide greater insight into the extent of pulmonary vascular disease present in a given patient when compared with steady state measurements such as PVR.[46]

Because not all laboratories have the equipment and expertise to perform invasive exercise testing, other investigators have advocated for alternative provocative maneuvers to improve sensitivity. Rapid saline infusion can distinguish HFpEF from healthy controls.[47] In the authors' laboratory, we infuse 10 mL/kg of prewarmed (40°C) saline at 150 mL per minute. Using this method, Fujimoto and colleagues[47] found that subjects with HFpEF displayed an increase in PCWP relative to volume infused that was significantly greater than age-matched healthy controls. Compared with exercise, saline infusion has little effect on heart rate or blood pressure and does not provide nearly as much physiologic data as exercise, in which more dramatic changes in loading, autonomic tone, and metabolic stress are present. As such, exercise remains the preferred stressor if available.

In patients referred for PH, it can often be challenging to distinguish euvolemic HFpEF from patients with primary pulmonary vascular disease (World Health Organization Group 1 PH). Consensus guidelines recommend provocative testing (exercise or saline infusion) in patients with PH and typical HFpEF risk factors.[48] Recently, Robbins and colleagues[49] reported data from their single-center series, wherein 22% of subjects with apparent Group 1 PH (ie, PH with PCWP <15 mm Hg) based on initial hemodynamic assessment developed an increase in PCWP to greater than 15 mm Hg after 0.5 L saline infused for 5 to 10 minutes. Although this suggests that a significant proportion of patients previously thought to have non–HF-related PH might in fact have early stage HFpEF, it is important to remember that approximately 20% of normal adults may develop PCWP greater than 15 mm Hg with acute saline infusion and it may be that using a higher cutoff (as is done with exercise testing) will avoid false-positive diagnosis of HFpEF.[42,47]

FUTURE DIRECTIONS

A possible explanation for the neutral results in earlier trials is the pathophysiological heterogeneity present in HFpEF.[50,51] More precise phenotyping before enrollment in trials may prove most effective to study more homogenous populations that would be expected to respond to therapeutic interventions more consistently. For example, subjects might be grouped hemodynamically, based on the presence or absence of pulmonary vascular disease, CO limitations with exercise, or by the nature of the increase in cardiac filling pressures (isolated left heart increase or increase in right and left heart pressures in tandem). Each of these groups might be optimally treated using different interventions. For example, pulmonary vasodilators in subjects with more severe pulmonary vascular disease[52]; systemic vasodilators in subjects with inadequate CO reserve; pericardial resection in subjects with symmetric, biventricular pressure elevation[53]; or creation of an interatrial shunt

when left atrial pressure greatly exceeds RAP.[54] Further study is required to determine whether hemodynamic phenotyping, either alone or in some combination with clinical, structural, and biomarker profiling, can improve treatment approaches for patients with HFpEF.

SUMMARY

Invasive hemodynamic assessment in HFpEF originated as a primary research tool to help in understanding the pathophysiology. Now, its role is expanding to the diagnostic arena in which invasive assessment offers a robust, sensitive, and specific way to diagnose or exclude HFpEF in patients with unexplained dyspnea and normal EF. In the future, invasive hemodynamic profiling may hold promise to more rigorously phenotype patients to individualized therapy and, potentially, deliver novel device-based structural interventions to improve morbidity and mortality in this growing cohort of people for whom there are few effective treatment options.

REFERENCES

1. Borlaug BA, Kass DA. Ventricular-vascular interaction in heart failure. Heart Fail Clin 2008;4(1):23–36.
2. Kass DA, Maughan WL, Guo ZM, et al. Comparative influence of load versus inotropic states on indexes of ventricular contractility: experimental and theoretical analysis based on pressure-volume relationships. Circulation 1987;76(6):1422–36.
3. Borlaug BA, Kass DA. Invasive hemodynamic assessment in heart failure. Heart Fail Clin 2009; 5(2):217–28.
4. Baicu CF, Zile MR, Aurigemma GP, et al. Left ventricular systolic performance, function, and contractility in patients with diastolic heart failure. Circulation 2005;111:2306–12.
5. Borlaug BA, Lam CS, Roger VL, et al. Contractility and ventricular systolic stiffening in hypertensive heart disease insights into the pathogenesis of heart failure with preserved ejection fraction. J Am Coll Cardiol 2009;54:410–8.
6. Opdahl A, Remme EW, Helle-Valle T, et al. Determinants of left ventricular early-diastolic lengthening velocity: independent contributions from left ventricular relaxation, restoring forces, and lengthening load. Circulation 2009;119:2578–86.
7. Cheng CP, Igarashi Y, Little WC. Mechanism of augmented rate of left ventricular filling during exercise. Circ Res 1992;70(1):9–19.
8. Kass DA. Assessment of diastolic dysfunction. Invasive modalities. Cardiol Clin 2000;18(3): 571–86.

9. De Tombe PP, Jones S, Burkhoff D, et al. Ventricular stroke work and efficiency both remain nearly optimal despite altered vascular loading. Am J Physiol 1993;264(6 Pt 2):H1817–24.

10. Hall JE, Guyton AC. Guyton and Hall textbook of medical physiology. 12th edition. Philadelphia: Saunders/Elsevier; 2011.

11. Abudiab MM, Redfield MM, Melenovsky V, et al. Cardiac output response to exercise in relation to metabolic demand in heart failure with preserved ejection fraction. Eur J Heart Fail 2013; 15(7):776–85.

12. Schwartzenberg S, Redfield MM, From AM, et al. Effects of vasodilation in heart failure with preserved or reduced ejection fraction implications of distinct pathophysiologies on response to therapy. J Am Coll Cardiol 2012;59(5):442–51.

13. van Heerebeek L, Borbély A, Niessen HW, et al. Myocardial structure and function differ in systolic and diastolic heart failure. Circulation 2006;113: 1966–73.

14. Kovacs G, Berghold A, Scheidl S, et al. Pulmonary arterial pressure during rest and exercise in healthy subjects: a systematic review. Eur Respir J 2009; 34(4):888–94.

15. Kawaguchi M, Hay I, Fetics B, et al. Combined ventricular systolic and arterial stiffening in patients with heart failure and preserved ejection fraction: implications for systolic and diastolic reserve limitations. Circulation 2003;107(5):714–20.

16. Zile MR, Baicu CF, Gaasch WH. Diastolic heart failure—abnormalities in active relaxation and passive stiffness of the left ventricle. N Engl J Med 2004; 350(19):1953–9.

17. Westermann D, Kasner M, Steendijk P, et al. Role of left ventricular stiffness in heart failure with normal ejection fraction. Circulation 2008;117(16):2051–60.

18. Prasad A, Hastings JL, Shibata S, et al. Characterization of static and dynamic left ventricular diastolic function in patients with heart failure with a preserved ejection fraction. Circ Heart Fail 2010; 3:617–26.

19. Zile MR, Gottdiener JS, Hetzel SJ, et al. Prevalence and significance of alterations in cardiac structure and function in patients with heart failure and a preserved ejection fraction. Circulation 2011;124(23): 2491–501.

20. Shah AM, Shah SJ, Anand IS, et al. Cardiac structure and function in heart failure with preserved ejection fraction: baseline findings from the echocardiographic study of the treatment of preserved cardiac function heart failure with an aldosterone antagonist trial. Circ Heart Fail 2014;7(1):104–15.

21. Borlaug BA, Nishimura RA, Sorajja P, et al. Exercise hemodynamics enhance diagnosis of early heart failure with preserved ejection fraction. Circ Heart Fail 2010;3(5):588–95.

22. Borlaug BA, Jaber WA, Ommen SR, et al. Diastolic relaxation and compliance reserve during dynamic exercise in heart failure with preserved ejection fraction. Heart 2011;97(12):964–9.

23. Wachter R, Schmidt-Schweda S, Westermann D, et al. Blunted frequency-dependent upregulation of cardiac output is related to impaired relaxation in diastolic heart failure. Eur Heart J 2009;30(24): 3027–36.

24. Borlaug BA, Melenovsky V, Russell SD, et al. Impaired chronotropic and vasodilator reserves limit exercise capacity in patients with heart failure and a preserved ejection fraction. Circulation 2006; 114(20):2138–47.

25. Haykowsky MJ, Brubaker PH, John JM, et al. Determinants of exercise intolerance in elderly heart failure patients with preserved ejection fraction. J Am Coll Cardiol 2011;58(3):265–74.

26. Borlaug BA, Olson TP, Lam CS, et al. Global cardiovascular reserve dysfunction in heart failure with preserved ejection fraction. J Am Coll Cardiol 2010;56(11):845–54.

27. Yu CM, Lin H, Yang H, et al. Progression of systolic abnormalities in patients with "isolated" diastolic heart failure and diastolic dysfunction. Circulation 2002;105(10):1195–201.

28. Brucks S, Little WC, Chao T, et al. Contribution of left ventricular diastolic dysfunction to heart failure regardless of ejection fraction. Am J Cardiol 2005; 95(5):603–6.

29. Kraigher-Krainer E, Shah AM, Gupta DK, et al. Impaired systolic function by strain imaging in heart failure with preserved ejection fraction. J Am Coll Cardiol 2014;63(5):447–56.

30. Maeder MT, Thompson BR, Brunner-La Rocca HP, et al. Hemodynamic basis of exercise limitation in patients with heart failure and normal ejection fraction. J Am Coll Cardiol 2010;56:855–63.

31. Lam CS, Roger VL, Rodeheffer RJ, et al. Pulmonary hypertension in heart failure with preserved ejection fraction: a community-based study. J Am Coll Cardiol 2009;53:1119–26.

32. Melenovsky V, Hwang S, Zakeri R, et al. Right heart dysfunction in heart failure with preserved ejection fraction in revision. Eur Heart J 2014. in press.

33. Lam CS, Roger VL, Rodeheffer RJ, et al. Cardiac structure and ventricular-vascular function in persons with heart failure and preserved ejection fraction from Olmsted County, Minnesota. Circulation 2007;115(15):1982–90.

34. Borlaug BA, Paulus WJ. Heart failure with preserved ejection fraction: pathophysiology, diagnosis, and treatment. Eur Heart J 2011;32(6):670–9.

35. Kuznetsova T, Herbots L, Lopez B, et al. Prevalence of left ventricular diastolic dysfunction in a general population. Circ Heart Fail 2009;2(2): 105–12.

36. Melenovsky V, Borlaug BA, Rosen B, et al. Cardiovascular features of heart failure with preserved ejection fraction versus nonfailing hypertensive left ventricular hypertrophy in the urban Baltimore community: the role of atrial remodeling/dysfunction. J Am Coll Cardiol 2007;49(2):198–207.

37. Ommen SR, Nishimura RA, Appleton CP, et al. Clinical utility of Doppler echocardiography and tissue Doppler imaging in the estimation of left ventricular filling pressures: a comparative simultaneous Doppler-catheterization study. Circulation 2000; 102(15):1788–94.

38. From AM, Lam CS, Pitta SR, et al. Bedside assessment of cardiac hemodynamics: the impact of noninvasive testing and examiner experience. Am J Med 2011;124(11):1051–7.

39. Anjan VY, Loftus TM, Burke MA, et al. Prevalence, clinical phenotype, and outcomes associated with normal B-type natriuretic peptide levels in heart failure with preserved ejection fraction. Am J Cardiol 2012;110(6):870–6.

40. Paulus WJ, Tschope C, Sanderson JE, et al. How to diagnose diastolic heart failure: a consensus statement on the diagnosis of heart failure with normal left ventricular ejection fraction by the Heart Failure and Echocardiography Associations of the European Society of Cardiology. Eur Heart J 2007; 28(20):2539–50.

41. Tolle JJ, Waxman AB, Van Horn TL, et al. Exercise-induced pulmonary arterial hypertension. Circulation 2008;118(21):2183–9.

42. Borlaug BA. Invasive assessment of pulmonary hypertension: time for a more fluid approach? Circ Heart Fail 2014;7(1):2–4.

43. Tyberg JV, Taichman GC, Smith ER, et al. The relationship between pericardial pressure and right atrial pressure: an intraoperative study. Circulation 1986;73(3):428–32.

44. Janicki JS. Influence of the pericardium and ventricular interdependence on left ventricular diastolic and systolic function in patients with heart failure. Circulation 1990;81(Suppl 2):II15–20.

45. Tedford RJ, Hassoun PM, Mathai SC, et al. Pulmonary capillary wedge pressure augments right ventricular pulsatile loading. Circulation 2012;125(2): 289–97.

46. Lewis GD, Bossone E, Naeije R, et al. Pulmonary vascular hemodynamic response to exercise in cardiopulmonary diseases. Circulation 2013; 128(13):1470–9.

47. Fujimoto N, Borlaug BA, Lewis GD, et al. Hemodynamic responses to rapid saline loading: the impact of age, sex, and heart failure. Circulation 2013;127(1):55–62.

48. Hoeper MM, Barbera JA, Channick RN, et al. Diagnosis, assessment, and treatment of non-pulmonary arterial hypertension pulmonary hypertension. J Am Coll Cardiol 2009;54(Suppl 1):S85–96.

49. Robbins IM, Hemnes AR, Pugh ME, et al. High prevalence of occult pulmonary venous hypertension revealed by fluid challenge in pulmonary hypertension. Circ Heart Fail 2014;7(1):116–22.

50. Shah SJ. Matchmaking for the optimization of clinical trials of heart failure with preserved ejection fraction: no laughing matter. J Am Coll Cardiol 2013;62(15):1339–42.

51. Borlaug BA. Heart failure with preserved and reduced ejection fraction: different risk profiles for different diseases. Eur Heart J 2013;34(19): 1393–5.

52. Bonderman D, Ghio S, Felix SB, et al. Riociguat for patients with pulmonary hypertension caused by systolic left ventricular dysfunction: a phase IIb double-blind, randomized, placebo-controlled, dose-ranging hemodynamic study. Circulation 2013;128(5):502–11.

53. Stray-Gundersen J, Musch TI, Haidet GC, et al. The effect of pericardiectomy on maximal oxygen consumption and maximal cardiac output in untrained dogs. Circ Res 1986;58(4):523–30.

54. Kaye D, Shah SJ, Borlaug BA, et al. Effects of an interatrial shunt on rest and exercise hemodynamics: results of a computer simulation in heart failure. J Card Fail 2014;20(3):212–21.

Exercise Physiology in Heart Failure and Preserved Ejection Fraction

Mark J. Haykowsky, PhD[a],*, Dalane W. Kitzman, MD[b]

KEYWORDS

- Heart failure and preserved ejection fraction • Exercise physiology • Physical conditioning

KEY POINTS

- Heart failure with preserved ejection fraction (HFPEF) is the most common and fastest growing form of heart failure.
- HFPEF is associated with markedly increased morbidity, mortality, and health care expenditures.
- The prognosis of HFPEF is worsening, its pathophysiology is poorly understood, and no medications have been proved to be effective.
- The primary chronic symptom in patients with HFPEF, even when well compensated, is severe exercise intolerance, measured objectively as decreased peak oxygen uptake (peak Vo_2).
- Recent advances in the pathophysiology of exercise intolerance in HFPEF suggest that noncardiac peripheral factors contribute to the reduced peak Vo_2, and are the major contributor to its improvement after supervised endurance exercise training.

INTRODUCTION

Heart Failure with Preserved Ejection Fraction: A Major Health Care Problem with No Proven Therapy

Heart failure (HF) with preserved ejection fraction (HFPEF) is a recently recognized disorder and the fastest growing form of HF.[1,2] HFPEF is nearly exclusively found in older persons, particularly women, in whom 90% of new HF cases are HFPEF.[3] HFPEF is associated with markedly increased morbidity, mortality, and health care expenditures.[4–7] Despite its importance, the prognosis of HFPEF is worsening, its pathophysiology is poorly understood, and no medication trials

have had positive effect on their primary end points.[2] Consequently, there are no evidence-based guideline recommendations for improving clinical outcomes in the growing population of elderly patients with HFPEF.

Exercise Intolerance is the Primary Symptom in Patients with HFPEF

The primary chronic symptom in patients with HFPEF, even when well compensated, is severe exercise intolerance, which can be measured objectively during whole body exercise as decreased peak Vo_2 (peak exercise oxygen uptake).[8–19] Specifically, peak Vo_2 in patients with

Dr M.J. Haykowsky is the Exercise Physiology team lead for the Alberta Heart study funded by Alberta Innovates Health Solutions (AIHS). Dr D.W. Kitzman research was funded by NIH grants R37AG18917 and P30AG21332.
[a] Faculty of Rehabilitation Medicine, Alberta Cardiovascular and Stroke Research Centre (ABACUS), Mazankowski Alberta Heart Institute, University of Alberta, 3-16 Corbett Hall, Edmonton, Alberta T6G-2G4, Canada; [b] Cardiology Section, Department of Internal Medicine, Wake Forest School of Medicine, Medical Center Boulevard, Winston-Salem, NC 27157-1045, USA
* Corresponding author.
E-mail address: mark.haykowsky@ualberta.ca

HFPEF is 40% lower than age-matched and sex-matched controls (**Fig. 1**). Reduced exercise tolerance is a strong determinant of prognosis and reduced quality of life.[10,20] A clear understanding of the pathophysiology of exercise intolerance is necessary to guide future therapies aimed at improving patients with HFPEF symptoms.

Pathophysiology of Exercise Intolerance in Patients with HFPEF

In accordance with the Fick principle, the amount of oxygen consumed per minute is equal to the product of cardiac output and arterial-venous oxygen content difference; therefore, the reduced peak Vo_2 in patients with HFPEF may be caused by decreased oxygen delivery to or impaired oxygen extraction by the exercising skeletal muscles (**Fig. 2**).[10] Cross-sectional studies by Borlaug and colleagues[16,17,19] have suggested that the lower peak Vo_2 in patients with HFPEF compared with age-matched healthy or comorbidity-matched controls without HF was associated with reduced peak cardiac output, which was caused primarily by blunted heart rate response, myocardial contractility, and peripheral vascular vasodilator reserve.[18] A series of studies by Kitzman and colleagues[8] extended these results by showing that the lower peak Vo_2 in older patients with HFPEF versus age-matched healthy controls was caused not only by reduced peak exercise cardiac output but also by an equal contribution of reduced systemic arterial-venous oxygen content difference.[12] Moreover, the change in arterial-venous oxygen content difference from rest to peak exercise was the strongest independent predictor of peak Vo_2 for both patients with HFPEF and controls.[12] Bhella and colleagues[15] confirmed that noncardiac peripheral factors play an important role in limiting exercise tolerance, because the reduced peak Vo_2 in older patients with HFPEF compared with age-matched healthy controls occurred despite no significant difference in peak exercise cardiac output between groups. Potential peripheral mechanisms that may limit exercise capacity include decreased skeletal muscle mass, reduced type I (oxidative fatigue-resistant) muscle fibers, and impaired blood flow to or extraction by the active skeletal muscles.[10]

Skeletal Muscle Mass and Oxygen Utilization and Exercise Intolerance in Patients with HFPEF

Most of the oxygen consumed during the transition from rest to peak cycle exercise occurs in the active muscles, therefore a loss in metabolically active tissue may contribute to exercise intolerance in patients with HFPEF.[14,21] Our group tested this hypothesis and compared lean body mass and peak Vo_2 in 60 older patients with HFPEF and 40 age-matched healthy controls.[14] Three novel findings were reported. First, the percent total lean body mass and percent leg lean mass were significantly lower in patients with HFPEF compared with healthy controls.[14] Second, peak Vo_2 indexed to total lean body mass or leg lean mass was significantly lower in elderly patients with HFPEF versus healthy controls.[14] Third, the change in peak Vo_2 with increasing percent leg lean mass was markedly reduced in patients with HFPEF compared with

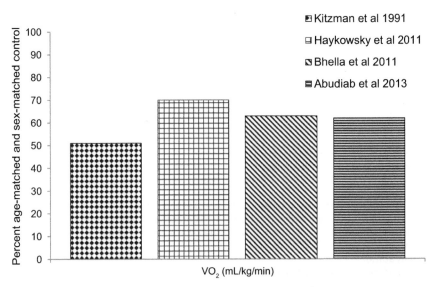

Fig. 1. Peak oxygen uptake in patients with HFPEF. (*Data from* Refs.[8,12,15,18])

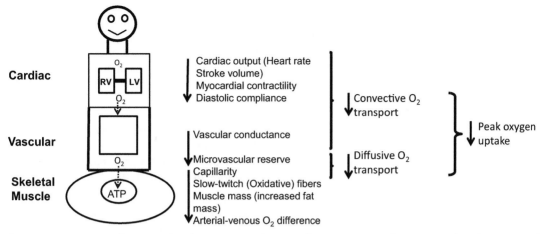

Fig. 2. Determinants of exercise intolerance in patients with HFPEF. ATP, adenosine triphosphate; LV, left ventricle; O_2, oxygen; RV, right ventricle.

healthy controls (HFPEF mean slope: 11 ± 5 mL O_2/min vs healthy controls mean slope: 36 ± 5 mL O_2/min, $P<.001$). Taken together, these findings show that older patients with HFPEF have decreased lean muscle mass; however, they also have abnormal O_2 utilization, which is independent of and in addition to the reduced muscle mass.

Impaired Muscle Blood Flow and Exercise Intolerance in Patients with HFPEF

In healthy older adults, the 11-fold increase in blood flow to the active muscles during the transition from rest to peak cycle exercise is caused by sympathetic-mediated redistribution of blood from nonexercising regions to the working muscles coupled with metabolic-mediated vasodilation in the exercising muscles.[22,23] Changes in central and peripheral arterial function may result in inefficient distribution of cardiac output to the active muscles and contribute to exercise intolerance in patients with HFPEF.[10]

Kitzman and colleagues[24] compared carotid arterial and proximal thoracic aortic distensibility in healthy younger (≤ 30 years) and older (≥ 60 years) individuals and older patients with HFPEF.[25] The novel finding of these studies was that carotid arterial distensibility and proximal thoracic aortic distensibility were reduced in older patients with HFPEF beyond the changes that occur with normal aging alone and both were directly related to peak V_{O_2}. These findings suggest that increased central arterial stiffness contributes to exercise intolerance in older patients with HFPEF and may be a potential therapeutic target.

Impaired peripheral arterial endothelial function may result in impaired exercise blood flow reserve

in patients with HFPEF. Haykowsky and colleagues[11] assessed brachial artery flow-mediated dilation in response to 5 minutes of cuff ischemia, a noninvasive measure of arterial endothelial function, in 47 younger and older healthy controls (mean age: 25 years and 70 years, respectively) and 66 older patients with HFPEF (mean age: 70 years). The major finding of this study was that brachial artery flow-mediated dilation was significantly reduced in healthy older compared with healthy young control participants; however, brachial artery flow-mediated dilation was not significantly different in patients with HFPEF compared with healthy age-matched older controls.[11] Hundley and colleagues,[26] using phase-contrast magnetic resonance imaging, measured the change in superficial femoral artery cross-sectional area and velocity at baseline and in response to 5 minutes of thigh cuff occlusion in elderly patients with HFPEF and age-matched healthy controls. The change in superficial femoral artery cross-sectional area and velocity were not significantly different between patients with HFPEF compared with healthy controls.[26] Taken together, large conduit arterial endothelial function is preserved and may not limit exercise tolerance in older patients with HFPEF. An important feature of these studies was exclusion of patients with any evidence of clinical atherosclerosis, which is known to independently reduce endothelial function.

Although conduit arterial endothelial function seems to be preserved in HFPEF, impaired microvascular function may limit exercise performance in older patients with HFPEF. Borlaug and colleagues,[16] using automated fingertip plethysmography in response to cuff ischemia and peak exercise as a measure of microvasculature reserve, reported that the change in finger blood flow in response to cuff occlusion or cycle exercise was reduced in elderly patients with HFPEF compared with age-matched healthy control participants but was not different in patients with HFPEF compared with hypertensive control participants without HF. A consequence of the blunted microvascular reserve is that it may be associated with decreased diffusive oxygen transport to the active muscle, which would reduce exercise tolerance. Borlaug and colleagues[16] found that systemic vascular conductance and microvascular reserve were positively related to peak Vo_2 in HFPEF.

Skeletal Muscle Composition, Fiber Type, and Capillarity and Exercise Intolerance in Patients with HFPEF

Increased intermuscular adipose has been reported in several conditions associated with severely reduced physical function, including HF with reduced ejection fraction and aging, and is potentially modifiable. Haykowsky and colleagues[27] recently examined the composition of thigh muscle and its relationship to peak Vo_2 in 23 older patients with HFPEF compared with 15 age-matched healthy controls. Despite no significant intergroup differences in total thigh area or subcutaneous adipose area, patients with HFPEF had significantly increased intermuscular adipose area (35.6 ± 11.5 vs 22.3 ± 7.6 cm^2, $P = .01$) and ratio of intermuscular adipose to skeletal muscle area (0.38 ± 0.10 vs 0.28 ± 0.09, $P = .007$).[27] In multivariate analyses, intermuscular adipose area and intermuscular adipose to muscle area (partial $r = -0.51$ and $r = -0.45$ respectively, $P<.01$ for both) were independent predictors of peak Vo_2.[27] Thus abnormal skeletal muscle composition contributes to the severely reduced exercise capacity in older patients with HFPEF and is a potential therapeutic target.

It is well established that patients with HF and reduced ejection fraction have multiple skeletal muscle abnormalities, including reduced percent type I (oxidative) fibers and oxidative enzymes, reduced volume density of mitochondria, and surface density of mitochondrial cristae.[28–31] Kitzman and colleagues[32] recently reported that compared with healthy controls, older patients with HFPEF showed a shift in skeletal muscle fiber type distribution with reduced percent slow-twitch type I fibers, type I/type II fiber ratio and capillary/fiber ratio, and these alterations are associated with their severely reduced peak exercise Vo_2. A consequence of the fiber type shift from oxidative to glycolytic fibers coupled with abnormal mitochondrial function is that it may impair oxidative metabolism during exercise. In a preliminary report,

Bhella and colleagues[15] found reduced leg muscle oxidative metabolism by magnetic resonance imaging during exercise in patients with HFPEF. Accordingly, interventions that reverse skeletal muscle oxidative dysfunction may result in a concomitant increase in peak Vo_2 in patients with HFPEF.

THERAPEUTIC OPTIONS AND CLINICAL OUTCOMES
Effects of Physical Conditioning on Exercise Tolerance in Patients with HFPEF

Kitzman and colleagues[33] performed the first single-center, single-blind, medically supervised, randomized controlled trial comparing the effects of 4 months of endurance exercise training versus attention control in 46 clinically stable older (mean age = 70 years) patients with HFPEF. The novel finding of this study was that 4 months of endurance exercise training increased peak Vo_2, ventilatory anaerobic threshold, distance walked in 6 minutes, improved physical quality of life without altering left ventricular mass, mass/volume ratio, ejection function, diastolic filling, or neuroendocrine function.[33]

In a follow-up analysis, the determinants of the training-related increase in peak Vo_2 were examined. There was a modest but significant increase in peak heart rate, but a modest decline in peak stroke volume, such that there was no significant change in peak cardiac output with training.[13] However, there was a significant training-related increase in peak arterial venous oxygen content difference, and in multivariate analysis,[13] this accounted for nearly 100% of the improvement in peak Vo_2. This finding indicated that the endurance exercise training-related improvement in peak Vo_2 was caused by peripheral adaptations.[13]

Kitzman and colleagues[34] performed a second, separate, randomized, attention-controlled, single-blind trial of exercise training, to determine if improved arterial function, measured either as carotid arterial stiffness or brachial artery flow-mediated dilation, improved with training and accounted for the training-related improvement in peak Vo_2. The study included 54 older patients with HFPEF (mean age = 70 years). The investigators found that 4 months of upper and lower extremity endurance exercise training resulted in a significant increase in peak Vo_2 without altering carotid arterial stiffness or brachial artery flow-mediated dilation.[34] This finding suggested, by elimination, that skeletal muscle adaptations may account for the training-related increase in peak Vo_2 in older patients with HFPEF.[34] In both trials, the change exercise capacity was clinically meaningful, because the baseline peak Vo_2 in patients with HFPEF randomly assigned to endurance exercise training was at or lower than the Vo_2 threshold required for independent living and was higher than this value after the 4-month intervention.[34]

Edelmann and colleagues[35] performed the first multicenter randomized controlled exercise trial comparing the effects of 3 months of combined endurance and strength training versus usual care on peak Vo_2, 6-minute walk distance, cardiac morphology, diastolic function, HF biomarkers, and quality of life in 64 clinically stable patients with HFPEF (mean age = 65 years). The major novel finding was that 3 months of endurance and strength training significantly improved peak Vo_2, ventilatory anaerobic threshold, quality of life, and resting measures of left atrial volume, early diastolic mitral annulus velocity, early transmitral inflow velocity to early diastolic mitral annulus velocity (E/e') ratio, and procollagen type I levels compared with usual care. Moreover, the increase in peak Vo_2 was correlated with the improvement in resting E/e'.[35] In contrast, Smart and colleagues[36] reported that the increase in peak Vo_2 after 4 months of moderate-intensity endurance exercise was not associated with a change in resting systolic and diastolic function or quality of life in 30 patients with HFPEF (mean age = 65 years).

Taken together, the few studies performed to date indicate that endurance exercise training with or without supplemental strength training is an effective nonpharmacologic therapy that improves clinically stable patients with HFPEF exercise tolerance. The improvement in peak Vo_2 seems to be primarily caused by favorable microvascular or skeletal muscle adaptations that increase diffusive oxygen transport or oxygen utilization by the working muscles.[10]

COMPLICATIONS AND CONCERNS
Diagnostic Usefulness of Exercise Stress Testing in HFPEF

Cardiopulmonary exercise (CPX) testing, with or without invasive hemodynamic monitoring, may enhance the diagnosis and treatment of patients with HFPEF, particularly those with early stage disease, in whom abnormalities in hemodynamic and cardiovascular reserve may occur only during incremental to peak exercise.[37] Moreover, noninvasive CPX testing with expired gas analysis is the gold-standard measure of aerobic (cardiorespiratory) fitness and provides important clinical information regarding risk stratification and prognosis, as well as an assessment of functional performance.[20] CPX testing can also identify abnormalities in individual patients that can have therapeutic implications, such as severe chronotropic incompetence and exaggerated blood pressure response to exercise.[20] CPX testing provides information (heart rate, power output, Vo_2, and rate of perceived exertion at the ventilation threshold and during peak exercise) that can be used by HF specialists and exercise specialists to prescribe endurance training programs for clinically stable patients with HFPEF as part of a comprehensive cardiac rehabilitation program.[20]

Safety of Supervised Exercise Training in Patients with HFPEF

The safety of supervised endurance training performed alone or combined with supplemental strength training was reported in 3 randomized controlled trails.[33–35] In all studies, no major adverse cardiac events were reported during the 3-month to 4-month training period; however, 20% of the patients with HFPEF in the combined endurance and strength training program conducted by Edelmann and colleagues[35] reported mild skeletal muscle discomfort with exercise. Thus, it seems that clinically stable older patients with HFPEF who do not have any contraindications to exercise testing or training can safely participate in a medically supervised 3-month to 4-month physical conditioning training program.

Although the efficacy of home-based exercise training after completed supervised training has not been studied in patients with HFPEF, findings from the HF-ACTION (Heart Failure and A Controlled Trial Investigating Outcomes of exercise traiNing) trial[38] suggest that 40% of patients with HF with reduced ejection fraction do not adhere to unsupervised exercise training. Adherence to home-based exercise training can be facilitated by several strategies during regular clinic visits to overcome barriers to exercise: provide information of the safety of exercise; discuss preferred modes of exercise and encourage activities that the patient prefers; discuss how exercise can fit into the lives of patients with HF; set realistic goals for increasing physical activity; provide information on how regular exercise improves symptoms; provide positive reinforcement for exercise adherence.[39]

FUTURE DIRECTIONS

Traditional exercise training programs for patients with HFPEF have primarily focused on moderate-intensity endurance exercise training; however, Tomczak and colleagues[40] found that an acute bout of high-intensity treadmill exercise (4-minute interval performed on a treadmill at 95% peak heart rate interspersed by a 3-minute recovery period performed at 76% peak heart rate, repeated 4 times) was associated with an increase in postexercise left and right ventricular ejection fraction in clinically stable HF patients with reduced ejection fraction. A recent systematic review and meta-analysis[41] extended these findings by reporting that vigorous to maximal aerobic interval exercise was superior to moderate-intensity continuous endurance training for improving peak Vo_2 in patients with HF with reduced ejection fraction.

The benefits and optimal intensity of strength training performed alone or in combination with endurance training to improve peak Vo_2, skeletal muscle morphology, and function remains unknown. Given these uncertainties, the recent National Heart, Lung, and Blood Institute working group on exercise as therapy for HF recommended future research regarding innovative exercise training modalities: what is the optimal training intensity (high-intensity vs moderate-intensity continuous exercise), mode (large vs small muscle mass training $\pm$ resistance training) and duration of training (short-term: 2–3 months vs 1 year) to improve cardiovascular and skeletal muscle function, health status, physical functional performance, and survival in patients with HF. (Fleg J, Copper LS, Borlaug BA, et al. Exercise training as therapy for heart failure: results from a national heart, lung, and blood working group. Submitted for publication.)

SUMMARY

The primary chronic symptom in patients with HFPEF, even when well compensated, is severe exercise intolerance. Recent advances in the pathophysiology of exercise intolerance in patients with HFPEF have suggested that noncardiac peripheral factors contribute to the reduced peak Vo_2, and are the major contributor to its improvement after endurance exercise training. Although the peripheral adaptations responsible for the increase in peak Vo_2 after endurance training are unknown, they may be the result of favorable changes in microvascular and skeletal muscle function that result in increased diffusive O_2 transport or greater oxygen utilization by the working muscles. There is no guideline-recommended therapy that improves clinical outcomes in patients with HFPEF. A greater understanding of the peripheral skeletal muscle vascular adaptations that occur with physical conditioning may allow for individually tailored exercise rehabilitation programs for patients with HFPEF to improve their primary chronic symptom, exercise intolerance. Furthermore, the identification of specific mechanisms that improve whole body and peripheral skeletal muscle oxygen uptake could establish potential therapeutic targets for medical therapies and a means to follow therapeutic response.

REFERENCES

1. Redfield MM. Understanding "diastolic" heart failure. N Engl J Med 2004;350:1930–1.
2. Owan TE, Hodge DO, Herges RM, et al. Trends in prevalence and outcome of heart failure with preserved ejection fraction. N Engl J Med 2006;355:251–9.
3. Gottdiener JS, Arnold AM, Aurigemma GP, et al. Predictors of congestive heart failure in the elderly: the cardiovascular health study. J Am Coll Cardiol 2000;35:1628–37.
4. Gottdiener JS, McClelland RL, Marshall R, et al. Outcome of congestive heart failure in elderly persons: influence of left ventricular systolic function. The Cardiovascular Health Study. Ann Intern Med 2002;137:631–9.
5. Liao L, Jollis JG, Anstrom KJ, et al. Costs for heart failure with normal vs reduced ejection fraction. Arch Intern Med 2006;166:112–8.
6. Ather S, Chan W, Bozkurt B, et al. Impact of noncardiac comorbidities on morbidity and mortality in a predominantly male population with heart failure and preserved versus reduced ejection fraction. J Am Coll Cardiol 2012;59:998–1005.
7. Senni M, Tribouilloy CM, Rodeheffer RJ, et al. Congestive heart failure in the community: trends in incidence and survival in a 10-year period. Arch Intern Med 1999;159:29–34.
8. Kitzman DW, Higginbotham MB, Cobb FR, et al. Exercise intolerance in patients with heart failure and preserved left ventricular systolic function: failure of the Frank-Starling mechanism. J Am Coll Cardiol 1991;17:1065–72.
9. Kitzman DW, Little WC, Brubaker PH, et al. Pathophysiological characterization of isolated diastolic heart failure in comparison to systolic heart failure. JAMA 2002;288:2144–50.
10. Haykowsky M, Brubaker P, Kitzman D. Role of physical training in heart failure with preserved ejection fraction. Curr Heart Fail Rep 2012;9:101–6.
11. Haykowsky MJ, Herrington DM, Brubaker PH, et al. Relationship of flow-mediated arterial dilation and exercise capacity in older patients with heart failure and preserved ejection fraction. J Gerontol A Biol Sci Med Sci 2013;68:161–7.
12. Haykowsky MJ, Brubaker PH, John JM, et al. Determinants of exercise intolerance in elderly heart failure patients with preserved ejection fraction. J Am Coll Cardiol 2011;58:265–74.

13. Haykowsky MJ, Brubaker PH, Stewart KP, et al. Effect of endurance training on the determinants of peak exercise oxygen consumption in elderly patients with stable compensated heart failure and preserved ejection fraction. J Am Coll Cardiol 2012;60:120–8.

14. Haykowsky MJ, Brubaker PH, Morgan TM, et al. Impaired aerobic capacity and physical functional performance in older heart failure patients with preserved ejection fraction: role of lean body mass. J Gerontol A Biol Sci Med Sci 2013;68:968–75.

15. Bhella PS, Prasad A, Heinicke K, et al. Abnormal haemodynamic response to exercise in heart failure with preserved ejection fraction. Eur J Heart Fail 2011;13:1296–304.

16. Borlaug BA, Olson TP, Lam CS, et al. Global cardiovascular reserve dysfunction in heart failure with preserved ejection fraction. J Am Coll Cardiol 2010;56:845–54.

17. Borlaug BA, Melenovsky V, Russell SD, et al. Impaired chronotropic and vasodilator reserves limit exercise capacity in patients with heart failure and a preserved ejection fraction. Circulation 2006;114: 2138–47.

18. Abudiab MM, Redfield MM, Melenovsky V, et al. Cardiac output response to exercise in relation to metabolic demand in heart failure with preserved ejection fraction. Eur J Heart Fail 2013;15:776–85.

19. Borlaug BA. Mechanisms of exercise intolerance in heart failure with preserved ejection fraction. Circ J 2013;78(1):20–32.

20. Guazzi M, Adams V, Conraads V, et al. EACPR/AHA scientific statement. Clinical recommendations for cardiopulmonary exercise testing data assessment in specific patient populations. Circulation 2012; 126:2261–74.

21. Mitchell JH, Blomqvist G. Maximal oxygen uptake. N Engl J Med 1971;284:1018–22.

22. Beere PA, Russell SD, Morey MC, et al. Aerobic exercise training can reverse age-related peripheral circulatory changes in healthy older men. Circulation 1999;100:1085–94.

23. Katz SD, Zheng H. Peripheral limitations of maximal aerobic capacity in patients with chronic heart failure. J Nucl Cardiol 2002;9:215–25.

24. Kitzman DW, Herrington DM, Brubaker PH, et al. Carotid arterial stiffness and its relationship to exercise intolerance in older patients with heart failure and preserved ejection fraction. Hypertension 2013;61: 112–9.

25. Hundley WG, Kitzman DW, Morgan TM, et al. Cardiac cycle-dependent changes in aortic area and distensibility are reduced in older patients with isolated diastolic heart failure and correlate with exercise intolerance. J Am Coll Cardiol 2001;38:796–802.

26. Hundley WG, Bayram E, Hamilton CA, et al. Leg flow-mediated arterial dilation in elderly patients with heart failure and normal left ventricular ejection fraction. Am J Physiol Heart Circ Physiol 2007;292: H1427–34.

27. Haykowsky MJ, Kouba EJ, Brubaker PH, et al. Skeletal muscle composition and its relation to exercise intolerance in older patients with heart failure and preserved ejection fraction. Am J Cardiol 2014; 113:1211–6.

28. Drexler H, Riede U, Munzel T, et al. Alterations of skeletal muscle in chronic heart failure. Circulation 1992;85:1751–9.

29. Sullivan MJ, Green HJ, Cobb FR. Skeletal muscle biochemistry and histology in ambulatory patients with long-term heart failure. Circulation 1990;81: 518–27.

30. Mancini DM, Coyle E, Coggan A, et al. Contribution of intrinsic skeletal muscle changes to 31P NMR skeletal muscle metabolic abnormalities in patients with chronic heart failure. Circulation 1989;80:1338–46.

31. Schaufelberger M, Eriksson BO, Grimby G, et al. Skeletal muscle alterations in patients with chronic heart failure. Eur Heart J 1997;18:971–80.

32. Kitzman DW, Nicklas B, Kraus WE, et al. Skeletal muscle abnormalities and exercise intolerance in older patients with heart failure and preserved ejection fraction. Am J Physiol Heart Circ Physiol 2014. [Epub ahead of print].

33. Kitzman DW, Brubaker PH, Morgan TM, et al. Exercise training in older patients with heart failure and preserved ejection fraction: a randomized, controlled, single-blind trial. Circ Heart Fail 2010;3: 659–67.

34. Kitzman DW, Brubaker PH, Herrington DM, et al. Effect of endurance exercise training on endothelial function and arterial stiffness in older patients with heart failure and preserved ejection fraction: a randomized, controlled, single-blind trial. J Am Coll Cardiol 2013;62:584–92.

35. Edelmann F, Gelbrich G, Dungen HD, et al. Exercise training improves exercise capacity and diastolic function in patients with heart failure with preserved ejection fraction: results of the EX-DHF (Exercise Training in Diastolic Heart Failure) pilot study. J Am Coll Cardiol 2011;58:1780–91.

36. Smart NA, Haluska B, Jeffriess L, et al. Exercise training in heart failure with preserved systolic function: a randomized controlled trial of the effects on cardiac function and functional capacity. Congest Heart Fail 2012;18:295–301.

37. Borlaug BA, Nishimura RA, Sorajja P, et al. Exercise hemodynamics enhance diagnosis of early heart failure with preserved ejection fraction. Circ Heart Fail 2010;3:588–95.

38. Keteyian SJ, Pina IL, Hibner BA, et al. Clinical role of exercise training in the management of patients with chronic heart failure. J Cardiopulm Rehabil Prev 2010;30:67–76.

39. Conraads VM, Deaton C, Piotrowicz E, et al. Adherence of heart failure patients to exercise: barriers and possible solutions: a position statement of the Study Group on Exercise Training in Heart Failure of the Heart Failure Association of the European Society Of Cardiology. Eur J Heart Fail 2012;14:451–8.

40. Tomczak CR, Thompson RB, Paterson I, et al. Effect of acute high-intensity interval exercise on postexercise biventricular function in mild heart failure. J Appl Physiol (1985) 2011;110: 398–406.

41. Haykowsky MJ, Liang Y, Pechter D, et al. A meta-analysis of the effect of exercise training on left ventricular remodeling in heart failure patients: the benefit depends on the type of training performed. J Am Coll Cardiol 2007;49:2329–36.

Natriuretic Peptides in Heart Failure with Preserved Ejection Fraction

A. Mark Richards, MB ChB, MD, PhD, FRACP, FRCP[a,b,]*,
James L. Januzzi Jr, MD[c],
Richard W. Troughton, MB ChB, PhD, FRACP[b]

KEYWORDS

- Heart failure • Cardiac natriuretic peptides • B-type natriuretic peptide
- N-terminal prohormone B-type natriuretic peptide • Diagnosis • Prognosis

KEY POINTS

- Threshold values of B-type natriuretic peptide (BNP) and N-terminal prohormone B-type natriuretic peptide (NT-proBNP) validated for diagnosis of undifferentiated acutely decompensated heart failure (ADHF) remain useful in patients with heart failure with preserved ejection fraction (HFPEF), with minor loss of diagnostic performance.
- BNP and NT-proBNP measured on admission with ADHF are powerfully predictive of in-hospital mortality in both HFPEF and heart failure with reduced EF (HFREF), with similar or greater risk in HFPEF as in HFREF associated with any given level of either peptide.
- In stable treated heart failure, plasma natriuretic peptide concentrations often fall below cut-point values used for the diagnosis of ADHF in the emergency department; in HFPEF, levels average approximately half those in HFREF.
- BNP and NT-proBNP are powerful independent prognostic markers in both chronic HFREF and chronic HFPEF, and the risk of important clinical adverse outcomes for a given peptide level is similar regardless of left ventricular ejection fraction.
- Serial measurement of BNP or NT-proBNP to monitor status and guide treatment in chronic heart failure may be more applicable in HFREF than in HFPEF.

INTRODUCTION

Timely diagnosis, early introduction of appropriate treatment, accurate risk stratification, and optimal titration of therapy are all key to the management of heart failure (HF). Plasma cardiac natriuretic peptides (NPs) are valuable aids in each of these elements of care. However, most data are derived from undifferentiated HF or HF with reduced ejection fraction (HFREF). The performance and best

Disclosures: Professor A.M. Richards is the recipient of speakers honoraria, consultancy fees and/or research grants (in cash or in kind) from Roche Diagnostics, Alere and Critical Diagnostics. Professor J.L. Januzzi is the recipient of speakers honoraria, consultancy fees, and/or research grants from Roche Diagnostics, Siemens, Thermo Fisher, Singulex, Critical Diagnostics, Zensun, Amgen, and Novartis. Professor R.W. Troughton is the recipient of grants and/or speakers honoraria/consulting fees from Roche Diagnostics and St. Jude Medical.

[a] Cardiac Department, Cardiovascular Research Institute, National University Heart Centre, National University of Singapore, 1E Kent Ridge Road, NUHS Tower Block, Level 9, Singapore 119228, Singapore; [b] Department of Medicine, Christchurch Heart Institute, University of Otago, Christchurch, 2 Riccarton Avenue, Christchurch 8140, New Zealand; [c] Cardiac Intensive Care Unit, Massachusetts General Hospital, Harvard Medical School, 55 Fruit Street, Boston, MA 02114, USA

* Corresponding author. Cardiac Department, Cardiovascular Research Institute, National University Heart Centre, National University of Singapore, 1E Kent Ridge Road, NUHS Tower Block, Level 9, Singapore 119228, Singapore.
E-mail addresses: mdcarthu@nus.edu.sg; mark.richards@cdhb.health.nz

heartfailure.theclinics.com

application of NPs in heart failure with preserved ejection fraction (HFPEF) is less certain. This uncertainty is not unimportant, as a substantial percentage of patients with HF presently have HFPEF. This review outlines the evidence for the use of NPs in the evaluation and management of HFPEF.

The bioactivity of atrial NP (ANP) and B-type NP (BNP) encompasses short-term and long-term hemodynamic, renal, neurohormonal, and trophic effects.[1] The relationship between cardiac hemodynamic load, plasma concentrations of ANP and BNP, and the cardioprotective profile of NP bioactivity have led to investigation of both biomarker and therapeutic potential of NPs in HF.

Use of parenteral human recombinant BNP received approval from the Food and Drug Administration for relief of symptoms of acutely decompensated heart failure (ADHF) and human ANP is used in Japan in the context of acute myocardial infarction.[2,3] However, the accumulated evidence does not support any significant advantage of BNP therapy over other treatments, and NP infusions are not recommended for routine use in ADHF, although they may be of value in defined niche applications.[4] Data on therapeutic value, or lack thereof, specifically in HFPEF are absent. Therefore, the remainder of this review is focused on the diagnostic, prognostic, and monitoring applications of measurement of plasma concentrations of NPs in HFPEF.

Single or serial measurement of plasma NPs, particularly the B-type peptides including BNP and its cosecreted amino-terminal congener N-terminal prohormone BNP (NT-proBNP), is currently endorsed within authoritative guidelines on the diagnosis and management of HF.[5,6] Best proven as an adjunct to the diagnosis of ADHF in patients presenting with new-onset breathlessness,[7,8] both BNP and NT-proBNP are also acknowledged as powerful independent prognostic markers in acute and chronic HF,[8–11] and serial measurement is gaining acceptance as a useful guide for titration of therapy and monitoring in chronic HF.[12–15] Despite the growing array of candidate biomarkers in HFPEF,[16,17] the B-type NPs are the best studied and have exhibited the strongest performance to date.

NATRIURETIC PEPTIDES AND THE DIAGNOSIS OF ADHF IN HFPEF

Landmark trials of the NPs, including the Breathing Not Properly and the International Collaborative on NT-proBNP (ICON) studies, defined optimal threshold values for BNP and NT-proBNP in diagnosing ADHF among heterogeneous populations of patients presenting to the emergency department (ED) with new-onset breathlessness.[7,8] From the Breathing Not Properly trial, among a subgroup of 452 patients with an adjudicated diagnosis of ADHF and with echocardiographic estimates of left ventricular ejection fraction (LVEF) obtained within 30 days of their presentation, 165 (36.5%) had HFPEF (LVEF >45%) and 287 (63.5%) HFREF.[18] Plasma BNP was lower in HFPEF than in HFREF (median 413 vs 821 pg/mL; P<.001). In distinguishing undifferentiated HF from non-HF cases, BNP 100 pg/mL had 90% sensitivity, 76% specificity, a negative predictive value of 89%, and 83% accuracy, and performed only slightly less well when applied specifically to HFPEF (sensitivity 86%, negative predictive value 96%, and overall accuracy 75%). The pattern of overall lower values of BNP or NT-proBNP in HFPEF compared with HFREF, together with a slightly weaker diagnostic performance, has been corroborated in other reports.[8,19,20] In a subgroup analysis from the ProBNP Investigation of Dyspnea in the ED (PRIDE) study among those with echo data available, peptide levels in HFPEF versus HFREF were 259 versus 592 pg/mL, respectively, for BNP, and 2848 versus 6196 pg/mL for NT-proBNP. The false-negative rate for both peptides was 7% in HFREF but was higher (20% for BNP and 9% for NT-proBNP) in HFPEF.[19,20]

> Plasma BNP and NT-proBNP thresholds (100 pg/mL and 300 pg/mL, respectively) used in the diagnosis of undifferentiated ADHF retain good diagnostic performance for acute HFPEF.

In 651 cases from ICON with echo available, 295 (45%) had LVEF greater than 50% and 358 had HFREF with LVEF less than 50%. NT-proBNP levels were lower in HFPEF (median 3070 pg/mL [interquartile range 1344–7974] vs 6356 pg/mL [2777–13,407]; P = .001). The optimal rule-out level of NT-proBNP for undifferentiated HF (300 pg/mL) was less sensitive for HFPEF with ADHF (84%) compared with HFREF cases (92%). **Table 1** displays the diagnostic test performance for BNP and NT-proBNP for ADHF for HFREF and HFPEF subgroups.

Of note, the use of plasma NPs in diagnostic applications requires awareness of the differential diagnosis of elevated NPs. Conditions, both cardiac and noncardiac, potentially elevating plasma NPs are listed in **Box 1**.

Table 1
Plasma B-type natriuretic peptides: diagnostic performance for acutely decompensated heart failure in the emergency department

Category of HF	Marker	Median (pg/mL)	Cut Point (pg/mL)	Sensitivity (%)	Specificity (%)	PPV (%)	NPV (%)	Ref.
All HF	BNP	675	100	90	73	75	90	7
	N-BNP	4639	300	99	60	79	89	8,19
HFREF	BNP	821	100	NR	NR	NR	NR	18
	N-BNP	6356	300	90	89	85	93	19,20
HFPEF	BNP	413	100	86	NR	NR	96	18
	N-BNP	3070	300	84	89	79	86	19,20
Non-HF	BNP	34						7,18
	N-BNP	108						8,19

The values refer to the performance of the cut-points (BNP 100 pg/mL and NT-proBNP 300 pg/mL) in discriminating between (1) undifferentiated HF and non-HF cases; (2) HFREF and non-HF cases; and (3) between HFPEF and non-HF cases.
Abbreviations: BNP, B-type natriuretic peptide; HF, heart failure; HFPEF, heart failure with preserved ejection fraction; HFREF, heart failure with reduced ejection fraction; N-BNP, NT-proBNP; NPV, negative predictive value; NR, not reported; PPV, positive predictive value.
Data from Refs.[7,8,18–20]

Box 1
Causes of increased plasma cardiac natriuretic peptides

CARDIAC

- Heart failure, acute and chronic
- Acute coronary syndromes
- Atrial fibrillation
- Valvular heart disease
- Cardiomyopathies
- Myocarditis
- Cardioversion
- Left ventricular hypertrophy

NONCARDIAC

- Age
- Female sex
- Renal impairment
- Pulmonary embolism
- Pneumonia (severe)
- Obstructive sleep apnea
- Critical illness
- Bacterial sepsis
- Severe burns
- Cancer chemotherapy
- Toxic and metabolic insults

CARDIAC STRUCTURAL AND FUNCTIONAL DETERMINANTS OF PLASMA NPS IN HFPEF

NP release is determined by cardiac chamber wall stress, a function of transmural distending pressure gradient, chamber radius, and wall thickness. Unit wall stress is less in concentrically hypertrophied HFPEF hearts than in dilated HFREF hearts. In part this underlies the lower levels of NPs observed in ADHF in HFPEF in comparison with HFREF.[8,18–20]

> Plasma NPs are related to multiple echo indicators of cardiac structure and function in both HFREF and HFPEF.

Imaging confirms associations of NP concentrations with many structural and functional measures in HFPEF.[21–23] In 160 patients presenting with HF, Iwanaga and colleagues[24] measured plasma BNP levels and performed echocardiography and cardiac catheterization to calculate systolic and diastolic wall stress. BNP correlated ($r^2 = 0.296$; $P<.001$) with left ventricular end-diastolic pressure (LVEDP). However, the correlation with end-diastolic wall stress (EDWS) ($r^2 = 0.887$ [$P<.001$]) was strikingly more powerful. In a subanalysis of 62 patients with HFPEF, r^2 was 0.143 for LVEDP and 0.704 for EDWS. End-diastolic pressures were similar, but EDWS was significantly higher in HFREF than in HFPEF

(P<.001), as were plasma BNP concentrations. BNP levels reflect left ventricular (LV) EDWS more than other ventricular parameters in both HFREF and HFPEF. The relationship of LV EDWS to plasma BNP may provide a better insight into interindividual differences in plasma NP values than other ventricular measures.

Plasma NPs are strongly correlated to diastolic dysfunction independent of LVEF, age, sex, body mass index, and renal function. Clear elevations occur in the most severe grade of diastolic dysfunction with restrictive LV filling when NT-proBNP greater than 600 pg/mL and BNP greater than 100 pg/mL are strong independent predictors of restrictive filling. Peptide levels correlate with E/E′ ratio in addition to indices of LV compliance and myocardial relaxation in both HFPEF and HFREF. Plasma peptide values are also related to left atrial (LA) dimensions and volume, with this relationship remaining strong in HFPEF while weakening in increasingly severe grades of systolic dysfunction. In both HFREF and HFPEF, plasma B peptides are inversely related to right ventricular (RV) ejection fraction, and positively related to RV size and estimated RV pressures.[22]

Systolic function is not normal in HFPEF. In an echocardiographic substudy of the PARAMOUNT trial, Kraigher-Krainer and colleagues[25] demonstrated that LV systolic longitudinal and circumferential strain were reduced in HFPEF compared with both normal controls and patients with hypertension free of HF. These abnormalities were modestly but significantly related to plasma NT-proBNP even after adjustment for age, sex, systolic and diastolic blood pressure, body mass index, LVEF, left atrial volume index (LAVI), E/E′, atrial fibrillation, and estimated glomerular filtration rate.

Echocardiography offers an invaluable adjunct to the diagnosis of HF in newly symptomatic patients when NPs fall into the gray zone between rule-out and rule-in values for acute HF (ie, between 100 and 500 pg/mL for BNP and 300 and 1800 pg/mL for NT-proBNP). Doppler estimates of E/E′ indicating raised filling pressures and/or the presence of a restrictive filling pattern can secure the diagnosis of HF irrespective of LVEF.[22]

Atrial fibrillation (AF) is common (~30%–40% prevalence) in acute and chronic HF. The presence of AF impairs the diagnostic performance of NPs (including mid-regional pro-ANP [MR-proANP]) in undifferentiated ADHF.[26] It is unknown whether AF affects the diagnostic performance of NPs more in ADHF with HFPEF or HFREF.

In chronic HF, AF may have a differential influence on plasma NPs in HFPEF compared with HFREF. Linssen and colleagues[27] studied 927 patients (36% with AF) with stable HF. AF was present in 35% (n = 215) HFREF and 40% (n = 121) HFPEF. In HFREF neither average plasma concentration of NT-proBNP nor prognosis differed between patients with AF and normal sinus rhythm, but in HFPEF AF raised peptide levels and was an independent predictor of death or HF hospitalization. McKelvie and colleagues[28] reported from the Irbesartan in HFPEF (I-PRESERVE) trial that the baseline characteristic most strongly associated with higher NT-proBNP levels in multivariate analyses was AF on electrocardiogram (ECG). Present in 26% of I-PRESERVE participants, AF was associated with median NT-proBNP of 903 pg/mL, compared with 257 pg/mL for those in sinus rhythm.

NP CONCENTRATIONS IN CHRONIC HFPEF AND HFREF

The Valsartan Heart Failure Therapy (Val-HeFT) and the I-PRESERVE trials have provided data defining typical plasma BNP levels in chronic HFREF and HFPEF, respectively.[9–11] Val-HeFT tested the efficacy of valsartan added to angiotensin-converting enzyme inhibition and other indicated HF therapy in stable HFREF (LVEF <40%; LV end-diastolic diameter/body surface area ≥2.9 cm/m²). In a neurohormonal substudy of 3916 patients, mean LVEF was 27% and median (range, quartiles 1–3) concentrations of NT-proBNP and BNP were 895 (375–985) pg/mL and 99 (41–242) pg/mL, respectively, at baseline. Half of the patients had baseline BNP levels lower than 100 pg/mL.

> BNP and NT-proBNP fall below ADHF thresholds in stable HFREF in approximately 50% and 20% of cases, respectively. Levels in stable HFPEF are even lower, approximately half those in HFREF.

I-PRESERVE, a randomized controlled therapeutic trial of the angiotensin-2 type 1 receptor blocker irbesartan, recruited patients with LVEF of 45% or greater, aged 60 years or older, in New York Heart Association (NYHA) functional class II to IV with an HF admission within 6 months, or NYHA III to IV with echocardiographic corroboration of cardiac dysfunction. In a subgroup (n = 3562) of this stable HFPEF population, the median plasma concentration of NT-proBNP was 341 pg/mL.[11] Of note, relatively low levels of BNP have been documented in HFPEF patients with increased filling pressures measured by cardiac catheterization. Anjan and colleagues[29] found that 29% of HFPEF cases assessed in this way had BNP levels less than 100 pg/mL.

The relatively low levels of BNP and NT-proBNP observed in early HF and in stable, treated patients mean that the signal-to-noise ratio for the marker is markedly diminished, and factors influencing peptide concentrations that are of little importance in ADHF become major potential confounders. These factors include the inverse relationship between body mass index and plasma NPs, which may give falsely reassuring NP levels in obese, ambulant patients. Noncardiac factors associated with rising plasma NP levels include age and renal function. All of these factors should be considered when interpreting plasma NP levels in nonacute settings. Hence, consistent with studies in ADHF, plasma concentrations of NT-proBNP in chronic HFREF are about twice those observed in HFPEF.

Table 2 lists typical median plasma BNP concentrations in both ADHF and chronic HF from selected trials and registries.

EARLY HEART FAILURE IN THE COMMUNITY

Several reports have assessed the performance of NT-proBNP in distinguishing LV hypertrophy or LVEF of less than 40% in asymptomatic or minimally symptomatic community-based participants.[30,31] The area under the curve for discrimination of LVEF less than 40% was approximately 0.90, similar to the sensitivity for ADHF. The threshold values of NT-proBNP yielding this performance were an order of magnitude lower than those applicable for the diagnosis of ADHF.

> Whereas BNPs have 90% sensitivity for asymptomatic LVEF of less than 40% in the community (a precursor state for HFREF), they offer no clear guide to the presence of early community-based HFPEF.

Unfortunately, no similar data are available on assessing community-based ambulatory patients with early-stage or minimally symptomatic HFPEF, which, in the absence of abnormal LVEF, has no easily acquired gold-standard diagnostic signature. Definition of early HFPEF may require invasive hemodynamic or echocardiographic Doppler assessment of response to exercise, which is clearly not an affordable strategy for mass screening. At present, a very low B-peptide value (ie, <30 pg/mL for BNP or 125 pg/L for NT-proBNP) may provide confidence that the likelihood of untreated HFPEF or HFREF is low.[5]

The higher average age and more prevalent comorbidities in HFPEF may further confound the diagnostic power of NPs in HFPEF outside of ED or hospitalized HF settings. Mason and colleagues[32] assessed the utility of biomarkers in the differential diagnosis of HF in older people in long-term care. For undifferentiated HF a BNP level of 115 pg/mL had sensitivity of 67% and a negative predictive value of 86%, and an NT-proBNP of 760 pg/mL had sensitivity of 62% and specificity of 87%. This is a far less useful performance than observed in the ED. For the subgroup adjudicated to have HFPEF, a BNP level of 110 pg/mL had sensitivity of only 63% and

Table 2
Median plasma concentrations of BNP in acute and chronic HFREF and HFPEF from selected registries and trials

Category of HF	Marker	Median (pg/mL)	N	Study/Trial
ADHF				
HFREF	BNP	821	287	Breathing Not Properly
	N-BNP	6356	358	ICON
	BNP	~1000	47,025	Get With the Guidelines
	BNP	1210	19,544	ADHERE Registry
HFPEF	BNP	413	165	Breathing Not Properly
	N-BNP	3070	295	ICON
	BNP	~550	38,955	Get With the Guidelines
	BNP	564	12,631	ADHERE Registry
Chronic HF				
HFREF	BNP	99	3916	Val-HeFT
	N-BNP	895	3916	Val-HeFT
HFPEF	N-BNP	339	3480	I-PRESERVE

Abbreviations: ADHF, acutely decompensated heart failure; N-BNP, NT-proBNP.
Data from Refs.[8,9,11,19,37,38]

specificity of 61% while values for an NT-proBNP level of 477 pg/mL were 68% and 58%, respectively.

NPS IN PUBLISHED GUIDELINES FOR DIAGNOSING HFPEF

Given the background offered herein, what do authoritative international guidelines have to say on NPs in the diagnosis of HFPEF?

> Guidelines recommend BNP and NT-proBNP as adjuncts to the diagnosis of acute and chronic HF and for risk stratification. Refinements for application to HFPEF are needed.

The 2013 American College of Cardiology Foundation/American Heart Association guidelines provide definitions of HFREF (LVEF <40%), HFPEF borderline (LVEF 41%–49%), and HFPEF (LVEF ≥50%).[6] High levels of recommendation (Class I) and evidence (Level A) are accorded to the B-type peptides for diagnostic and prognostic applications in both hospitalized and ambulatory HF, and a lesser level of support for their potential role in titrating therapy (Class IIa, evidence level B) and as part of a treatment guidance strategy to reduce HF death and admissions (Class IIb, evidence level B). However, these guidelines offer no specific cut-points or algorithms including plasma NPs, and there is no discussion of the possibly differing optimal thresholds and relative utility of NPs in HFREF in comparison with HFPEF.

The 2007 and 2012 European Society of Cardiology guidelines have offered evolving NP thresholds within diagnostic algorithms (**Fig. 1**).[5,33] The 2007 guidelines suggest that diagnosis of HFPEF requires symptoms or signs of HF, LVEF greater than 50%, LV end-diastolic volume index less than 97 mL/m^2, together with further support from either invasive hemodynamic measurements (pulmonary capillary wedge pressure >12 mm Hg or LVEDP >16 mm Hg) or from further echocardiographic indices (E/E′ >15, or if E/E′ >8 but <15 then supporting evidence from E/A ratio <0.5 or deceleration time <280 milliseconds or ARd-Ad index >30 milliseconds, LAVI >40 mL/m^2 or LV mass index >122 g/m^2 in women; >149 g/m^2 in men or AF). Paulus and colleagues[33] suggested plasma B peptides could be incorporated in this algorithm coupled with E/E′ greater than 8 to secure the diagnosis if BNP is greater than 200 pg/mL or NT-proBNP is greater than 220 pg/mL. However, from the preceding discussion it is very clear that these NP cut-points are far too high to offer any proper sensitivity for many acute HFPEF cases and, probably, most stable ambulant HFPEF. The 2012 version provided simplified diagnostic rules for HFREF and HFPEF (**Box 2**). With respect to NPs the guidelines state "A normal natriuretic peptide level in an untreated patient virtually excludes significant cardiac disease, making an echocardiogram unnecessary...." "For patients presenting with acute onset or worsening of symptoms, the optimal exclusion cut-off is 300 pg/mL for NT-proBNP and 100 pg/mL for BNP (see **Fig. 1**). In one other study MR-proANP at a cut-off point of 120 pmol/L, was shown to be noninferior to these thresholds for BNP and NT-proBNP in the acute setting."

The guidelines make the crucial distinction between acute and nonacute presentations. "For patients presenting in a nonacute way the optimal exclusion cut-off point is 125 pg/mL for NT-proBNP and 35 pg/mL for BNP. The specificity and sensitivity of BNP and NT-proBNP for the diagnosis of HF are lower in nonacute patients." The common set of NP thresholds recommended for both HFPEF and HFREF will inevitably produce a significant percentage of false negatives, especially for BNP and especially in the HFPEF group. The algorithm requires prospective validation and revision to better identify optimal NP cut-points which will differ between HFREF and HFPEF.

NPS AND PROGNOSIS IN HFPEF

The literature on plasma BNPs since the discovery of BNP in 1988[34] and NT-proBNP in 1995[35] consistently confirms the powerful relationship between plasma NPs and outcomes in HF. These peptides are the most powerful performers in multivariate models relating assorted candidate predictors to clinical outcomes including all-cause mortality, cardiovascular mortality, new-onset HF, recurrent HF decompensation events, and HF mortality in varied populations including ADHF, chronic HF, acute and chronic coronary heart disease, ambulant asymptomatic community-based populations, and heterogeneous populations of severely ill patients.[7–11,36–39]

> The prognostic power of NPs is similar in HFREF and HFPEF.
>
> Defined levels of BNP and NT-proBNP correlate with similar short-term and long-term risks of important clinical adverse outcomes in both HFREF and HFPEF.

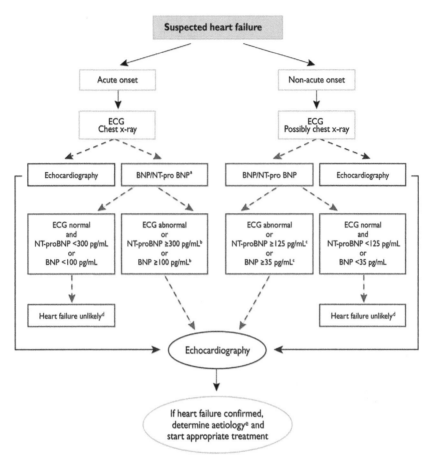

Fig. 1. Diagnostic algorithm for suspected heart failure presenting either acutely or nonacutely. [a] In the acute setting, mid-regional pro–atrial natriuretic peptide may also be used (cutoff point 120 pmol/L; ie, <120 pmol/L = heart failure unlikely). [b] Other causes of elevated natriuretic peptide levels in the acute setting are an acute coronary syndrome, atrial or ventricular arrhythmias, pulmonary embolism, and severe chronic obstructive pulmonary disease with elevated right heart pressures, renal failure, and sepsis. Other causes of an elevated natriuretic level in the nonacute setting are old age (>75 years), atrial arrhythmias, left ventricular hypertrophy, chronic obstructive pulmonary disease, and chronic kidney disease. [c] Exclusion cutoff points for natriuretic peptides are chosen to minimize the false-negative rate while reducing unnecessary referrals for echocardiography. [d] Treatment may reduce natriuretic peptide concentration, and natriuretic peptide concentrations may not be markedly elevated in patients with heart failure with preserved ejection fraction. [e] See text and **Table 2**. BNP, B-type natriuretic peptide; ECG, electrocardiogram; NT-proBNP, N-terminal prohormone of B-type natriuretic peptide. (*From* McMurray JJ, Adamopoulos S, Anker SD, et al. The task force for the diagnosis and treatment of acute and chronic heart failure 2012 of the European Society of Cardiology. ESC guidelines for the diagnosis and treatment of acute and chronic heart failure 2012. Eur Heart J 2012;33:1787–847; with permission.)

NPs and In-Hospital Mortality in ADHF with and Without Preserved LVEF

Hsich and colleagues,[40] reporting on approximately 100,000 patients admitted with ADHF included in the "Get with the Guidelines" initiative, noted the relationship between BNP and risk of in-hospital mortality was the same among 3 strata of LVEF (<40%, n = 47,025; 40%–50%, n = 13,950; >50%, n = 38,955). These investigators analyzed 6 subgroups according to sex and reduced, borderline, or preserved EF. Men with reduced EF were used as the reference. In-hospital mortality was calculated for each of the 6 subgroups and stratified by those above and below the median BNP value.

The median BNP overall was 816 pg/mL (interquartile range 380–1670 pg/mL). BNP levels were slightly higher in women than in men (median for LVEF <40%: women 1259 pg/mL [606–2413], men 1113 pg/mL [535–2130]; median for LVEF 40%–50%: women 821 pg/mL [412–1574], men

732 pg/mL [366–1420]; median for LVEF >50%: women 559 pg/mL [279–1075], men 540 pg/mL [253–1064]). In-hospital mortality overall was 2.7%. In each stratum of LVEF mortality was higher in those with supra-median BNP levels (adjusted hazard ratios 1.18–1.52 with no difference across

the 6 LVEF/sex subgroups), with rates slightly higher in patients with LVEF greater than 50% in comparison with those with LVEF less than 50%.

Although hazard ratios for in-hospital mortality above and below median values are similar across gender and LVEF subgroups, the absolute value of those median values varies across a 2.5-fold range (from 540 pg/mL in men with HFPEF to 1259 pg/mL in women with HFREF) among those subgroups. Hence men with LVEF higher than 50% with BNP greater than 540 pg/mL had the same risk of in-hospital mortality as men with reduced LVEF and BNP above 1113 pg/mL. In this large data set, inspection of unadjusted risk of in-hospital mortality plotted against admission BNP as continuous variables (**Fig. 2**) provides a simple "ready reckoner" for the clinician (**Table 3**): plasma concentrations of 500, 1000, 2000, and 4000 pg/mL correspond to risk of in-hospital death of approximately 1.9%, 2.0%, 3.2%, and 4.7%, respectively in HFREF and approximately 1.8%, 2.9%, 4.5%, and 4.7%, respectively in HFPEF with only minor differences between the sexes. Thus, risk is well matched between HFREF and HFPEF at 500 pg/mL and 4000 pg/mL, but exhibits a steeper association with increasing mortality in HFPEF in the 1000 to 2000 pg/mL range.

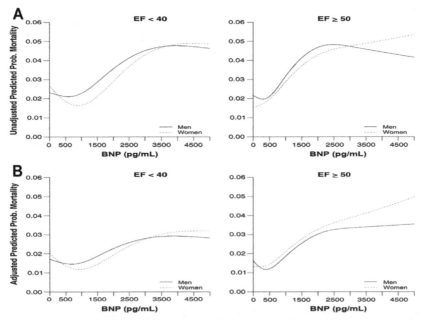

Fig. 2. Unadjusted (*A*) and adjusted (*B*) in-hospital mortality in patients hospitalized with acute decompensated heart failure plotted according to admission plasma BNP. BNP, B-type natriuretic peptide; EF, ejection fraction. (*From* Hsich EM, Grau-Sepulveda MV, Hernandez AF, et al. Relationship between sex, ejection fraction, and B-type natriuretic peptide levels in patients hospitalized with heart failure and associations with in-hospital outcomes: findings from the Get with the Guideline—Heart Failure registry. Am Heart J 2013;166:1063–71; with permission.)

Table 3
Approximate (unadjusted) risk of in-hospital mortality during hospitalization for ADHF according to admission plasma BNP

BNP (pg/mL)	500	1000	2000	4000
Risk of In-Hospital Mortality (%)				
HFREF	1.9	2.0	3.2	4.7
HFPEF	1.8	2.9	4.5	4.7

Data from Hsich EM, Grau-Sepulveda MV, Hernandez AF, et al. Relationship between sex, ejection fraction, and B-type natriuretic peptide levels in patients hospitalized with heart failure and associations with in-hospital outcomes: findings from the Get with the Guideline—Heart Failure registry. Am Heart J 2013;166:1063–71.

In the Acute Decompensated HF National Registry (ADHERE), higher in-hospital mortality is again associated with higher BNP in analyses from more than 48,000 ADHF admissions stratified by quartiles of LVEF and BNP.[41] Risk of in-hospital mortality increased stepwise per quartile at 1.4%, 2.8%, 3.2%, and 6.4% in quartiles 1 to 4, respectively, in those with LVEF less than 40% (n = 19,544) and at 1.6%, 2.3%, 3.0%, and 4.9% in quartiles 1 to 4 in those with LVEF of 50% or higher (n = 11,631) (**Fig. 3**). As expected, BNP levels overall (and therefore quartile thresholds) were lower in HFPEF compared with HFREF, but the relationships of BNP versus risk overlapped. Risk in HFREF quartile 2 (622–1201 pg/mL) at 2.8% was similar to that in HFPEF quartile 3 (565–1069 pg/mL), at 3.0%.

NPs and Prognosis in Chronic Stable HFPEF and HFREF

Van Veldhuisen and colleagues[42] divided 615 patients with HF (>18 years of age, NYHA II–IV with evidence of underlying structural heart disease) according to LVEF. Over 18 months, 171 (28%) patients died. When stratified according to LVEF above and below 40% and then further stratified according to BNP level 0 to 250 pg/mL (n = 180), 251 to 750 pg/mL (n = 238), and greater than 750 pg/mL (n = 197), mortality increased with BNP, but for any stratum of BNP mortality was strikingly similar whether LVEF was higher or lower than 40% (**Fig. 4**).

The prognostic performance of both NT-proBNP and BNP in chronic stable HFREF has been addressed in several reports from Val-HeFT.[9–11,43] In multivariate models adjusting for 20 or more acknowledged demographic, biochemical, clinical, and imaging predictors of outcome in HF, both BNP and NT-proBNP are consistently identified as strong individual independent predictors of all-cause mortality, composite end points of morbidity and mortality, and HF hospitalizations. Of note, BNP outperforms other neurohormonal markers including norepinephrine, aldosterone, and endothelin.[43] Increments in NT-proBNP of 500 pg/mL were

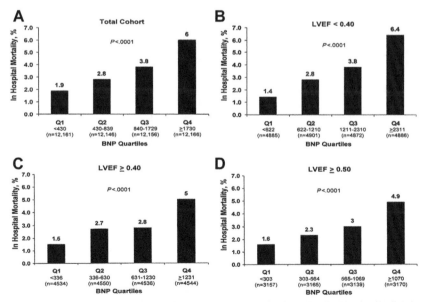

Fig. 3. (*A–D*) In-hospital mortality by quartile of admission B-type natriuretic peptide (BNP) after hospitalization for acute decompensated heart failure, divided according to left ventricular ejection fraction (LVEF). (*From* Fonarow GC, Peacock WF, Phillips CO, et al. Admission B-type natriuretic peptide levels and in-hospital mortality in acute decompensated heart failure. J Am Coll Cardiol 2007;49(19):1943–50; with permission.)

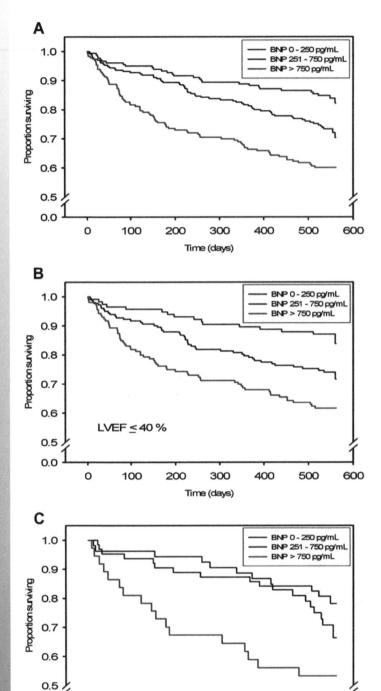

Fig. 4. All-cause mortality curves in chronic heart failure divided according to levels of B-type natriuretic peptide (BNP): 0–250 pg/mL (*black*), 251–750 pg/mL (*blue*) and greater than 750 pg/mL (*red*), plotted for all cases (*A*), left ventricular ejection fraction (LVEF) 40% or less (*B*), and LVEF greater than 40% (*C*). Mortality curves for each level of BNP are similar regardless of LVEF. (*From* van Veldhuisen DJ, Linssen GM, Jaarsma T, et al. B-type natriuretic peptide and prognosis in heart failure patients with preserved and reduced ejection fraction. J Am Coll Cardiol 2013;61(14):1498–506; with permission.)

associated with increments of 3.0% to 3.8% in the risk of all-cause mortality, morbidity and mortality, and HF hospitalizations. Corresponding increases in risk for increments of 50 pg/mL in BNP fell between 5.4% and 5.7%.[9] Overall, in the Val-HeFT neurohormonal substudy (n = 3916), a median NT-proBNP level of 895 pg/mL was associated with a mortality of 19.4% at 23 months' follow-up (ie, crude annualized mortality of ~10.1%). Division of the Val-HeFT population into deciles by levels of NT-proBNP and BNP display a 4- to 5-fold change in risk of key end points including all-cause mortality, a composite mortality/morbidity end point, and hospitalization for HF (**Fig. 5**).

From I-PRESERVE, Komajda and colleagues[10] have defined the relationship of baseline plasma NT-proBNP levels with outcomes in 4128 HFPEF patients incurring 1515 episodes of the primary end point of all-cause mortality or cardiovascular admission, 881 deaths, and 716 episodes of HF death or HF hospitalization. In a Cox multivariable model adjusted for 58 variables, NT-proBNP emerged as the strongest independent predictor of 3-year outcomes, which could be risk stratified across septiles of NT-proBNP from 8.1% to 59.9% for the primary end point, 2.7% to 36.5% for risk of death, and 2.1% to 38.9% for risk of the composite end point HF death or HF hospitalization. Hence NT-proBNP incorporated with standard predictors allowed fine-grained prediction of key clinical outcomes across a wide range, from very high to very low risk. Findings from I-PRESERVE were also assessed by Anand and colleagues.[11] Overall, in I-PRESERVE a median baseline NT-proBNP of 339 pg/mL was associated with 21.1% mortality at 49.5 months (ie, a crude annualized mortality of 5.1%). Division of the I-PRESERVE population by quartiles of NT-proBNP (**Fig. 6**) displayed a 4- to 6-fold increase

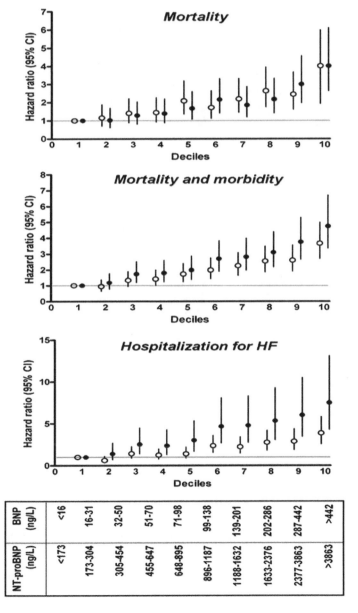

Fig. 5. Hazard ratios per decile of plasma B-type natriuretic peptide (BNP) (*open circles*) and plasma N-terminal prohormone of BNP (NT-proBNP) (*closed circles*) (decile 1 as reference) for mortality (*upper*), mortality and morbidity (*middle*), and hospitalization for heart failure (HF) (*lower*) in patients with HFREF participating in Val-HeFT. CI, confidence interval. (*From* Masson S, Latini R, Anand IS, et al. Direct comparison of B-type natriuretic peptide (BNP) and amino-terminal proBNP in a large population of patients with chronic and symptomatic heart failure: the valsartan heart failure (Val-HeFT) data. Clin Chem 2006;52:1528–38; with permission.)

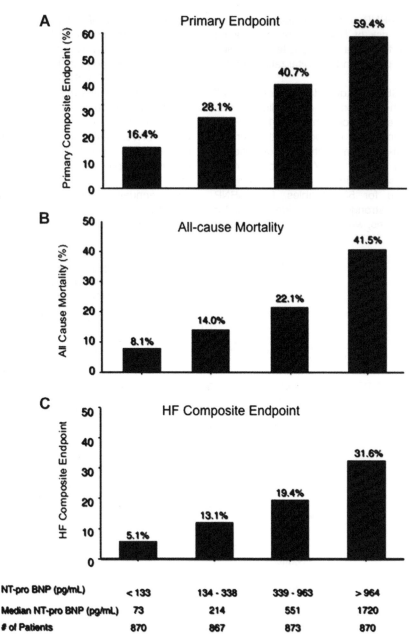

Fig. 6. Event rates per quartile of plasma NT-proBNP for the primary end point (*A*), all-cause mortality (*B*), and composite heart failure (HF) end point (*C*) in the I-PRESERVE trial. (*From* Anand IS, Rector TS, Cleland JG, et al. Prognostic value of baseline plasma amino-terminal pro-brain natriuretic peptide and its interactions with irbesartan treatment effects in patients with heart failure and preserved ejection fraction: findings from the I-PRESERVE trial. Circ Heart Fail 2011;4:569–77; with permission.)

from lowest to highest quartile levels of clinical end points, including all-cause mortality and HF end points.

As a convenient approximation, clinicians can assume that in stable or chronic HFREF, typical NT-proBNP levels in the range of 800 to 1000 pg/mL are associated with approximately 10% annual mortality, and in stable HFPEF typical

levels of 300 to 500 pg/mL are associated with approximately 5% annual mortality.

ARE SERIAL MEASUREMENTS OF NPS USEFUL FOR GUIDING THERAPY IN HFPEF?

The associations between plasma BNPs and both cardiac function and clinical prognosis has provided the rationale for a series of controlled trials of hormone-guided therapy in chronic HF.[5,6,12–15] These trials have tested the hypothesis that directing therapy to drive plasma NT-proBNP or BNP down toward normal according to repeated measurement of plasma NT-proBNP or BNP, in addition to standard-of-care management of HF, will improve clinical outcomes. Repeated meta-analyses have consistently reported significant beneficial effects of the guided strategy on total mortality (>20% reduction), with the more recent meta-analyses indicating a reduction in HF hospitalizations (>20% reduction) as well.[14,15] The Guiding Evidence Based Therapy Using Biomarker Intensified Treatment (GUIDEIT) trial (ClinicalTrials.gov NCT01685840) is under way, and will provide definitive data on application of the strategy in HFREF.

> Serial measurement of NPs for guiding treatment titration and improving outcomes is effective in HFREF but may not be as applicable in HFPEF.

Trials of hormone-guided treatment in chronic HF have included approximately 2000 patients.[14,15] Most participants (>90%) have had HFREF and, hence, our ability to assess the likely utility of this approach in HFPEF is severely limited. The TIME-CHF investigators have provided the only dedicated report on this issue.[44] TIME-CHF recruited patients 60 years of age or older with dyspnea (NYHA class II or more) and a history of admission for HF within the last 12 months, and NT-proBNP levels of 400 pg/mL or higher in those younger than 75 years and 800 pg/mL or higher in those older than 75. Both HFREF and HFPEF subjects were recruited, but these subgroups have been reported separately. In the 499 HFREF participants in TIME-CHF the average age was 77 years, mean LVEF about 30%, and plasma concentrations of NT-proBNP approximately 4000 pg/mL. Mortality (hazard ratio 0.68 [0.45–1.02], $P = .06$) and HF admissions (hazard ratio 0.68 [0.50–0.92], $P = .01$) were improved, and this was more apparent in those younger than 75 years (mortality hazard ratio 0.41 [0.19–0.87], $P = .01$).[13]

Recently, results from the 123 HFPEF participants in TIME-CHF have been published.[44] Their average age was 80 years and LVEF 56%, and NT-proBNP levels (~2200 pg/mL) were lower than in HFREF participants in TIME-CHF (~4000 pg/mL). Worryingly, NT-proBNP–guided treatment was associated with worse clinical outcomes in HFPEF, with significant interactions between LVEF stratum and management strategy

for survival (HFPEF hazard ratio 1.82 [0.83–4.01] vs HFREF 0.68 [0.45–1.02]; $P = .03$ for interaction) and HF hospitalization-free survival (HFPEF hazard ratio 1.64 [0.89–3.0] vs HFREF 0.68 [0.5–0.92]; $P = .01$ for interaction).

This discouraging signal from a single report on a small sample of HFPEF patients cannot be regarded as definitive, and corroboration in independent and larger samples is required. However, the pattern is consistent with the absence of proven therapies for HFPEF. If there is no proven therapy in HFPEF, titrating doses of ineffective therapy against plasma NP concentrations is likely to be futile. Moreover, the results from TIME-CHF raise the specter of harm from this approach in HFPEF. The pronounced sensitivity of ventricular filling pressures, systemic arterial pressure, and renal perfusion pressure in response to relatively subtle changes in circulating volume and pressures, such as those induced by vasodilator and diuretic drugs in patients with small, stiff HFPEF hearts, may underlie this result.

Daily plasma BNP concentrations have been obtained using a finger-prick point-of-care technology in both HFREF and HFPEF participants in the recently reported HF Assessment with B-type Natriuretic Peptide in the Home (HABIT) study.[45] Unlike the relatively slow evolving trends over days or weeks in plasma BNP observed in HFREF patients, a subset of HFPEF patients, without clinical ADHF, exhibited rapid spikes and falls in plasma BNP with clear elevation well above the normal range alternating with falls to frankly normal values, occurring at intervals of hours to 1 or 2 days only (**Fig. 7**). Again this may reflect the steeper relationship between shifts in circulating volumes and changes in intracardiac pressures that occur in HFPEF, compared with HFREF. This pattern may render marker-guided titration of therapy inapplicable to at least a subgroup of HFPEF.

INSIGHTS INTO NPS IN HFPEF FROM RANDOMIZED CONTROLLED THERAPEUTIC TRIALS

The data yielded by 2 large trials, Val-HeFT and I-PRESERVE, on typical plasma concentrations of the BNPs in chronic HFREF and chronic HFPEF, respectively, and their respective relationships to prognosis, have been discussed earlier in this review.[9,10]

> Randomized controlled trials of therapy in HFPEF suggest that plasma NT-proBNP is a valid surrogate end point.

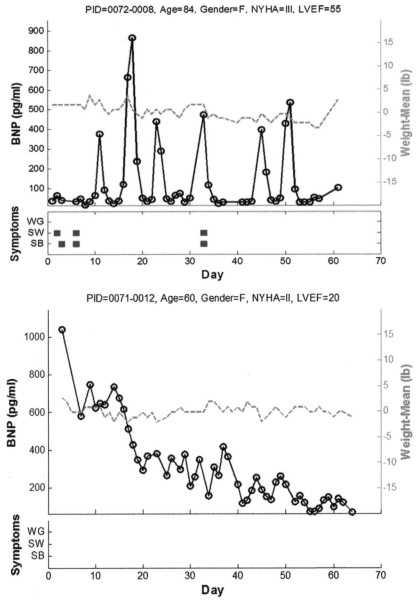

Fig. 7. Serial daily pin-prick BNP readings in a patient with HFPEF (*upper*) and another with HFREF (*lower*) without clinical evidence of acute decompensated heart failure in either case. Volatile spiking of plasma BNP from the normal to the acute heart failure range is observed in the HFPEF case, with cycles occurring over brief periods of 1 to 3 days. Upper axes show BNP (*left axis, blue*) and weight minus mean (*right axis, green*). Lower axes show symptoms (*red squares*) where SW is a day of swelling, SB is a day of shortness of breath, and WG is a day of weight gain (5 lb within 3 days). HFPEF, heart failure with preserved ejection fraction; HFREF, heart failure with reduced ejection fraction; LVEF, left ventricular ejection fraction; NYHA, New York Heart Association functional class. (*From* Maisel A, Barnard D, Jaski B, et al. Primary results of the HABIT trial (heart failure assessment with BNP in the home). J Am Coll Cardiol 2013;61(16):1726–35; with permission.)

In general, because elevated BNP or NT-proBNP are associated with higher risk, marker thresholds are included in selection criteria for inclusion in therapeutic trials to enrich the trial population and provide adequate event rates to help ensure the trial is powered to detect any clinically significant effects of the experimental therapy on key clinical end points. The corollary is the added expectation that benefit will be more apparent and more easily detected in those with higher marker levels. In this regard, I-PRESERVE yielded an unexpected result: benefit of treatment with irbesartan was associated with baseline NT-proBNP plasma concentrations below the median (339 pg/mL). This relationship between submedian NT-proBNP levels with therapeutic benefit was retained even after adjustment for 20 covariates, and was observed for the primary end point of all-cause mortality plus prespecified cardiovascular hospitalizations (hazard ratio 0.74 [0.60–0.90], P = .003), all-cause mortality (hazard ratio 0.75 [0.56–0.99], P = .046) and HF death or hospitalization (hazard ratio 0.57 [0.41–0.80], P = .001).[11] Does this mean that irbesartan is only of benefit in earlier or milder stages of HFPEF? The result is surprising, but is derived from a large data set and is consistent across clinical end points. It casts doubt on the exact role, if any, of angiotensin-receptor antagonists in HFPEF, and it is confusing with respect to use of peptides for case-selection purposes in therapeutic trials. This finding requires corroboration.

Another trial, Aldo-DHF, tested 25 mg spironolactone versus placebo in HFPEF (>50 years, LVEF ≥50% and NYHA class II or III, diastolic dysfunction on echo of grade I or higher, and peak oxygen uptake [Vo_2] of 25 mL/kg/min or less).[46] Treatment reduced E/E′ and LV mass without improving symptoms or maximum Vo_2. NT-proBNP, a secondary end point, declined with spironolactone more than in the placebo group at 6 and 12 months of treatment (P = .03). It is notable that baseline levels of NT-proBNP were not markedly elevated, with median values of 165 and 152 pg/mL in the placebo and spironolactone group, respectively. These levels are half those seen in I-PRESERVE, and may reflect patient selection. Of note, a history of an episode of frank cardiac decompensation was not required for inclusion and, therefore, this trial may have selected for mild HF.

In the Prospective Comparison of ARNI with ARB on Management of HFPEF (PARAMOUNT) study, 149 patients (LVEF ≥45%, NYHA class II–III, and NT-proBNP >400 pg/mL with a documented history of HF) were randomized to receive either valsartan or a novel drug (LCZ696) combining angiotensin-receptor blockade with neprilysin inhibition (NEPI).[47] Neprilysin (EC 3.4.24.11) enzymatically cleaves the ring structure of mature bioactive carboxy-terminal bioactive ANP, BNP, and C-type NP. NEPI is thought to exert therapeutic effects via delayed NP clearance and increased plasma NP concentrations. NT-proBNP is not a neprilysin substrate and, therefore, falling plasma levels still faithfully reflect cardiac decompression with associated reductions in cardiac release of NPs. About 80% had an LVEF greater than 50%. The primary end point was decline in NT-proBNP over 12 weeks of treatment. Median NT-proBNP decreased from 783 pg/mL to 605 pg/mL in those on LCZ696, compared with 862 to 835 pg/mL in the valsartan group (P = .005). In addition, LCZ696 significantly reduced left atrial volumes and improved NYHA functional class. This population is clearly different to that recruited to Aldo-DHF, with NT-proBNP levels even higher than those recorded in I-PRESERVE and actually approximating values observed in HFREF participants in Val-HeFT (median 895 pg/mL). In contrast to I-PRESERVE, there was no interaction of baseline NT-proBNP levels with response to therapy.

The long-awaited results of the TOPCAT (Treatment of Preserved Cardiac Function Heart Failure With an Aldosterone Antagonist) trial (NCT00094302)[48] have been presented in major meetings but are yet to be published. This trial of spironolactone in HFPEF recruited 3445 patients older than 50 years with HF signs and symptoms, and either a history of hospitalization with HF in the past 12 months (n = 2480) or elevated plasma B-type peptide levels (ie, BNP >100 pg/mL or NT-proBNP >360 pg/mL, n = 965). Although no improvement in all-cause mortality or sudden cardiac death was observed, rates of HF hospitalization were improved. Of note, outcomes were more clearly improved in the subset of patients selected according to the nominated BNP or NT-proBNP thresholds.

SUMMARY

Data on BNP and NT-proBNP specifically in HFPEF are scant in comparison with undifferentiated acute HF and certainly less well defined than in patients with HFREF.

Plasma NPs are useful in HFPEF for:

1. Diagnosis in ADHF

2. Prognosis

3. As a surrogate end point in therapeutic trials

Plasma NPs are not currently applicable in HFPEF for:

1. Community screening for early HFPEF

2. Excluding HFPEF in stable treated patients

3. Guiding treatment in chronic HFPEF by serial measurement

Population screening using BNP or NT-proBNP to detect early HFPEF is unlikely to be fruitful. In chronic HF, BNP or NT-proBNP are equally strong independent predictors of important adverse end points in both HFREF and HFPEF. Across the span of plasma levels for both peptides, a 4- to 6-fold range of risk in both phenotypes and absolute levels of BNP and NT-proBNP are associated with similar levels of risk in HFREF and HFPEF. Change in BNP levels may be a valid surrogate end point in therapeutic trials in HFPEF. Whether trial case selection according to BNP values is an effective strategy to enrich trial populations for treatment "responders" is unclear. Guided treatment of chronic HFPEF according to serial NP measurements may be less useful in HFPEF than in HFREF. Plasma BNP or NT-proBNP is on average lower (about half) in both ADHF and chronic HF in HFPEF when compared with HFREF. However, the elevation of BNP or NT-proBNP concentrations in HFPEF with ADHF still provides sufficient signal to noise to provide good diagnostic performance. Acute elevations measured at the time of hospitalization for ADHF are associated with similar risks of in-hospital mortality in both HFREF and HFPEF. In early HFPEF or in stable, treated HFPEF, plasma NP levels will be lower than in HFREF and may well be normal in many cases, and diagnostic cut-points are not well defined. On a background of near normal levels, confounding factors including obesity, age, and renal function are important, and may preclude the use of NPs to rule out compensated HFPEF.

REFERENCES

1. Espiner EA, Richards AM. Atrial natriuretic peptide. An important factor in sodium and blood pressure regulation. Lancet 1989;333:707–10.
2. O'Connor CM, Starling RC, Hernandez AF, et al. Effect of nesiritide in patients with acute decompensated heart failure. N Engl J Med 2011;365:32–43.
3. Saito Y. Roles of atrial natriuretic peptide and its therapeutic use. J Cardiol 2010;56:262–70.
4. Mentzer RM, Oz MC, Sladen RN, et al. Effects of perioperative nesiritide in patients with left ventricular dysfunction undergoing cardiac surgery. The NAPA trial. J Am Coll Cardiol 2007;49:716–26.
5. McMurray JJ, Adamopoulos S, Anker SD, et al. ESC guidelines for the diagnosis and treatment of acute and chronic heart failure 2012. The task force for the diagnosis and treatment of acute and chronic heart failure 2012 of the European Society of Cardiology. Developed in collaboration with the Heart Failure Association (HFA) of the ESC. Eur Heart J 2012; 33:1787–847. http://dx.doi.org/10.1093/eurheartj/ehs104.
6. Yancy CW, Jessup M, Bozkurt B, et al. 2013 ACCF/AHA guideline for the management of heart failure: a report of the American College of Cardiology Foundation/American Heart Association task force on

practice guidelines. Circulation 2013;128:e240–327. http://dx.doi.org/10.1161/CIR. 0b013e31829e8776.
7. Maisel AS, Krishnaswamy P, Nowak RM, et al. Rapid measurement of B-type natriuretic peptide in the emergency diagnosis of heart failure. N Engl J Med 2002;347:161–7.
8. Januzzi JL, van Kimmenade R, Lainchbury J, et al. NT-proBNP testing for diagnosis and short-term prognosis in acute destabilized heart failure: an international pooled analysis of 1256 patients the International Collaborative of NT-proBNP Study. Eur Heart J 2006;27:330–7.
9. Masson S, Latini R, Anand IS, et al. Direct comparison of B-type natriuretic peptide (BNP) and amino-terminal proBNP in a large population of patients with chronic and symptomatic heart failure: the valsartan heart failure (Val-HeFT) data. Clin Chem 2006;52:1528–38.
10. Komajda M, Carson PE, Hetzel S, et al. Factors associated with outcome in heart failure with preserved ejection fraction findings from the irbesartan in heart failure with preserved ejection fraction study (I- PRESERVE). Circ Heart Fail 2011;4:27–35.
11. Anand IS, Rector TS, Cleland JG, et al. Prognostic value of baseline plasma amino-terminal pro-brain natriuretic peptide and its interactions with irbesartan treatment effects in patients with heart failure and preserved ejection fraction: findings from the I-PRESERVE trial. Circ Heart Fail 2011;4:569–77.
12. Lainchbury JG, Troughton RW, Strangman KM, et al. N-terminal Pro-B-type natriuretic peptide-guided treatment for chronic heart failure results from the BATTLESCARRED (NT-proBNP–assisted treatment to lessen serial cardiac readmissions and death) trial. J Am Coll Cardiol 2010;55:53–60.
13. Pfisterer M, Buser P, Rickli H, et al. (TIME-CHF) randomized trial elderly patients with congestive heart failure the trial of intensified vs standard medical therapy in BNP-guided vs symptom-guided heart failure therapy. JAMA 2009;301:383–92.
14. Savarese G, Trimarco B, Dellegrottaglie S, et al. Natriuretic peptide-guided therapy in chronic heart failure: a meta-analysis of 2,686 patients in 12 randomized trials. PLoS One 2013;8:58287. http://dx.doi.org/10.1371/journal.pone.0058287.
15. Troughton RW, Frampton CM, Brunner-La Rocca HP, et al. Effect of B-type natriuretic peptide-guided treatment of chronic heart failure on total mortality and hospitalization: an individual patient meta-analysis. Eur Heart J 2014. http://dx.doi.org/10.1093/eurheartj/ehu090.
16. O'Meara E, de Denus S, Rouleau J-L, et al. Circulating biomarkers in patients with heart failure and preserved ejection fraction. Curr Heart Fail Rep 2013;10:350–8.
17. Cheng JM, Akkerhuis KM, Battes LC, et al. Biomarkers of heart failure with normal ejection

fraction: a systematic review. Eur J Heart Fail 2013; 15:1350–62.

18. Maisel AS, McCord J, Nowak RM, et al. Bedside B-type natriuretic peptide in the emergency diagnosis of heart failure with reduced or preserved ejection fraction results from the breathing not properly multinational study. J Am Coll Cardiol 2003;41:2010–7.

19. Januzzi JL, Camargo CA, Anwaruddin S, et al. The N-terminal Pro-BNP Investigation of Dyspnea in the Emergency Department (PRIDE) study. Am J Cardiol 2005;95:948–54.

20. O'Donoghue M, Chen A, Baggish AI, et al. The effects of ejection fraction on N-terminal ProBNP and BNP levels in patients with acute CHF: analysis from the ProBNP Investigation of Dyspnea in the Emergency Department (PRIDE) study. J Card Fail 2005;11(Suppl 5):S9–14.

21. Troughton RW, Prior DL, Pereira JJ, et al. Plasma BNP levels in systolic heart failure: the importance of left ventricular diastolic and right ventricular function. J Am Coll Cardiol 2004;43:416–22.

22. Troughton RW, Richards AM. B-type natriuretic peptides and echocardiographic measures of cardiac structure and function. JACC Cardiovasc Imaging 2009;2:216–25.

23. Jaubert MP, Armero S, Bonello L, et al. Predictors of B-type natriuretic peptide and left atrial volume index in patients with preserved left ventricular systolic function: an echocardiographic-catheterization study. Arch Cardiovasc Dis 2010;103:3–9.

24. Iwanaga Y, Nishi I, Furuichi S, et al. B-type natriuretic peptide strongly reflects diastolic wall stress in patients with chronic heart failure comparison between systolic and diastolic heart failure. J Am Coll Cardiol 2006;47:742–8.

25. Kraigher-Krainer E, Shah AM, Gupta DK, et al. Impaired systolic function by strain imaging in heart failure with preserved ejection fraction. J Am Coll Cardiol 2014;63:447–56.

26. Richards AM, Di Somma S, Mueller C, et al. Atrial fibrillation impairs the diagnostic performance of cardiac natriuretic peptides in dyspneic patients: results from the biomarkers in acute heart failure (BACH) study. JACC Heart Fail 2013;1:192–9.

27. Linssen GC, Rienstra M, Jaarsma T, et al. Clinical and prognostic effects of atrial fibrillation in heart failure patients with reduced and preserved left ventricular ejection fraction. Eur heart J 2011;13:1111–20.

28. McKelvie RS, Komajda M, Mc Murray J, et al. Baseline plasma NT-proBNP and clinical characteristics: results from the irbesartan in heart failure with preserved ejection fraction trial. J Card Fail 2010;16:128–34.

29. Anjan VY, Loftus TM, Burke MA, et al. Prevalence, clinical phenotype, and outcomes associated with normal B-type natriuretic peptide levels in heart failure with preserved ejection fraction. Am J Cardiol 2012;110:870–6.

30. Hildebrandt P, Collinson PO, Doughty RN, et al. Age-dependent values of N-terminal pro-B-type natriuretic peptide are superior to a single cutpoint for ruling out suspected systolic dysfunction in primary care. Eur Heart J 2010;31:1881–9.

31. Costello-Boerrigter LC, Boerrigter G, Redfield RM, et al. Amino-terminal Pro-B-type natriuretic peptide and B-type natriuretic peptide in the general community. Determinants and detection of left ventricular dysfunction. J Am Coll Cardiol 2006; 47:345–53.

32. Mason JM, Hancock HC, Close H, et al. Utility of biomarkers in the differential diagnosis of heart failure in older people: findings from the heart failure in care homes (HFinCH) diagnostic accuracy study. PLoS One 2013;8:e53560.

33. Paulus WJ, Tschöpe C, Sanderson JE, et al. How to diagnose diastolic heart failure: a consensus statement on the diagnosis of heart failure with normal left ventricular ejection fraction by the Heart Failure and Echocardiography Associations of the European Society of Cardiology. Eur Heart J 2007;28: 2539–50.

34. Sudoh T, Kangawa K, Minamino N, et al. A new natriuretic peptide in porcine brain. Nature 1988; 332:78–81.

35. Hunt PJ, Yandle TG, Nicholls MG, et al. The amino-terminal portion of pro-brain natriuretic peptide (Pro-BNP) circulates in human plasma. Biochem Biophys Res Commun 1995;214:1175–83.

36. Wang TJ, Larsen MG, Levy D, et al. Plasma natriuretic peptide levels and the risk of cardiovascular events and death. N Engl J Med 2004;350:655–63.

37. McDonagh TA, Cunningham AD, Morrison CE, et al. Left ventricular dysfunction, natriuretic peptides, and mortality in an urban population. Heart 2001; 86:21–6.

38. Baptista R, Jorge E, Sousa E, et al. B type natriuretic peptide predicts long-term prognosis in a cohort of critically ill patients. Heart Int 2011;6:e18. http://dx.doi.org/10.4081/hi. 2011.e18.

39. Kucher N, Printzen G, Goldhaber SZ. Prognostic role of brain natriuretic peptide in acute pulmonary embolism. Circulation 2003;107:2545–7.

40. Hsich EM, Grau-Sepulveda MV, Hernandez AF, et al. Relationship between sex, ejection fraction, and B-type natriuretic peptide levels in patients hospitalized with heart failure and associations with in-hospital outcomes: findings from the Get with the Guideline—Heart Failure registry. Am Heart J 2013; 166:1063–71.

41. Fonarow GC, Peacock WF, Phillips CO, et al. Admission B-type natriuretic peptide levels and in-hospital mortality in acute decompensated heart failure. J Am Coll Cardiol 2007;49:1943–50.

42. van Veldhuisen DJ, Linssen GC, Jaarsma T, et al. B-type natriuretic peptide and prognosis in heart failure patients with preserved and reduced ejection fraction. J Am Coll Cardiol 2013;61:1498–506.

43. Latini R, Masson S, Anand I, et al. The comparative prognostic value of plasma neurohormones at baseline in patients with heart failure enrolled in Val-HeFT. Eur Heart J 2004;25:292–9.

44. Maeder MT, Rickenbacher P, Rickli H, et al. N-terminal pro brain natriuretic peptide-guided management in patients with heart failure and preserved ejection fraction: findings from the trial of intensified versus standard medical therapy in elderly patients with congestive heart failure (TIME-CHF). Eur J Heart Fail 2013;15:1148–56.

45. Maisel A, Barnard D, Jaski B, et al. Primary results of the HABIT trial (heart failure assessment with BNP in the home). J Am Coll Cardiol 2013;61:1726–35.

46. Edelmann F, Wachter R, Schmidt AG, et al. Effect of spironolactone on diastolic function and exercise capacity in patients with heart failure with preserved ejection fraction. The Aldo-DHF randomized controlled trial. JAMA 2013;309:781–91.

47. Solomon SD, Zile M, Pieske B, et al. The angiotensin receptor neprilysin inhibitor LCZ696 in heart failure with preserved ejection fraction: a phase 2 double-blind randomised controlled trial. Lancet 2012;380:1387–95.

48. Desai AS, Lewis EF, Li R, et al. Rationale and design of the treatment of preserved cardiac function heart failure with an aldosterone antagonist trial: a randomized, controlled study of spironolactone in patients with symptomatic heart failure and preserved ejection fraction. Am Heart J 2011;162:966–72.

Novel Biomarkers in Heart Failure with Preserved Ejection Fraction

Kevin S. Shah, MD[a], Alan S. Maisel, MD[b],*

KEYWORDS

- Heart failure • Biomarkers • Preserved ejection fraction • Diagnosis • Prognosis

KEY POINTS

- Heart failure with preserved ejection fraction (HFPEF) is a common subtype of congestive heart failure for which therapies to improve morbidity and mortality have been limited thus far.
- Numerous biomarkers have emerged over the past decade demonstrating prognostic significance in HFPEF, including natriuretic peptides, galectin-3, soluble ST2, and high-sensitivity troponins.
- These markers reflect the multiple mechanisms implicated in the pathogenesis of HFPEF, and future research will likely use these markers to not only help determine heart failure phenotypes but also target specific therapies.

BACKGROUND

Heart failure (HF) is a global epidemic, defined as an abnormality of cardiac function leading to the inability to deliver oxygen at a rate adequate to meet the requirements of tissues.[1] It is truly a clinical syndrome of symptoms and signs resulting from this cardiac abnormality. Over the past decade, further characterization into 2 entities has occurred: HF with preserved ejection fraction (HFPEF) and HF with reduced ejection fraction (HFREF). HFPEF, previously termed diastolic HF, encompasses the syndrome of HF with a preserved ejection fraction. Cutoffs for this ejection fraction typically are from 45% to 50%. The prevalence of HF is upward of 1% to 2% of the adult population, with an increased prevalence found in elderly and female patients.[2] Multiple studies have shown that the prevalence of HFPEF is actually comparable with the number of patients with HFREF.[3,4] As expected, most deaths from HFPEF are cardiovascular, comprising 51% to 70% of mortality. Typical causes of death include sudden

death and HF death.[5] However, there tend to be some epidemiologic differences between patients with HFPEF and HFREF. Patients diagnosed with HFPEF tend to be older, female, and obese.[6,7] In patients with HFPEF, comorbidities including hypertension, diabetes mellitus, arrhythmias, and renal dysfunction are common.[8–13] Theories remain as to whether HFPEF is primarily a manifestation of impaired ventricular relaxation, or a combination of uncontrolled comorbidities that predisposes to the signs and symptoms of HF.

PATHOPHYSIOLOGY

The pathophysiology of HFPEF is controversial and remains poorly understood. Originally, HFPEF was thought to be a primary manifestation of diastolic dysfunction of the left ventricle. However, patients with HFREF are known to also commonly have impaired ventricular relaxation.[14,15] As already mentioned, the primary mechanism of left ventricular (LV) dysfunction is based on structural remodeling and endothelial dysfunction,

a Department of Internal Medicine, University of California, San Diego, 402 Dickinson Street, Suite 380, San Diego, CA 92103-8425, USA; b Cardiology Section (9111-A), VA San Diego Healthcare System, 3350 La Jolla Village Drive, San Diego, CA 92161, USA
* Corresponding author.
E-mail address: amaisel@ucsd.edu

Heart Failure Clin 10 (2014) 471–479
http://dx.doi.org/10.1016/j.hfc.2014.04.005
1551-7136/14/$ – see front matter Published by Elsevier Inc.

heartfailure.theclinics.com

lending itself to LV stiffness, and increased left atrial pressure. This pressure change is what drives pulmonary venous congestion and subsequent symptomatology.[16–20] The ventricular stiffness commonly seen in HFPEF is attributed to multiple mechanisms, including fibrosis, excessive collagen deposition, cardiomyocyte stiffness, and slow LV relaxation.[21–23] Aside from LV dysfunction, HFPEF has been described as a clinical syndrome in which multiple comorbidities likely play role in the clinical manifestations.[24–26] Multiple other mechanisms, including inflammation driven by comorbidities and fibrosis, have also been thought to be linked to the creation of LV dysfunction seen in HFPEF.[27–29] Clinicians' incomplete understanding of all of the pathophysiologic mechanisms driving HFPEF is a primary reason why the role of biomarkers will likely be 2-fold: to assist in understanding the pathophysiology, and to help target therapies to improve morbidity and mortality.

THERAPY

Results from the few randomized controlled trials attempting to find effective therapeutic agents for patients with HFPEF have been limited and mostly discouraging. What has been established as effective includes primarily managing decompensated HFPEF with diuretics to improve fluid status and symptom control. With respect to angiotensin-converting enzyme inhibitors, the PEP-CHF trial demonstrated no significant mortality or rehospitalization benefit with perindopril.[30] The CHARM-Preserved trial showed no mortality benefit with the angiotensin-receptor blocker (ARB) candesartan, but fewer rehospitalizations were attained.[31] The I-PRESERVE trial showed no mortality or rehospitalization benefit with the ARB irbesartan.[32] β-Blockers are recommended in HF guidelines, primarily with the role of controlling tachyarrhythmias. β-Blockers have shown improvement in diastolic dysfunction, and mixed results in terms of mortality and readmission.[33]

Statin therapy has shown some clinical benefit in HFPEF, but only from observational data thus far.[34] As mentioned earlier, therapeutic agents have shown mixed results in HFPEF, with no medication demonstrating an unambiguous mortality benefit. This finding is in sharp contrast with the positive trial results published in patients with systolic dysfunction, or HF with reduced ejection fraction (HFREF). The primary role of biomarkers in trials will serve to create stratified therapies, and biomarkers may ultimately play a role as surrogate end points, reflecting improvement of the disease state.

BIOMARKERS
Natriuretic Peptides

The natriuretic peptides (NPs) are the cornerstone biomarker in congestive HF (CHF). Many of the details of the role of NPs are covered in an article by Florea and Anand.[35] The Breathing Not Properly trial originally helped establish the role of B-type natriuretic peptide (BNP) in the diagnosis of CHF.[36] BNP and the N-terminal prohormone BNP (NT-proBNP) have been shown in numerous trials to be an excellent tool for ruling out CHF as a cause of acute dyspnea. Aside from a strong negative predictive value, NPs correlate with HF severity, prognostication, outpatient CHF management, and screening.[37] When attempting to use NPs specifically to distinguish between HFPEF and HFREF, results have shown that NPs do not have a particular cutoff, but are typically elevated in HFPEF in comparison with patients without HF. These levels of NPs in HFPEF are typically lower than levels in patients with HFREF.[38–40] In a cohort of 615 subjects with CHF, median BNP values stratified by ejection fraction are shown in **Table 1**.[41] These results demonstrate lower baseline BNP levels in patients with HFPEF, regardless of which cutoff is used for preserved ejection fraction. This same study demonstrated that although BNP levels are lower in HFPEF than in HFREF, for a given BNP level the prognosis in HFPEF is as

---

Table 1
BNP values across CHF patients stratified by ejection fraction

	All Patients (n = 615)	LVEF ≤20% (n = 132)	LVEF 21%–30% (n = 199)	LVEF 31%–40% (n = 129)	LVEF 41%–50% (n = 81)	LVEF >50% (n = 74)	P value
BNP (pg/mL)	463 (212–918)	534 (275–1130)	502 (243–1120)	447 (215–798)	424 (179–828)	256 (112–598)	<.001

Abbreviations: BNP, B-type natriuretic peptide; CHF, congestive heart failure; LVEF, left ventricular ejection fraction.
From van Veldhuisen D, Linssen GC, Jaarsma T, et al. B-type natriuretic peptide and prognosis in heart failure patients with preserved and reduced ejection fraction. J Am Coll Cardiol 2013;61(14):1501; with permission.

poor as for HFREF (**Fig. 1**). This finding is unique in that it demonstrates that NP is a powerful indicator of HF severity, regardless of ejection fraction. At present there is no precise cutoff level for the diagnosis of HFPEF. The role of NPs in the future will likely be multifactorial, including titration of medication, outpatient monitoring, and prognostication to identify patients with HFPEF at highest risk.

High-Sensitivity Troponin

The role of troponin and, specifically, high-sensitivity troponin T (hsTnT) in CHF is a vibrant area of research. As the sensitivity of assays for troponin has improved, this biomarker is growing past a marker solely for use in the acute coronary syndrome. Patients with decompensated HF and elevated troponin are known to have higher in-hospital mortality, independently of other predictive variables.[42] Troponin release found in

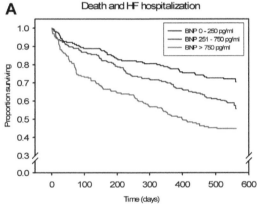

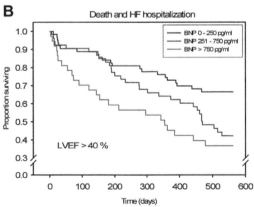

Fig. 1. Subjects with HFPEF have increased long-term mortality when stratified by BNP. Panel *(A)* represents all patients with HF and panel *(B)* represents those with preserved EF. (*From* van Veldhuisen D, Linssen GC, Jaarsma T, et al. B-type natriuretic peptide and prognosis in heart failure patients with preserved and reduced ejection fraction. J Am Coll Cardiol 2013; 61(14):1502; with permission.)

decompensated HF is thought to have multiple mechanisms, including subendocardial ischemia, a manifestation of inflammation, oxidative stress, and the renin-angiotensin-aldosterone system. Detection of troponin in patients with HF may identify patients thought to be at higher risk for mortality and rehospitalization. hsTnT has been shown to be elevated in patients with HF, regardless of the presence of coronary artery disease and independent of ejection fraction.[43–46] Specifically, studies have demonstrated that hsTnT levels are significantly higher in HFREF than HFPEF.[47] These findings help to distinguish and elucidate the pathophysiology of HFPEF. Some investigators believe that HFREF may primarily represent a myocardial-specific disorder, whereas HFPEF may represent a systemic or metabolic condition.[47] More specifically, HFPEF is likely a manifestation of a systemic inflammatory state, causing oxidative stress and eventual stiffness/hypertrophy.[29] The future of hsTnT in HFPEF and HF will likely be a combination of recognition of baseline levels in patients presenting with acute coronary syndrome (ACS) and also utilizing levels to help risk-stratify and prognosticate patients with chronic HF.

Galectin-3

Galectins are a family of proteins, soluble β-galactoside-binding lectins, which have multiple roles in the human body.[48] Galectins bind to cell-surface glycans and catalyze a variety of cellular processes, including fibrosis and inflammation.[49] Animal models have demonstrated that myocardial galectin-3 is upregulated in hearts that eventually develop HF.[50] Levels of galectin-3 correlate well with markers of cardiac extracellular matrix turnover in patients with known diagnoses of HF.[51] Many of the mechanisms thought to be partially at play in the development of HFPEF, including inflammation, fibrogenesis, and fibroblast proliferation, have been linked to elevated galectin-3 levels.[52,53] In patients presenting with acute dyspnea in the emergency department, patients ultimately diagnosed with HF have elevated levels of galectin-3.[54] Similarly, in patients presenting with ACS, those with elevated galectin-3 levels are at higher risk for developing subsequent HF.[55] Thus, galectin-3 is thought to be a marker indicating which patients are at high risk for developing HF, given its role in the mechanisms behind HF. In patients with chronic HF, galectin-3 levels are a significant predictor of mortality, even after adjustment for typical covariates including age, sex, severity of HF, and renal dysfunction.[56] Changes in levels (baseline and 4 months) of galectin-3 also have been shown to predict mortality, morbid events, and HF hospitalizations.[56] Large cohort retrospective analyses have confirmed the value of changes in galectin-3 levels.[57] Galectin-3 levels are also shown to be inversely related to renal function in patients with and without HF.[58] Clinicians' ability to use galectin-3 specifically in HFPEF relies on understanding the pathophysiology of myocardial stiffness and impaired relaxation. Specifically, the greatest potential for galectin-3 in HFPEF may lie in the powerful connection between aldosterone and HFPEF.[59] Myocardial fibrosis can be induced by chronic aldosterone administration in animal models.[60] These models have demonstrated that elevated levels of aldosterone will exacerbate cardiac fibrosis through activation of inflammation along with fibrosis. Thus, inhibition of these processes via eplerenone (a mineralocorticoid receptor antagonist) may improve outcomes in HFPEF, and galectin-3 could potentially serve as a surrogate biomarker for fibrosis in this scenario. Future trials incorporating galectin-3 as a surrogate end point in HFPEF are currently in development. Findings from the Coordinating study evaluating Outcomes of Advising and Counseling in Heart failure (COACH) trial demonstrated that in patients hospitalized for decompensated HF, galectin-3 values were similar in patients with HFPEF and HFREF; however, interestingly, an identical increase in galectin-3 levels represented a stronger risk for all-cause mortality and HF hospitalization in those with HFPEF.[56] Galectin-3 is a biomarker with high potential for early detection, HF phenotyping, and therapeutic targeting of HFPEF.[60–62]

Soluble ST2

Soluble ST2 is a form of the interleukin-1 receptor member, ST2. With respect to the ST2 receptor, the binding ligand itself is interleukin (IL)-33. When IL-33 is bound to ST2, the physiologic response is cardioprotective. Measurement of the biomarker soluble ST2 has been demonstrated to be a reflection of cardiac fibrosis and pathophysiologic remodeling.[63,64] In one retrospective analysis of patients with severe HF of nonischemic etiology (with reduced ejection fraction), changes in levels of ST2 were proved to be a predictor of mortality.[65] In addition, in patients with LV dysfunction after acute myocardial infarction, ST2 predicted LV functional recovery.[66] In undifferentiated patients with dyspnea, ST2 levels predicted 1-year mortality in those ultimately diagnosed with HF and those who were not.[67,68] Recently, ST2 was shown to outperform galectin-3 in 5-year mortality prediction in a cohort with chronic HFREF.[69]

Levels of the marker are also shown to correlate with HF severity, LV ejection fraction (LVEF), and additional abnormalities seen on echocardiography.[70] Of importance, ST2 concentrations have been shown to be lower in HFPEF than HFREF, but still remain an independent predictor of mortality, regardless of the LVEF.[71] Recently, on analysis of 447 subjects with acutely decompensated heart failure, levels of ST2 had moderate positive correlations with troponin, C-reactive protein, and NT-proBNP; however, the levels of ST2 were not significantly different in HFPEF versus HFREF.[47] ST2's ability to distinguish between HFPEF and HFREF demonstrated a modest area under the curve by receiver-operating characteristic analysis of 0.662. **Fig. 2** shows survival curves for 1-year

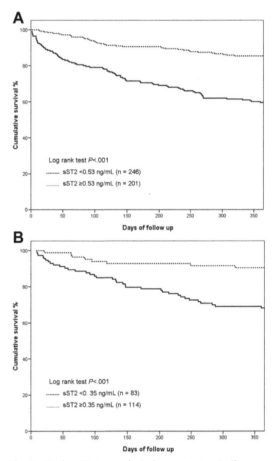

Fig. 2. Kaplan-Meier analysis demonstrates similar separation of survival rate based on ST2 levels in patients with HF (A) and specifically HFPEF (B), through 1-year follow-up. (*From* Manzano-Fernández S, Mueller T, Pascual-Figal D, et al. Usefulness of soluble concentrations of interleukin family member ST2 as predictor of mortality in patients with acutely decompensated heart failure relative to left ventricular ejection fraction. Am J Cardiol 2011;107(2):263; with permission.)

mortality according to ST2 in 3 panels: all patients, preserved, and reduced ejection fraction.

The role of ST2 in the pathogenesis of HF is multifactorial, given its relationship to myocardial strain as a possible mediator of myocardial hypertrophy and fibrosis.[72,73] Given the marker's prognostic significance regardless of ejection fraction, this may reflect the activity of cardiac remodeling, regardless of LVEF. It has been established that remodeling is a pivotal mechanism behind the pathophysiology of HFPEF.[74,75] The future role of ST2 in HFPEF will also likely be to prognosticate patients with HFPEF and eventually seek out therapies that specifically work toward driving down levels of the biomarker in an attempt to improve long-term outcomes.

Renal Biomarkers

Although the role of novel renal biomarkers has not been fully explored specifically in HFPEF, they likely have an impactful role in the assessment and management of acute kidney injury (AKI) and the cardiorenal syndrome. Two biomarkers are briefly discussed here: neutrophil gelatinase-associated lipocalin (NGAL) and cystatin C. NGAL is a 25-kDa protein in the lipocalin family of proteins with a role in inflammation and immune modulation.[76–78] Of importance to the clinician, levels of NGAL in serum and urine increase in the setting of renal failure and may provide a complementary role to traditional serum creatinine.[79–81] Cystatin C is a 13.3-kDa member of the cystatin family of protease inhibitors, which is free filtered and not reabsorbed at the glomeruli. Studies have demonstrated its comparability with creatinine in assessing glomerular filtration rate (GFR)[82] and its dynamic increase before AKI.[83] Both cystatin C and NGAL may have a role in assessment of the cardiorenal syndrome, as their early increase before a decrease in GFR may help in acute HF management decisions, including decisions regarding diuretics and potentially nephrotoxic medications that have cardioprotective effects.

FUTURE DIRECTIONS

The future of biomarkers and their utility in HF is very promising, starting with the potential for using biomarkers as end points in trials. Biomarkers serve as surrogates for various pathophysiologic mechanisms, and there are potential benefits in using them as trial end points.[84] Advantages include the ability to obtain quick and early data, as well as possibly better understand the nature of the disease.[76] However, the counterargument against using biomarkers as trial end points includes whether treatment effects on a biomarker reliably predict effects on a clinically meaningful end point. **Table 2** lists a summary of contemporary and novel

Table 2
Novel biomarkers in congestive heart failure and potential roles in management

Biomarker	Pathophysiology	Potential Role in HFPEF
Copeptin	Stress marker and fluid homeostasis as a precursor to antidiuretic hormone	Prognostic marker in chronic heart failure and role as a target for therapies with vasopressin antagonism
Endothelin-1	Produced by the endothelium in response to vascular stress and inflammation, leading to vasoconstriction and cardiac remodeling	Predictor of mortality; unclear role in management
Galectin-3	Fibrosis and inflammation	Predictor of mortality; possible role as a target for aldosterone antagonism
GDF-15 (growth differentiation factor)	Myocyte stretch marker	Predictor of mortality in HFPEF; unclear role in management
Hs-cTn (high-sensitivity cardiac troponin)	Cardiac muscle contraction proteins released after necrosis	Predictor of mortality; possible utility in serial monitoring in outpatient setting
MR-proADM (mid-regional proadrenomedullin)	Vasodilation in response to stress	Predictor of mortality; unclear role in management
ST2	Increased in response to fibrosis and inflammation	Predictor of mortality; possible role as a target for β-blocker therapy

Abbreviation: HFPEF, heart failure with preserved ejection fraction.

biomarkers in CHF, some of which are not specifically detailed in this overview. The other potential for novel biomarkers will be to help possibly identify HFPEF phenotypes that may or may not respond to certain therapies. Patients with elevated levels of certain biomarkers may be prone to having an improved response to certain pharmacologic therapies. In this respect, the aim of biomarker utilization would be not only to further comprehend pathophysiology but also to identify which patients would benefit most from specific therapy.

REFERENCES

1. McMurray JJ, Adamopoulos S, Anker SD, et al. ESC guidelines for the diagnosis and treatment of acute and chronic heart failure 2012: the task force for the diagnosis and treatment of acute and chronic heart failure 2012 of the European Society of Cardiology. Developed in collaboration with the Heart Failure Association (HFA) of the ESC. Eur J Heart Fail 2012;14:803–69.

2. Mosterd A, Hoes AW. Clinical epidemiology of heart failure. Heart 2007;93:1137–46.

3. Vasan RS, Benjamin EJ, Levy D. Prevalence, clinical features and prognosis of diastolic heart failure: an epidemiologic perspective. J Am Coll Cardiol 1995;26:1565–74.

4. Owan TE, Redfield MM. Epidemiology of diastolic heart failure. Prog Cardiovasc Dis 2005;47:320–32.

5. Chan MM, Lam CS. How do patients with heart failure with preserved ejection fraction die? Eur J Heart Fail 2013;15(6):604–13.

6. Heart Failure Society of America, Lindenfeld J, Albert NM, et al. HFSA 2010 comprehensive heart failure practice guideline. J Card Fail 2010;16(6): e1–194.

7. Hunt SA, Abraham WT, Chin MH, et al. 2009 Focused update incorporated into the ACC/AHA 2005 guidelines for the diagnosis and management of heart failure in adults: a report of the American College of Cardiology Foundation/American Heart Association task force on practice guidelines: developed in collaboration with the International Society for Heart and Lung Transplantation. Circulation 2009;119:e391–479.

8. Lee DS, Gona P, Vasan RS, et al. Relation of disease pathogenesis and risk factors to heart failure with preserved or reduced ejection fraction: insights from the Framingham Heart Study of the National Heart, Lung, and blood Institute. Circulation 2009;119:3070–7.

9. Bursi F, Weston SA, Redfield MM, et al. Systolic and diastolic heart failure in the community. JAMA 2006;296:2209–16.

10. Bhatia RS, Tu JV, Lee DS, et al. Outcome of heart failure with preserved ejection fraction in a population-based study. N Engl J Med 2006;355: 260–9.

11. Fonarow GC, Stough WG, Abraham WT, et al. Characteristics, treatments, and outcomes of patients with preserved systolic function hospitalized for heart failure: a report from the OPTIMIZE-HF Registry. J Am Coll Cardiol 2007;50:768–77.

12. Yancy CW, Lopatin M, Stevenson LW, et al. Clinical presentation, management, and in-hospital outcomes of patients admitted with acute decompensated heart failure with preserved systolic function: a report from the Acute Decompensated Heart Failure National Registry (ADHERE) Database. J Am Coll Cardiol 2006; 47:76–84.

13. Lenzen MJ, Scholte op Reimer WJ, Boersma E, et al. Differences between patients with a preserved and a depressed left ventricular function: a report from the EuroHeart Failure Survey. Eur Heart J 2004;25:1214–20.

14. Sanderson JE. Heart failure with a normal ejection fraction. Heart 2007;93:155–8.

15. McMurray J, Pfeffer MA. New therapeutic options in congestive heart failure: part II. Circulation 2002;105:2223–8.

16. Paulus WJ, Tschope C, Sanderson JE, et al. How to diagnose diastolic heart failure: a consensus statement on the diagnosis of heart failure with normal left ventricular ejection fraction by the Heart Failure and Echocardiography Associations of the European Society of Cardiology. Eur Heart J 2007;28: 2539–50.

17. Tschoepe C, Westermann D. Heart failure with normal ejection fraction. Pathophysiology, diagnosis, and treatment. Herz 2009;34:89–96.

18. Lam CS, Lyass A, Kraigher-Krainer E, et al. Cardiac structure and ventricular-vascular function in persons with heart failure and preserved ejection fraction from Olmsted County, Minnesota. Circulation 2007;115:1982–90.

19. Zile RM, Baicu CF, Gaasch WH. Diastolic heart failure—abnormalities in active relaxation and passive stiffness of the left ventricle. N Engl J Med 2004; 350:1953–9.

20. Borlaug BA, Paulus WJ. Heart failure with preserved ejection fraction: pathophysiology, diagnosis, and treatment. Eur Heart J 2011;32:670–9.

21. Weber KT, Brilla CG, Janicki JS. Myocardial fibrosis: functional significance and regulatory factors. Cardiovasc Res 1993;27:341–8.

22. van Heerebeek L, Borbely A, Niessen HW, et al. Myocardial structure and function differ in systolic and diastolic heart failure. Circulation 2006;113: 1966–73.

23. Sohn DW, Kim HK, Park JS, et al. Hemodynamic effects of tachycardia in patients with relaxation abnormality: abnormal stroke volume response as

an overlooked mechanism of dyspnea associated with tachycardia in diastolic heart failure. J Am Soc Echocardiogr 2007;20:171–6.

24. Ather S, Chan W, Bozkurt B, et al. Impact of noncardiac comorbidities on morbidity and mortality in a predominantly male population with heart failure and preserved versus reduced ejection fraction. J Am Coll Cardiol 2012;59: 998–1005.

25. Maurer MS, Hummel SL. Heart failure with a preserved ejection fraction: what is in a name? J Am Coll Cardiol 2011;58:275–7.

26. Mohammed SF, Borlaug BA, Roger VL, et al. Comorbidity and ventricular and vascular structure and function in heart failure with preserved ejection fraction: a community based study. Circ Heart Fail 2012;5:710–9.

27. van Heerebeek L, Franssen CP, Hamdani N, et al. Molecular and cellular basis for diastolic dysfunction. Curr Heart Fail Rep 2008;4:13–21.

28. Borbely A, van Heerebeek L, Paulus WJ. Transcriptional and posttranslational modifications of titin: implications for diastole. Circ Res 2009;104:12–4.

29. Paulus WJ, Tschöpe C. A novel paradigm for heart failure with preserved ejection fraction: comorbidities drive myocardial dysfunction and remodeling through coronary microvascular endothelial inflammation. J Am Coll Cardiol 2013;62(4):263–71.

30. Cleland JG, Tendera M, Adamus J, et al. The perindopril in elderly people with chronic heart failure (PEP-CHF) study. Eur Heart J 2006;27:2338–45.

31. Yusuf S, Pfeffer MA, Swedberg K, et al. Effects of candesartan in patients with chronic heart failure and preserved left-ventricular ejection fraction: the CHARM-Preserved Trial. Lancet 2003;362: 777–81.

32. Massie BM, Carson PE, McMurray JJ, et al. Irbesartan in patients with heart failure and preserved ejection fraction. N Engl J Med 2008;359:2456–67.

33. Flather MD, Shibata MC, Coats AJ, et al. Randomized trial to determine the effect of nebivolol on mortality and cardiovascular hospital admission in elderly patients with heart failure (SENIORS). Eur Heart J 2005;26:215–25.

34. Fukuta H, Sane DC, Brucks S, et al. Statin therapy may be associated with lower mortality in patients with diastolic heart failure. Circulation 2005;112: 357–63.

35. Florea VG, Anand IS. Biomarkers. Heart Fail Clin 2012;8(2):207–24.

36. Maisel AS, Krishnaswamy P, Nowak RM, et al, Breathing Not Properly Multinational Study Investigators. Rapid measurement of B-type natriuretic peptide in the emergency diagnosis of heart failure. N Engl J Med 2002;347(3):161–7.

37. Maisel AS, Daniels LB. Breathing not properly 10 years later: what we have learned and what we still need to learn. J Am Coll Cardiol 2012; 60(4):277–82.

38. Daniels LB, Maisel AS. Natriuretic peptides. J Am Coll Cardiol 2007;50:2357–68.

39. Januzzi JL Jr, Rehman SU, Mohammed AA, et al. Use of amino-terminal pro-B-type natriuretic peptide to guide outpatient therapy of patients with chronic left ventricular dysfunction. J Am Coll Cardiol 2011;58:1881–9.

40. Parekh N, Maisel AS. Utility of B-natriuretic peptide in the evaluation of left ventricular diastolic function and diastolic heart failure. Curr Opin Cardiol 2009; 24:155–60.

41. van Veldhuisen DJ, Linssen GC, Jaarsma T, et al. B-type natriuretic peptide and prognosis in heart failure patients with preserved and reduced ejection fraction. J Am Coll Cardiol 2013;61(14): 1498–506.

42. Peacock WF 4th, De Marco T, Fonarow GC, et al, ADHERE Investigators. Cardiac troponin and outcome in acute heart failure. N Engl J Med 2008;358(20):2117–26.

43. Kociol RD, Pang PS, Gheorghiade M, et al. Troponin elevation in heart failure prevalence, mechanisms, and clinical implications. J Am Coll Cardiol 2010;56:1071–8.

44. Latini R, Masson S, Anand IS, et al. Prognostic value of very low plasma concentrations of troponin T in patients with stable chronic heart failure. Circulation 2007;116:1242–9.

45. Sato Y, Yamada T, Taniguchi R, et al. Persistently increased serum concentrations of cardiac troponin T in patients with idiopathic dilated cardiomyopathy are predictive of adverse outcomes. Circulation 2001;103:369–74.

46. Dinh W, Nickl W, Futh R, et al. High sensitive troponin T and heart fatty acid binding protein: novel biomarker in heart failure with normal ejection fraction? A cross-sectional study. BMC Cardiovasc Disord 2011;11:41.

47. Santhanakrishnan R, Chong JP, Ng TP, et al. Growth differentiation factor 15, ST2, high-sensitivity troponin T, and N-terminal pro brain natriuretic peptide in heart failure with preserved vs. reduced ejection fraction. Eur J Heart Fail 2012;14(12):1338–47.

48. Dumic J, Dabelic S, Flögel M. Galectin-3: an open-ended story. Biochim Biophys Acta 2006;1760: 616–35.

49. Yang RY, Rabinovich GA, Liu FT. Galectins: Structure, function and therapeutic potential. Expert Rev Mol Med 2008;13:e17–39.

50. Sharma UC, Pokharel S, van Brakel TJ, et al. Galectin-3 marks activated macrophages in failure-prone hypertrophied hearts and contributes to cardiac dysfunction. Circulation 2004; 110:3121–8.

51. Lin YH, Lin LY, Wu YW, et al. The relationship between serum galectin-3 and serum markers of cardiac extracellular matrix turnover in heart failure patients. Clin Chim Acta 2009;409:96–9.

52. Calvier L, Miana M, Reboul P, et al. Galectin-3 mediates aldosterone-induced vascular fibrosis. Arterioscler Thromb Vasc Biol 2013;33:67.

53. Yu L, Ruifrok WP, Meissner M, et al. Genetic and pharmacological inhibition of galectin-3 prevents cardiac remodeling by interfering with myocardial fibrogenesis. Circ Heart Fail 2013;6:107–17.

54. van Kimmenade RR, Januzzi JL Jr, Ellinor PT, et al. Utility of amino-terminal pro-brain natriuretic peptide, galectin-3, and apelin for the evaluation of patients with acute heart failure. J Am Coll Cardiol 2006;48:1217–24.

55. Lok DJ, Van Der Meer P, de la Porte PW, et al. Prognostic value of galectin-3, a novel marker of fibrosis, in patients with chronic heart failure: data from the DEAL-HF study. Clin Res Cardiol 2010;99:323–8.

56. Anand IS, Rector TS, Kuskowski M, et al. Baseline and serial measurements of galectin-3 in patients with heart failure: relationship to prognosis and effect of treatment with valsartan in the Val-HeFT. Eur J Heart Fail 2013;15(5):511–8.

57. van der Velde AR, Gullestad L, Ueland T, et al. Prognostic value of changes in galectin-3 levels over time in patients with heart failure: data from CORONA and COACH. Circ Heart Fail 2013;6:219–26.

58. Gopal DM, Kommineni M, Ayalon N, et al. Relationship of plasma galectin-3 to renal function in patients with heart failure: effects of clinical status, pathophysiology of heart failure, and presence or absence of heart failure. J Am Heart Assoc 2012;1:e000760.

59. Azibani F, Benard L, Schlossarek S, et al. Aldosterone inhibits antifibrotic factors in mouse hypertensive heart. Hypertension 2012;59:1179–87.

60. Brilla CG. Aldosterone and myocardial fibrosis in heart failure. Herz 2000;25(3):299–306.

61. de Boer RA, Lok DJ, Jaarsma T, et al. Predictive value of plasma galectin-3 levels in heart failure with reduced and preserved ejection fraction. Ann Med 2011;43:60–8.

62. de Boer RA, Edelmann F, Cohen-Solal A, et al. Galectin-3 in heart failure with preserved ejection fraction. Eur J Heart Fail 2013;15(10):1095–101.

63. Sanada S, Hakuno D, Higgins LJ, et al. IL-33 and ST2 comprise a critical biomechanically induced and cardioprotective signaling system. J Clin Invest 2007;117:1538–49.

64. Weinberg EO, Shimpo M, De Keulenaer GW, et al. Expression and regulation of ST2, an interleukin-1 receptor family member, in cardiomyocytes and myocardial infarction. Circulation 2002;3:2961–6.

65. Weinberg EO, Shimpo M, Hurwitz S, et al. Identification of serum soluble ST2 receptor as a novel heart failure biomarker. Circulation 2003;107:721–6.

66. Weir RA, Miller AM, Murphy GE, et al. Serum soluble ST2: a potential novel mediator in left ventricular and infarct remodeling after acute myocardial infarction. J Am Coll Cardiol 2010;55:243–50.

67. Januzzi JL Jr, Peacock WF, Maisel AS, et al. Measurement of the interleukin family member ST2 in patients with acute dyspnea: results from the PRIDE (Pro-Brain Natriuretic Peptide Investigation of Dyspnea in the Emergency Department) study. J Am Coll Cardiol 2007;50:607–13.

68. Mueller T, Dieplinger B, Gegenhuber A, et al. Increased plasma concentrations of soluble ST2 are predictive for 1-year mortality in patients with acute destabilized heart failure. Clin Chem 2008;54:752–6.

69. Bayes-Genis A, de Antonio M, Vila J, et al. Head-to-head comparison of 2 myocardial fibrosis biomarkers for long-term heart failure risk stratification: ST2 versus galectin-3. J Am Coll Cardiol 2014;63(2):158–66.

70. Shah RV, Chen-Tournoux AA, Picard MH, et al. Serum levels of the interleukin-1 receptor family member ST2, cardiac structure and function, and long-term mortality in patients with acute dyspnea. Circ Heart Fail 2009;2:311–31.

71. Manzano-Fernández S, Mueller T, Pascual-Figal D, et al. Usefulness of soluble concentrations of interleukin family member ST2 as predictor of mortality in patients with acutely decompensated heart failure relative to left ventricular ejection fraction. Am J Cardiol 2011;107(2):259–67.

72. Seki K, Sanada S, Kudinova AY, et al. Interleukin-33 prevents apoptosis and improves survival after experimental myocardial infarction through ST2 signaling. Circ Heart Fail 2009;2:684–91.

73. Mann DL, Bristow MR. Mechanisms and models in heart failure: the biomechanical model and beyond. Circulation 2005;111:2837–49.

74. Sugihara N, Genda A, Shimizu M, et al. Diastolic dysfunction and its relation to myocardial fibrosis in essential hypertension. J Cardiol 1988;18:353–61.

75. Borbely A, van der Velden J, Papp Z, et al. Cardiomyocyte stiffness in diastolic heart failure. Circulation 2005;111:774–81.

76. Kjeldsen L, Johnsen AH, Sengeløv H, et al. Isolation and primary structure of NGAL, a novel protein associated with human neutrophil gelatinase. J Biol Chem 1993;268:10425–32.

77. Flower DR. The lipocalin protein family: structure and function. Biochem J 1996;318:1–14.

78. Goetz DH, Willie ST, Armen RS, et al. Ligand preference inferred from the structure of neutrophil gelatinase associated lipocalin. Biochemistry 2000;39:1935–41.

79. Kusaka M, Kuroyanagi Y, Mori T, et al. Serum neutrophil gelatinase-associated lipocalin as a

predictor of organ recovery from delayed graft function after kidney transplantation from donors after cardiac death. Cell Transplant 2008;1(2):129–34.

80. Cruz DN, De Cal M, Garzotto F, et al. Plasma neutrophil gelatinase-associated lipocalin is an early biomarker for acute kidney injury in an adult ICU population. Intensive Care Med 2010;36(3):444–51.

81. Devarajan P. NGAL in acute kidney injury: from serendipity to utility. Am J kidney Dis 2008; 52(3):395.

82. Dharnidharka VR, Kwon C, Stevens G. Serum cystatin C is superior to serum creatinine as a marker of kidney function: a meta-analysis. Am J Kidney Dis 2002;40:221–6.

83. Herget-Rosenthal S, Marggraf G, Hüsing J, et al. Early detection of acute renal failure by serum cystatin C. Kidney Int 2004;66:1115–22.

84. Fleming TR, Powers JH. Biomarkers and surrogate endpoints in clinical trials. Stat Med 2012;31(25): 2973–84.

Comorbidities and Differential Diagnosis in Heart Failure with Preserved Ejection Fraction

Ross T. Campbell, MB ChB, John J.V. McMurray, MD*

KEYWORDS

- Prognosis • Comorbidity • HF-PEF • HF-REF

KEY POINTS

- Many patients presenting with the signs and/or symptoms of HF may have an alternative diagnosis.
- Symptoms should not be solely attributed to comorbidities as patients can also have more than one condition contributing to their symptoms.
- An alternative diagnosis, particularly heart failure with reduced ejection fraction, should be considered before arriving at the diagnosis of HF-PEF as this could dramatically alter treatment options that are available.

INTRODUCTION

Heart failure (HF) is common, affecting 1% to 2% of the general population,[1–3] with the prevalence rising to more than 10% in those aged more than 80 years.[1,4] HF has a high morbidity and reduced life expectancy, with 5- and 10-year survival rates of 50% and 10% reported in epidemiologic studies.[5,6] HF can broadly be divided into 2 groups: HF with reduced ejection fraction (HF-REF) and HF with preserved ejection fraction (HF-PEF). There is a suggestion that HF-PEF accounts for almost half of all patients with HF and that prognosis is equally poor between groups,[7,8] although a recent meta-analysis of 41,972 patients showed HF-REF to have a worse prognosis.[9] The main difference between these 2 groups is response to treatment. Where HF-REF has several evidence-based therapies proved to improve survival, no treatment has been shown to do so

in HF-PEF. The HF-PEF phenotype also differs from HF-REF, with HF-PEF patients being older, more often women, obese, and with more comorbidities. HF-PEF diagnosis is challenging and essentially a diagnosis of exclusion, with comorbidities potentially making the diagnosis more difficult. This article describes the comorbidities commonly associated with HF-PEF, the potential influence of these comorbidities on morbidity and mortality, and the differential diagnosis.

COMORBIDITIES

Any description of the comorbidities in HF-PEF would ideally be based on cohorts of patients without selection bias, who have a confirmed diagnosis of HF-PEF. Furthermore, as the diagnosis of HF-PEF is difficult and one of exclusion, any study describing this population would ideally be prospective and use echocardiography and

Funding: R.T.C. is supported by a British Heart Foundation project grant. All authors have no relationships relevant to the contents of this paper to disclose.
BHF Cardiovascular Research Centre, University of Glasgow, Glasgow, Scotland, UK
* Corresponding author. Institute of Cardiovascular and Medical Sciences, BHF Glasgow Cardiovascular Research Centre, University of Glasgow, Glasgow G12 8TA, UK.
E-mail address: john.mcmurray@glasgow.ac.uk

natriuretic peptides to confirm the diagnosis. Unfortunately, there are no such studies, possibly reflecting the evolving diagnostic criteria of HF-PEF. There are, however, several large epidemiologic/community cohorts,[10–15] hospital cohorts,[7,8,16–24] and randomized controlled clinical trials (RCTs)[25–37] available (**Table 1**). Many of these studies used different inclusion criteria and definitions of HF-PEF, reflecting different eras of recruitment. However, useful comparisons and observations can still be made from the large number of patients enrolled in these different settings. The most obvious comparison would be with HF-REF patients. Patients with HF-PEF are consistently older, regardless of whether the cohort is based in the community, hospital, or an RCT. Another striking difference in demographics is the proportion of female patients, with HF-PEF having much higher prevalence of women. Women generally accounted for more than half of HF-PEF patients, whereas the converse is true in HF-REF. Of the HF-PEF studies with more than 1000 participants, only 4 studies had less than 50% women. These were the DIG (Digoxin Investigation Group) ancillary trial,[31] CHARM (Candesartan in Heart failure: Assessment of Reduction in Mortality and Morbidity)-preserved trial,[36] the DIAMOND-CHF (Danish Investigations of Arrhythmia and Mortality) study,[16] and the population-based study by Ather and colleagues.[12] Even then, women accounted for a much higher proportion compared with HF-REF in the DIG (41% vs 23%), CHARM (40% vs 26%), and DIAMOND-CHF (49% vs 33%) cohorts. One notable exception is the study by Ather and colleagues, with only 9% women, although this is not unexpected as this was a study of Veterans. Again the proportion of women was higher in the HF-PEF group compared to HF-REF (9% vs 4%). There are other similarities between the different HF-PEF cohorts other than age and sex, namely type and frequency of comorbidities.

CARDIOVASCULAR COMORBIDITIES
Hypertension

Hypertension (HT) is the most common comorbidity associated with HF-PEF (see **Table 1**). Community cohorts report HT prevalence between 44% and 86%, with a higher proportion of HF-PEF with HT than HF-REF. Hospital cohorts and registries report similarly high proportions of HT, up to 80%. Again, HT would appear more common in hospitalized HF-PEF patients compared to HF-REF. Tribouilloy and colleagues[20] reported a marked difference between HF-PEF and HF-REF (74% vs 48%). Only the DIAMOND-CHF registry

reported less than 50% HT.[16] RCTs report even higher proportions of HT, with the recent I-PRESERVE (Irbesartan in Heart Failure with Preserved Systolic Function) and TOPCAT (Treatment of Preserved Cardiac Function Heart Failure with an Aldosterone Antagonist) trials reporting HT prevalence of 88% and 91%, respectively.[28,30] Although HT was also common in the HF-REF arms of several comparison studies, there was a much higher prevalence in HF-PEF.

The high prevalence of HT is not surprising, given increased left ventricular (LV) stiffness and impaired LV relaxation, often associated with concentric left ventricular hypertrophy (LVH), resulting in impaired diastolic dysfunction are thought to be key components in the pathophysiologic process of HF-PEF.[38] Indeed, the presence of LVH is now a component of the European Society of Cardiology Guidelines diagnostic pathway for HF-PEF.[39]

There would appear to be more to HF-PEF than old age, female sex, HT, and LVH. Comparisons can be made between large RCTs of HT and HF-PEF, which reported heart failure hospitalization (HFH) and overall mortality rates per 1000 patient years (**Table 2**).[31,40–50] Four HT trials enrolled elderly cohorts with mostly women: the HYVET (Hypertension in the Very Elderly Trial) trial had a mean age of 84 years, with 60% women[41]; the ANBP-2 (Second Australia National Blood Pressure) trial had a mean age of 72 years, with 51% women[45]; the LIFE (Losartan Intervention for Endpoint reduction in hypertension) trial had a mean age of 67 years, with 54% women[43]; and the STOP-2 (Swedish Trial in Old Patients with Hypertension) trial had a mean age of 76 years, with 67% women.[40] The 3 HF-PEF trials enrolled similar proportions of female patients and were also elderly: the DIG ancillary trial had a mean age of 67 years, with 41% women; the CHARM-preserved trial had a mean age of 67 years, with 40% women; and the I-PRESERVE trial had a mean age of 72 years, with 60% women. These 3 trials had a high prevalence of HT, 60%, 64%, and 68%, respectively. Despite the HT trials enrolling older patients with more HT, the overall mortality rates and HF hospitalization rates were still higher in the HF-PEF trials (see **Table 2**).

Although abnormal LV geometry and mass are thought to be important in the pathogenesis of HF-PEF, this does not wholly account for the morbidity and mortality. Despite similar LV mass in HT patients with LVH, HF-PEF patients have been shown to have worse diastolic function, lower LV cavity size, and stroke volume.[51] Both I-PRESERVE and LIFE published echocardiography substudies, with LIFE reporting a higher LV

Table 1
Comorbidities in HF-PEF and HF-REF cohorts

Study	n	Age	Women (%)	HT (%)	DM (%)	AF (%)	MI (%)	PCI/CABG (%)	Angina (%)	CVA/TIA (%)	CKD[a] (%)	Anaemia[b] (%)	Hyper-lipidemia (%)	COPD/Asthma (%)	Obesity (%)	Other
Community HF Cohorts																
Framingham[10]																
HF-PEF	220	80	65	59	22	29	37[c]	—	—	—	—	—	—	—	BMI 27 Kg/m²	—
HF-REF	314	78	40	56	27	22	63[c]	—	—	—	—	—	—	—	BMI 27 Kg/m²	—
Olmstead County[11]																
HF-PEF	308	77	57	86	36	31	36	—	—	—	11[d]	53	77	38	30	—
HF-REF	248	73	42	81	38	32	50	—	—	—	9[d]	49	80	30	29	—
Veterans[12]																
HF-PEF	2843	71	9	71	45	35	27	—	—	21	49	33	—	34	51	28% PVD, 22% cancer
HF-REF	6599	70	4	62	40	35	40	—	—	21	52	28	—	27	37	28% PVD, 19% cancer
ECHOES[13]																
HF-PEF	230	76	52	44	11	—	20	—	34	—	—	—	—	—	—	—
HF-REF	219	71	31	41	20	—	55	—	52	—	—	—	—	—	—	—
CHS[14]																
HF-PEF	170	75	56	60	27	15	58[c]	—	—	—	—	—	—	—	—	—
HF-REF	60	74	37	57	23	5	78[c]	—	—	—	—	—	—	—	—	—
SHS[15]																
HF-PEF	50	64	84	76	70	—	20[c]	—	—	—	—	—	—	—	—	—
HF-REF	45	~63	47	89	66	—	38[c]	—	—	—	—	—	—	—	—	—
Hospital HF Cohorts																
GWTG[23]																
HF-PEF	40,354	78	63	80	46	34	44[c]	—	—	15	52	22	43	33	33	11.9% PVD

(continued on next page)

Table 1
(continued)

Study	n	Age	Women (%)	HT (%)	DM (%)	AF (%)	MI (%)	PCI/CABG (%)	Angina (%)	CVA/TIA (%)	CKD[a] (%)	Anaemia[b] (%)	Hyper-lipidemia (%)	COPD/Asthma (%)	Obesity (%)	Other
HF-REF	55,083	70	36	72	40	28	52[c]	—	—	13	48	14	44	27	25	11.5% PVD
New York[22] HF Registry	619	72	73	78	40	23	43[c]	—	—	—	5 (dialysis)	—	—	25	46	10% hypo-thyroid
MAYO AHF[8]																
HF-PEF	2167	74	66	63	33	41	53[c]	—	—	—	—	—	—	—	41	—
HF-REF	2429	72	35	48	34	29	64[c]	—	—	—	—	—	—	—	36	—
EFFECT[7]																
HF-PEF	880	75	66	55	32	32	17	2/6	23	15	22[e]	21[f]	16	6	—	11% PVD, 6% dementia
HF-REF	1570	72	37	49	39	24	39	3/13	28	15	19[e]	10[f]	22	13	—	15% PVD, 5% dementia
Worchester AHF[21]																
HF-PEF	612	76	68	69	34	—	34	—	—	16	60	—	21	31	35	16% PVD
HF-REF	814	74	46	64	40	—	54	—	—	18	64	—	24	26	27	21% PVD
Tribouilloy et al[20]																
HF-PEF	368	76	53	74	26	36	9	—	—	5	—	—	—	20	—	20% cancer, 11% PVD
HF-REF	294	71	38	48	26	31	18	—	—	5	—	—	—	21	—	21% cancer, 20% PVD
MEDICARE[24]																
HF-PEF	6754	80	71	69	37	36	21	7/14	—	17	—	—	—	34	—	8% dementia
HF-REF	12,956	78	49	61	40	30	38	11/28	—	18	—	—	—	31	—	8% dementia
ADHERE[19]																
HF-PEF	26,322	74	62	77	45	21	24	—	—	—	26	—	—	31	—	17% PVD
HF-REF	25,865	70	40	69	40	17	36	—	—	—	26	—	—	27	—	17% PVD

Study (n)	n	Age	Women (%)	HT (%)	DM (%)	AF (%)	MI (%)	PCI/CABG (%)	Angina (%)	CVA/TIA (%)	CKD[a] (%)	Anaemia[b] (%)	Hyper-lipidemia (%)	COPD/Asthma (%)	Obesity (%)	Other
OPTIMIZE[18]																
HF-PEF	21,149	75	62	76	43	33[g]	38[h]	—	—	—	—	—	32	—	—	—
HF-REF	20,118	70	38	66	39	28[g]	54[h]	—	—	—	—	—	34	—	—	—
EURO HF[17]																
HF-PEF	3148	71	55	59	26	25	59[c]	12	—	16	5	—	—	—	—	—
HF-REF	3685	67	29	50	28	23	69[c]	18	—	14	6	—	—	—	—	—
DIAMOND-CHF[16]																
HF-PEF	2218	73	49	25	13	26	25	—	—	—	60	—	—	26	—	—
HF-REF	3022	71	33	23	19	23	46	—	—	—	77	—	—	19	—	—
Randomized controlled clinical trials HF-PEF																
CHARM[34-36]																
HF-PEF	3023	67	40	64	28	29	44	19/22	53	9	35	27	—	—	38	7% cancer
HF-REF	4576	65	26	49	29	26	58	15/25	51	9	37	23	—	—	27	—
PEP-CHF[33]	850	75	56	79	21	20	27	9/5	—	—	—	—	—	—	BMI ~ 27.5 Kg/m²	—
DIG[31,32]																
HF-PEF	988	67	41	60	29	N/A	50	-/-	30	—	49	—	—	—	34	—
HF-REF	6800	64	23	45	28	N/A	65	-/-	27	—	45	—	—	—	24	—
I-PRESERVE[30]	4133	72	60	88	27	29	24	13	40	10	31	15	—	—	41	—
SENIORS[29]																
HF-PEF	752	76	50	78	24	36	34	2/4	—	CVA in past 3 mo excluded	Significant renal dysfunction excluded	19	47	—	—	—
HF-REF	1359	76	30	53	27	34	49	5/12	—	—	—	19	45	—	—	—
TOPCAT[28]	3445	69	52	91	32	35	26	15/13	47	8	39 eGFR <30 mL/min/73 m² excluded	Hemoglobin <11 g/dL excluded	60	12/6	55	9% PVD
ALDO-DHF[27]	422	67	52	92	17	5	40[c]	—	—	—	—	—	65	3 (FEV1 <80 and vital capacity <80 excluded)	BMI ~ 29 Kg/m²	—

(continued on next page)

Table 1
(continued)

Study (n)	n	Age	Women (%)	HT (%)	DM (%)	AF (%)	MI (%)	PCI/CABG (%)	Angina (%)	CVA/TIA (%)	CKD[a] (%)	Anaemia[b] (%)	Hyper-lipidemia (%)	COPD/Asthma (%)	Obesity (%)	Other
J-DHF[26]	245	72	42	80	31	48	26[c]	—	—	12	—	—	41	—	BMI ~24 Kg/m²	—
DOSE[25]																
HF-PEF	81	74	42	84	47	70	46[c]	—	—	—	—	—	—	—	BMI 34 Kg/m²	—
HF-REF	219	66	20	80	53	48	63[c]	—	—	—	—	—	—	—	BMI 31 Kg/m²	—
RELAX-AHF[37]																
HF-PEF	281	75	58	93	46	61	43[c]	—	—	14	—	—	—	16	BMI 30 Kg/m²	—
HF-REF	810	71	31	84	47	48	57[c]	—	—	14	—	—	—	16	BMI 29 Kg/m²	—

Abbreviations: AF, atrial fibrillation; BMI, body mass index; CABG, coronary artery bypass graft; COPD, chronic obstructive pulmonary disease; CVA, cerebrovascular accident; DM, diabetes mellitus; HT, hypertension; PCI, percutaneous coronary intervention; PVD, peripheral artery disease; TIA, transient ischemic attack.
a CKD, chronic kidney disease (eGFR<60 mL/min/1.73 m²).
b WHO criteria hemoglobin less than 13 in men and less than 12 g/dL in women.
c Coronary artery disease/ischemic heart disease.
d Severely reduced renal function.
e Creatinine greater than 150 mmol/L.
f Hemoglobin less than 10 g/dL.
g Atrial arrhythmia.
h Ischemic etiology.

Table 2
Baseline characteristics and outcomes in cardiovascular and HF-PEF randomized controlled clinical trials

Study	n	Age	Women (%)	HT (%)	DM (%)	AF (%)	MI (%)	PCI/CABG (%)	Angina (%)	CVA/TIA (%)	Obesity (%)	HFH Rate (per 1000 pt y)	Mortality (per 1000 pt y)
HF-PEF													
DIG-Preserved[31]	988	67	41	60	29	N/A	50	-/-	30	—	34	73	76
I-PRESERVE[50]	4133	72	60	88	27	29	24	13	40	10	41	43	53
CHARM-preserved[50]	3023	67	40	64	28	29	44	19/22	53	9	38	69	54
Hypertension													
ALLHAT[46]	33,357	67	47	100	36	—	25[a]	13	—	—	BMI 30 Kg/m²	11.5	28.7
ANBP-2[45]	6083	72	51	100	7	—	8[a]	—	—	5	BMI 27 Kg/m²	5.5	15.7
LIFE[43,44]	9193	67	54	100	13	4	6	—	10	8	BMI 28 Kg/m²	7.1	17.3
VALUE[42]	15,313	67	42	92	32	—	46[a]	—	—	20	BMI 28 Kg/m²	11	25.6
HYVET[41]	3845	84	61	90	7	—	3	—	—	7	BMI 25 Kg/m²	5.3	47.2
STOP-2[40]	6614	76	77	100	11	5	3	—	8[a]	4	BMI 27 Kg/m²	16.4	33
Diabetes													
ACCORD[47]	10,251	62	39	—	100	—	—	—	—	—	BMI 32 Kg/m²	7.5	11.4
Ischaemic heart disease													
ACTION[48]	7665	63	20	52	15	—	51	45	100	—	23	4.6	16.4
Atrial Fibrillation													
ACTIVE I[49]	9016	70	39	88	20	100	—	—	—	13	BMI ~ 29 Kg/m²[b]	32[b]	50[b]

[a] Coronary artery disease/ischemic heart disease.
[b] Placebo arm of ACTIVE I.

Abbreviations: AF, atrial fibrilliation; BMI, body mass index; CABG, coronary artery bypass graft; COPD, chronic obstructive pulmonary disease; CVA, cerebrovascular accident; DM, diabetes mellitus; HF, heart failure; HFH, heart failure hospitalization; HF-PEF, heart failure with preserved ejection fraction; HF-REF, heart failure with reduced ejection fraction; HT, hypertension; PCI, percutaneous coronary intervention; PVD, peripheral artery disease; TIA, transient ischaemic attack.

mass than I-PRESERVE.[52,53] Again, I-PRESERVE had higher rates of overall mortality and HF hospitalization.

Atrial Fibrillation

Atrial fibrillation (AF) is another common comorbidity associated with HF-PEF and is reported in approximately one-third of patients, regardless of the setting studied (see **Table 1**). Community cohorts report prevalence between 15% and 35%, hospitalized cohorts between 21% and 41%, and RCTs between 29% and 70%. AF is similarly common in HF-REF, although most cohorts that included HF-PEF and HF-REF reported higher proportions of AF in HF-PEF. AF would appear to be more common in acute HF. The DOSE (Diuretics Optimization Strategies Evaluation) study recruited patients with acute decompensated HF, with both HF-PEF and HF-REF, and reported much higher prevalence of AF in both groups compared to other HF cohorts.[25] Again, HF-PEF had a higher prevalence of AF than HF-REF, 69% versus 48%, respectively. A similarly high proportion of AF in those with HF-PEF was reported in the RELAX-AHF (RELAXin in Acute Heart Failure) trial, with 61% of patients with HF-PEF and 48% of patients with HF-REF.[37] Another recent acute HF trial, which recruited both HF-PEF and HF-REF, was the CARRESS-HF (Cardiorenal Rescue Study in Acute Decompensated Heart Failure) trial.[54] AF was reported in 54% of all patients recruited. Whether the prevalence of AF in HF-PEF is as high as reported in the DOSE, RELAX-AHF, or CARRESS-HF study remains to be shown with prospective, unselective cohorts using screening with echocardiography and natriuretic peptides.

The high prevalence of AF is not surprising given there are several ways in which AF could theoretically contribute to the pathophysiologic processes in HF-PEF or be caused by HF-PEF itself.[55] AF is associated with increased left atrial (LA) size, which in turn can cause mitral valve annulus dilatation and mitral regurgitation leading to HF. Conversely, high filling pressures associated with a stiff noncompliant ventricle found in HF-PEF could lead to LA enlargement and thus cause AF. AF causes a loss of atrial contraction with an associated reduction in the active phase of diastolic filling, resulting in reduced cardiac output.[56] AF is also associated with increased LV fibrosis,[57] which is thought to contribute to the pathologic development of diastolic dysfunction. Another potential explanation for the high prevalence of AF in HF-PEF is that AF is common in elderly, with more than 9% of those aged more

than 80 years affected,[58] and as described earlier HF-PEF patients are frequently elderly.

One AF study that reported outcomes per 1000 patient years, allowing comparison to HF-PEF studies, is the ACTIVE-I (Atrial Fibrillation Clopidogrel Trial with Irbesartan for Prevention of Vascular Events) trial, which recruited 9016 patients with AF and other cardiovascular risk factors.[49] ACTIVE-I participants had a mean age of 70 years, were 39% women, and included 32% with HF and 88% HT. There were similar overall mortality rates between ACTIVE-I and the HF-PEF studies, although HF hospitalization rates were less in ACTIVE-I. Whether AF is causal, coincidental, or a consequence of HF-PEF is unclear. Regardless of EF, AF was associated with adverse cardiovascular outcomes in the CHARM program.[59]

Coronary and Peripheral Artery Disease

Cardiovascular comorbidities are prevalent in both HF-PEF and HF-REF, although ischemic heart disease (IHD) is much more so in HF-REF (see **Table 1**). Prevalence of previous myocardial infarction (MI) ranged from 9% to 50% in HF-PEF and 18% to 65% in HF-REF. The number of HF-PEF patients who had previously undergone revascularization (either surgical or percutaneous) was therefore understandably higher in HF-REF. Many studies only reported prevalence of IHD (including previous MI, angina, and revascularization). IHD was reported in 20% to 59% of HF-PEF patients and 38% to 78% of HF-REF patients. Peripheral arterial disease was documented in 8 studies, with similar proportions in patients with HF-PEF and HF-REF of 9% and 28%. Cerebrovascular disease, either previous stroke or transient ischemic attack, would appear to be equally prevalent in both HF groups (5%–21%) and similar to the proportion with peripheral artery disease. The presence of hyperlipidemia is reported variably and the proportion of patients with hyperlipidemia is also variable, with 16% to 77% and 22% to 80% of HF-PEF and HF-PEF, respectively.

The high prevalence of IHD and previous MI in HF-REF is expected given the clearly defined role MI plays in cardiac remodeling and dilation, leading to reduced EF and cardiac output.[60] However, whether IHD is a bystander in HF-PEF or contributes to pathogenesis of this condition is unclear. Ischemia increases LV end-diastolic pressures and myocardial stiffness, which alters the pressure-volume curve of the LV causing an upward shift. Some would speculate that underlying ischemia (silent) could explain some of the symptoms experienced in HF-PEF, namely breathlessness. The ACTION (A Coronary disease Trial Investigating Outcome with Nifedipine) trial allows for comparison between an ischemic population and HF-PEF RCTs.[48] The ACTION trial recruited 7665 patients, all with angina and a mean age of 63 years. Patients with known HF and LVEF less than 40% were excluded. Despite this very high proportion of IHD, rate of HFH was less compared to similar populations in HF-PEF (see **Table 2**). Other cardiovascular problems such as chronotropic incompetence and dynamic mitral regurgitation could also cause the HF-PEF syndrome, although prospective studies assessing the prevalence of these problems are not available.

NONCARDIOVASCULAR COMORBIDITY
Diabetes Mellitus

Diabetes mellitus (DM) is variably reported in HF studies between 11% and 70% (see **Table 1**). Community cohorts report prevalence of 11% to 70%, with hospital cohorts and RCTs reporting 13% to 46% and 17% to 47%, respectively. The SHS (Strong Heart Study), a population-based echocardiographic survey of Native Americans, which enrolled 3184 participants, reported an extremely high proportion of DM in HF-PEF and HF-REF (70% and 66%).[15] This potentially reflects the small sample size of patients with HF and perhaps genetic susceptibility of the study population as 50% of the whole cohort had DM. DM was more common in HF-REF compared to HF-PEF, although 7 out of 20 studies with both groups reported the converse. In the Framingham Health Study, participants were followed-up with serial echocardiograms.[61] Diabetes was associated with a steeper increase in LV mass and LV wall thickness compared to age and sex-adjusted controls in the study.[62] As discussed earlier, abnormal LV mass and geometry potentially play a role in the pathogenesis of HF-PEF.

Whether DM accounts for the morbidity and mortality associated with HF-PEF is unclear. A subgroup analysis of the CHARM program showed that a diagnosis of DM was associated with a poorer outcome, regardless of EF with a greater relative risk related to diabetes in HF-PEF compared to HF-REF.[63] So does diabetes account for the morbidity and mortality seen in HF-PEF? Comparison of HFH and overall mortality between a large diabetes trial and HF-PEF RCT would suggest otherwise. The ACCORD (Action to Control Cardiovascular Risk in Diabetes) trial enrolled 10,251 participants with DM, with a mean age of 63 years and 39% women.[47] Despite a higher proportion of DM in ACCORD, patients with similar

demographics in HF-PEF RCTs again had worse outcomes (**Table 2**).

Obesity

Review of any study of HF-PEF, in any setting, reveals a high prevalence of obesity and more so than HF-REF (see **Table 1**). Obesity is present in 30% to 51% of community and hospital cohorts of HF-PEF. RCTs of HF-PEF enrolled even higher proportions of obesity. Of note, the recent TOP-CAT trial enrolled 3445 patients with signs and symptoms of HF, an EF greater than 45%, and required a hospitalization in the previous year for which treatment of HF was given or raised natriuretic peptides. Fifty-five percent of the patients enrolled in TOPCAT were obese. Obesity can cause several symptoms found in HF-PEF, namely fatigue, dyspnea, and ankle swelling. Obesity is also known to cause obstructive sleep apnea in some, which in turn can result in pulmonary hypertension (PHT) and cor pulmonale. Furthermore, obstructive sleep apnea can be associated with several abnormalities/comorbidities found in HF-PEF such as HT, LVH, diastolic impairment, and AF.[64] Even patients without obstructive sleep apnea have been shown to have impaired diastolic function compared to normal controls.[65] Whether obesity is a cause of HF-PEF, a comorbidity, or merely a differential diagnosis remains to be seen.

Chronic Obstructive Pulmonary Disease and Pulmonary Hypertension

Chronic lung disease (either chronic obstructive pulmonary disease [COPD] or asthma) is reported in several community and hospitalized HF cohorts (see **Table 1**). Prevalence varies between 6% and 38% in HF-PEF and 13% and 31% in HF-REF. Generally, HF-PEF had a higher proportion of chronic lung disease than HF-PEF, although not always. COPD is another potentially important comorbidity in HF-PEF as many of the symptoms experienced are similar, and many signs found in COPD associated with secondary PHT are similar to HF. Lam and colleagues[66] performed a subgroup analysis of 203 HF-PEF and 719 HT control subjects from the Olmstead County cohort who had measurable pulmonary artery systolic pressure. PHT was present in 83% of the HF-PEF patients and 8% of the HT controls, and the presence of PHT was associated with worse survival in HF-PEF. The investigators also performed a secondary analysis, excluding HF-PEF patients with a diagnosis of COPD or known significant lung disease from both groups. Despite this, HF-PEF still had a higher proportion of PHT (82% vs 8%), and was still a strong predictor of mortality. This suggests that PHT may be involved in the pathophysiological process of HF-PEF or is a consequence or HF-PEF. Another possibility is that of undiagnosed pulmonary disease or primary PHT given this was not a prospective cohort. Undiagnosed lung disease seems less likely as all patients had spirometry performed in addition to echocardiography, but is possible in the absence of invasive investigations. Unfortunately, data are not available on the proportion of patients with COPD and secondary PHT in prospective, unselected HF cohorts, using the current diagnostic criteria for HF-PEF.

Chronic Kidney Disease and Anemia

The presence of chronic kidney disease (CKD), often determined by an estimated glomerular filtration rate of less than 60 mL/min/1.73 m^2, is variably reported in the available HF cohorts (see **Table 1**). The proportion of CKD ranges from 5% to 60% in HF-PEF and 6% to 77% in HF-REF, with no clear difference between the 2 groups. A high prevalence of CKD is not surprising for several reasons. Firstly, as previously discussed, risk factors for renal impairment or CKD are common in both HF-PEF and HF-REF, namely diabetes and HT. Secondly, HF itself is thought to contribute to CKD in the so-called cardiorenal syndrome. Reduced cardiac output, with subsequent reduced renal perfusion, as well as renal congestion, are thought to cause renal impairment. Also, several treatments for HF-REF can themselves worsen renal function, namely inhibition of the renin-angiotensin-aldosterone system. Regardless of EF, renal impairment is associated with poorer outcomes. A subgroup analysis of the CHARM study found the presence of CKD to be an independent predictor of adverse outcome (mortality, CV mortality, and HF hospitalization), regardless of EF.[67]

Prevalence of anemia varies between 15% and 53% in HF-PEF and 10% and 49% in HF-REF and would appear to be more common in HF-PEF. The cause of anemia was described by Ezekowitz and colleagues,[68] who analyzed the records of 12,065 patients discharged with a diagnosis of HF in Alberta, Canada. Anemia was present in 17%. Twenty-one percent had iron deficiency, 8% had other deficiencies, 13% had assorted other causes, and 58% had anemia of chronic disease. Anemia was an independent prognostic factor for mortality. This article did not provide a breakdown regarding EF and outcome. The CHARM and SENIORS (Study of Effects of Nebivolol Intervention on Outcomes and Rehospitalization in Seniors with Heart Failure) trials provide some insight into this, as both included HF-PEF and HF-REF. Subgroup analyses of both of these studies showed that the presence of anemia, regardless of EF, is associated with poor outcomes.[69,70] Although there is a suggestion that treating iron deficiency in anemic HF patients (with reduced EF) improves symptoms,[71] there is no evidence that increasing hemoglobin level improves survival.[72]

Other Comorbidities

Other comorbidities documented in the HF cohorts reviewed are cancer and dementia (see **Table 1**). Cancer prevalence ranges between 7% and 22%, with similar proportions in both HF-PEF and HF-REF, although it should be noted that most of the cohorts reviewed did not describe prevalence of cancer and for many RCTs this was an exclusion criteria. Dementia is generally a condition of the elderly and therefore not surprising that community and hospital cohorts of HF report prevalence between 6% and 8% (see **Table 1**). Prevalence of HT, AF, and CKD could also be influenced by the older age seen in HF-PEF populations, although this is difficult to quantify without age adjusted prevalence data. Although not strictly a comorbidity, is likely that physical deconditioning may mimic the symptoms of HF-PEF.

Influence of Comorbidities on Development of HF-PEF

The authors have seen that HF-PEF is associated with several comorbidities and that some of these co-morbidities may contribute to the pathophysiology of the condition, in particular HT and AF. Are these comorbidities themselves associated with increased risk of developing HF-PEF? The PREVEND (Prevention of Renal and Vascular End-stage Disease) study recruited 8592 participants from Groningen, The Netherlands, between 1997 and 1998.[73] Participants' cardiovascular and renal risk factors were thoroughly described at baseline. Participants were followed-up for 11 years and incident cases of HF described, of which there were 374 (125 HF-PEF). Risk factors for developing HF, HF-PEF, and HF-REF were detailed. Female gender, AF, increased urinary albumin excretion, and cystatin C were associated with significantly greater risk of developing HF-PEF. Not surprisingly, previous MI and male gender were associated with increased risk of HF-REF, but not HF-PEF. Older age conveyed a risk of HF development, although there was a much stronger association with development of HF-PEF versus HF-REF. Diabetes, HT, and obesity were all associated with HF risk. Interestingly, there was no statistical difference between risk of HF-PEF and HF-REF for these factors.

The Framingham Heart Study (FHS) population (n = 6340) were followed-up between 1981 and 2008 and incident cases of HF described (n = 457).[74] Older age, DM, and valvular heart disease were all associated with risk of developing HF. AF, higher body mass index (BMI), and smoking were associated with increased risk of HF-PEF. Male gender, total cholesterol, heart rate, cardiovascular disease, left bundle branch block, HT, and LVH were associated with development of HF-REF.

Another analysis of participants in the FHS (n = 1038) who had baseline echocardiography assessed the influence of cardiac and non-cardiac co-morbidities on incidence of HF-PEF and HF-REF, after adjustment for age, sex BMI, blood pressure, HT, cholesterol, DM, prior myocardial infarction, and valvular heart disease.[75] Unsurprisingly, asymptomatic left ventricular systolic dysfunction was associated with greater risk of developing HF-REF and asymptomatic diastolic dysfunction was associated with greater risk of HF-PEF. Anaemia and chronic kidney disease were risk factors for development of HF-REF, whereas airflow obstruction was associated with greater risk of developing HF-PEF.

Most of the findings in both of these studies are consistent with the observed comorbidities in HF cohorts. One anomaly was that HT was associated with greater risk of developing HF-REF than HF-PEF.

Influence of Comorbidities on Hospitalization and Death

As previously discussed, there is a suggestion that mortality in HF-PEF is similar to HF-REF, although a recent meta-analysis performed by the MAGGIC group would suggest that HF-REF has a poorer prognosis.[9] Comparison between HF-PEF and HF-REF in RCTs would also suggest that HF-REF has the worse prognosis and higher rates of HFH. Patients with HF-PEF are more likely to die from non-CV causes than HF-REF. Death attributed to HF is less common in HF-PEF also. Both DIG and CHARM reported cause of death in both groups. CHARM-preserved trial had 21% HF death versus 27% in CHARM-Reduced trial[76]; patients with preserved EF in DIG had 28% HF death versus 36% in patients with reduced EF.[32] Despite similar demographics, patients enrolled in HF-PEF RCTs had worse outcomes compared to HT, DM, and angina RCTs. Only the AF trial ACTIVE-I had outcomes comparable to the HF-PEF RCTs.[50] The influence of different comorbidities

on outcomes in a large ambulatory (albeit predominantly male) HF population was analyzed by Ather and colleagues.[12] Proportions of various comorbidities were in keeping with other studies, as described earlier. Patients with HF-PEF were more likely to have multiple comorbidities, and this was associated with higher rates of non-CV hospitalization and death. Although almost all individual comorbidities were associated with higher hazard ratio for mortality in both HF-PEF and HF-REF, only COPD had statistically significant higher hazard ratio in HF-PEF (1.61 in HF-PEF vs 1.23 in HF-REF, P = 0.01). The high proportion of comorbidities (especially non-CV comorbidities), with associated higher rates of non-CV outcomes, has been suggested as an explanation for why all pharmacologic RCTs in HF-PEF have failed to show an improvement in overall mortality or HF hospitalization.[12]

DIFFERENTIAL DIAGNOSIS

HF-PEF is essentially a diagnosis of exclusion, and the diagnosis is often made difficult by the number of comorbidities patients with HF-PEF. Furthermore, the signs and symptoms of HF are nonspecific (**Table 3**).[39] The differential diagnosis also varies depending on how the patient with HF-PEF present. Patients with HF-PEF broadly present in 1 of 2 ways: acutely with symptoms of HF and signs of congestion (both peripheral and pulmonary) or with symptoms of breathlessness and fatigue, sometimes without significant signs on examination.

Signs of HF are understandably more prevalent in patients presenting to hospital with acute decompensated HF (**Table 4**).[77] Common findings include peripheral edema and rales. Less common findings include elevated jugular venous distention, third heart sound, hepatojugular reflux, and radiological evidence of pulmonary congestion. The DOSE study reported very high proportions of signs in both HF-PEF and HF-REF, including very high proportions of peripheral edema and jugular venous distention (99% and 95% respectively), perhaps reflecting the inclusion criteria for the study that required at least one sign of HF to be present. Hospital cohorts report edema in about 66% to 73% of patients with HF-PEF, and this would appear to be a more common finding in HF-PEF versus HF-REF. A similar observation is made of the presence of pulmonary rales. Patients in the community and those presenting to outpatient clinics are likely to have symptoms of HF but fewer signs. This trend can be seen in the RCTs of HF-PEF, which reported the presence of signs at baseline (see **Table 4**). The differential

Table 3
Signs and symptoms commonly found in heart failure

Symptoms	Signs
Typical	**More specific**
Ankle swelling	Elevated jugular venous pressure
Orthopnea	Hepatojugular reflux
Paroxysmal nocturnal dyspnea	Third heart sound (gallop rhythm)
Reduced exercise tolerance	Laterally displaced apical impulse
Breathlessness	Cardiac murmur
Fatigue, tiredness, increased time to recover after exercise	
Less Typical	**Less Specific**
Nocturnal cough	Peripheral edema (ankle, sacral, scrotal)
Wheezing	Pulmonary crepitations
Weight gain (>2 kg/wk)	Reduced air entry and dullness to percussion at lung bases (pleural effusion)
Weight loss (in advanced heart failure)	Tachycardia
Bloated feeling	Irregular pulse
Loss of appetite	Tachypnea (>16 breaths/min)
Confusion (especially in the elderly)	Hepatomegaly
Depression	Ascites
Palpitations	Tissue wasting (cachexia)
Syncope	

Adapted from McMurray JJ, Adamopoulos S, Anker SD, et al. ESC Guidelines for the diagnosis and treatment of acute and chronic heart failure 2012: the task force for the diagnosis and treatment of acute and chronic heart failure 2012 of the European Society of Cardiology. Developed in collaboration with the Heart Failure Association (HFA) of the ESC. Eur Heart J 2012;33(14):1795; with permission.

diagnosis of HF-PEF presenting acutely can generally be divided into cardiac causes, respiratory causes, high-output state, or extracardiac volume overload (**Fig. 1**). The differential diagnosis in patients presenting to the outpatient department is similar, but also includes other causes for breathlessness including obesity and physical deconditioning (**Fig. 2**).

Cardiac Disease

The most obvious cardiac cause to consider is HF-REF, with overestimation of EF. Patients with HF-PEF are more commonly obese and suffer from AF, both making accurate assessment of EF difficult. Care should be taken with this initial assessment as this will determine treatment options available. Consideration of alternative imaging methods should be considered in patients with poor echocardiographic windows to ensure HF-REF is not underdiagnosed. Other common cardiac conditions that can present with signs and symptoms of HF include valve disease, pericardial disease (constriction/restriction and pericardial effusion), hypertrophic cardiomyopathy,

intracardiac shunt, and acute coronary syndrome complicated by acute pulmonary edema. Detailed and systematic echocardiography can usually distinguish between these different diagnoses; however, further imaging modalities or invasive investigations with right and left heart catheterization and even myocardial biopsy may be required. In the outpatient setting, ischemia without anginal pain should be considered a potential diagnosis; this is particularly relevant given the high burden of IHD and diabetes often found in these patients. As ischemia and other cardiovascular problems such as chronotropic incompetence and dynamic mitral regurgitation may also result in the HF-PEF syndrome, exercise testing and stress electrocardiography may be useful and should be considered in the outpatient setting.

Respiratory Disease

Respiratory disease must be considered before a diagnosis of HF-PEF is made. However, distinguishing respiratory disease from HF-PEF is challenging, particularly given the overlap between HF-PEF and PHT.[66] HF-PEF itself can cause

Table 4
Examination findings: HF-PEF versus HF-REF

Study	JVP (%)	S3 (%)	Peripheral Edema (%)	Pulmonary Rales (%)	CXR- Pulmonary Edema (%)	CXR- Pleural Effusions (%)	Hepatojugular Reflux (%)
Hospital HF Cohorts							
EFFECT[7]							
HF-PEF	58	8	66	84	47	41	8
HF-REF	61	13	57	84	52	46	8
ADHERE[19]							
HF-PEF	—	—	69	69	—	—	—
HF-REF	—	—	63	67	—	—	—
OPTIMIZE[18]							
HF-PEF	33	—	68	65	—	—	—
HF-REF	26	—	62	63	—	—	—
WORCESTER[21]							
HF-PEF	—	—	73	—	—	—	—
HF-REF	—	—	70	—	—	—	—
RCTs HF-PEF							
DOSE[25]							
HF-PEF	95	13	99	69	—	—	—
HF-REF	90	3	94	56	—	—	—
RELAX-AHF[37]							
HF-PEF	73	—	80	—	100[a]	—	—
HF-REF	77	—	79	—	100[a]	—	—
I-PRESERVE[30]	~8	~7	~24	~28	~40	—	—
CHARM[77]							
HF-PEF	~7	~5	~30	~15	~3	—	—
HF-REF	~10	~17	~24	~16	~4	—	—
TOPCAT[28]	18	—	60	15	28[b]	—	—
ALDO-HF[27]	—	—	39	—	—	—	—

Abbreviations: CXR, chest radiograph; JVP, jugular venous pressure; HF-PEF, heart failure with preserved ejection fraction; HF-REF, heart failure with a reduced ejection fraction.
[a] Pulmonary congestion on CXR was one of the inclusion criteria.
[b] Pulmonary congestion or pleural effusions.

PHT and as previously described, COPD and chronic lung disease are prevalent in HF-PEF, which can result in cor pulmonale with right ventricular dilatation and dysfunction, and this in turn can cause many of the signs seen in HF, particularly distended jugular veins and peripheral edema. Natriuretic peptides, although extremely useful in diagnosing HF, will often be in the 'gray zone' for patients with cor pulmonale (brain natriuretic peptide [BNP] 100–400 pg/mL).[78] In both acute and outpatient settings, the physician should attempt to exclude significant respiratory disease or other causes of PHT (**Box 1**).[79] Investigations that may prove helpful include lung function testing, ventilation perfusion scanning, high-resolution computed tomography (CT) scanning, and sleep studies. Ultimately, to fully exclude respiratory disease or PHT, invasive investigation may be required with right heart catheterization.

Other Diagnoses

Any condition that results in extracardiac volume overload can mimic the symptoms and signs of HF. Many of these conditions can be diagnosed with simple blood tests and urinalysis, such as nephrotic syndrome. Other conditions such as high output states seen in anemia, arteriovenous fistula, and extracardiac shunting require more

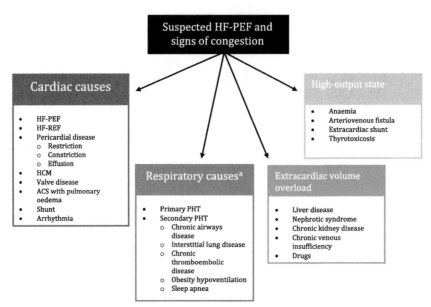

Fig. 1. Differential diagnosis in suspected HF-PEF + signs of congestion. ACS, acute coronary syndrome; HCM, hypertrophic cardiomyopathy, HF-REF, heart failure with reduced ejection fraction; HF-PEF, heart failure with preserved ejection fraction; PHT, pulmonary hypertension. [a] For full list of respiratory differential diagnoses, see **Box 1**.

consideration and careful attention to the patients past medical history. In the outpatient setting, consideration should be given to more mundane diagnoses such as obesity and physical deconditioning, especially when the only presenting feature is breathlessness and fatigue.

Case 1

A 61-year-old man presented acutely to hospital with New York Heart Association (NYHA) class IV breathlessness, paroxysmal nocturnal dyspnea (PND), orthopnea, and peripheral edema. He had a past medical history of HT, chronic AF, CKD,

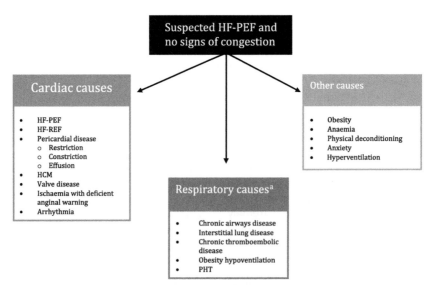

Fig. 2. Differential diagnosis in suspected HF-PEF + no signs of congestion. ACS, acute coronary syndrome; HCM, hypertrophic cardiomyopathy, HF-REF, heart failure with reduced ejection fraction; HF-PEF, heart failure with preserved ejection fraction; PHT, pulmonary hypertension. [a] For full list of respiratory differential diagnoses, see **Box 1**.

Box 1
Causes and classification of pulmonary hypertension (Dana Point, 2008)

1. Pulmonary arterial hypertension (PAH)

    1.1. Idiopathic

    1.2. Heritable

        1.2.1. BMPR2

        1.2.2. ALK1, endoglin (with or without hereditary hemorrhagic telangiectasia)

        1.2.3. Unknown

    1.3. Drugs and toxins induced

    1.4. Associated with (APAH)

        1.4.1. Connective tissue diseases

        1.4.2. HIV infection

        1.4.3. Portal hypertension

        1.4.4. Congenital heart disease

        1.4.5. Schistosomiasis

        1.4.6. Chronic hemolytic anemia

    1.5. Persistent pulmonary hypertension of the newborn

2. Pulmonary venoocclusive disease and/or pulmonary capillary hemangiomatosis

3. Pulmonary hypertension due to left heart disease

    3.1. Systolic dysfunction

    3.2. Diastolic dysfunction

    3.3. Valvular disease

4. Pulmonary hypertension due to lung diseases and/or hypoxia

    4.1. Chronic obstructive pulmonary disease

    4.2. Interstitial lung disease

    4.3. Other pulmonary diseases with mixed restrictive and obstructive pattern

    4.4. Sleep-disordered breathing

    4.5. Alveolar hypoventilation disorders

    4.6. Chronic exposure to high altitude

    4.7. Developmental abnormalities

5. Chronic thromboembolic pulmonary hypertension

6. PH with unclear and/or multifactorial mechanisms

    6.1. Hematological disorders: myeloproliferative disorders, splenectomy

    6.2. Systemic disorders: sarcoidosis, pulmonary Langerhans cell histiocytosis, lymphangioleiomyomatosis, neurofibromatosis, vasculitis

    6.3. Metabolic disorders: glycogen storage disease, Gaucher disease, thyroid disorders

    6.4. Others: tumoral obstruction, fibrosing mediastinitis, chronic renal failure on dialysis

Abbreviations: ALK-1, activin receptorlike kinase 1 gene; APAH, associated pulmonary arterial hypertension; BMPR2, bone morphogenetic protein receptor, type 2; HIV, human immunodeficiency virus; PAH, pulmonary arterial hypertension.

Adapted from Galiè N, Hoeper MM, Humbert M, et al. Guidelines for the diagnosis and treatment of pulmonary hypertension: the task force for the diagnosis and treatment of pulmonary hypertension of the European Society of Cardiology (ESC) and the European Respiratory Society (ERS), endorsed by the International Society of Heart and Lung Transplantation (ISHLT). Eur Heart J 2009;30(20):2497; with permission.

and obesity (BMI = 43). On examination, he had gross edema to the abdomen with associated ascites, raised jugular venous pressure (JVP), normal heart sounds, and reduced air entry on auscultation of the chest. BNP was mildly raised at 365 pg/mL, as was troponin I at 0.2 μg/mL. Electrocardiogram (ECG) showed AF, rate 90 bpm. Chest radiograph (CXR) was congested, with upper lobe diversion. A preliminary diagnosis of HF was made on clinical findings and a transthoracic echocardiogram (TTE) organized. This was limited by body habitus, but revealed undilated LV with estimated EF greater than 50%; mild LVH (mass 108 g/m^2); severely dilated right ventricle (RV) with evidence of pressure and volume overload; moderately dilated LA (biplane volume not possible); no significant left-sided valve disease; moderate tricuspid valve (TV) incompetence; severe PHT (estimated RV systolic pressure 67 mm Hg); and low LV filling pressure (E/é 6.7).

Given the low LV filling pressure, preserved EF, and RV enlargement with PHT, a diagnosis of HF was deemed unlikely and other causes of PHT investigated. CT chest did not demonstrate any evidence of pulmonary embolic disease. However, the patient was noted to be intermittently hypoxic. Arterial blood gas analysis showed chronic type II respiratory failure (H$^+$ 36 nmol/L, Pco$_2$ 8.0 kPa, Po$_2$ 7.5 kPa, So$_2$ 84.3%, HCO$_3$ 40.8 mmol/L). Sleep studies confirmed nocturnal hypoventilation without significant obstructive or central sleep apnea; therefore, a diagnosis of obesity hypoventilation syndrome with cor pulmonale and severe PHT was made. The patient was successfully treated with nocturnal noninvasive ventilation and his edema successfully treated with diuretics (with a net loss of 40 kg in weight).

Case 2

A 69-year-old woman presented to hospital in a similar fashion to case 1, with NYHA III breathlessness, orthopnea, PND, and extensive edema. Past medical history was also similar with HT, AF, and obesity. Examination demonstrated elevated JVP, RV heave, third heart sound, gross edema to the abdomen, and clinical pleural effusions. BNP was mildly elevated at 471 pg/mL. ECG showed AF, rate 80 bpm. CXR showed cardiomegaly, pleural effusions, and upper lobe venous diversion. TTE showed undilated LV with preserved EF (>50%); severely dilated RV and right atrium; severely enlarged LA (44.8 mL/m²); mild LVH (LV mass 90.4 g/m²); no significant left-sided valve disease; moderate TV incompetence with severe PHT (RV systolic pressure estimated at 80 mm Hg); and LV filling pressure was borderline (E/é 13.0).

Ventilation-perfusion imaging did not reveal any evidence of chronic thromboembolic disease, and lung function testing demonstrated a mild-moderate obstructive picture. Further investigation was carried out with right heart catheterization, which demonstrated a high wedge pressure at 20 mm Hg and therefore not in keeping with a purely respiratory cause of the PHT. Therefore, the likely diagnosis in this case was a combination of HF-PEF and COPD causing PHT and cor pulmonale.

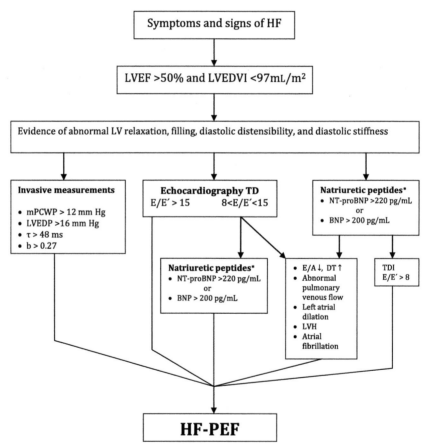

Fig. 3. Diagnostic pathway in suspected HF-PEF with signs of heart failure. b, constant of left ventricular chamber stiffness; DT, deceleration time; E, early mitral valve flow velocity; E/A, ratio of early (E) to late (A) mitral valve flow velocity; E', early TD lengthening velocity; LVEDP, left ventricular end-diastolic pressure; LVEDVI, left ventricular end-diastolic volume index; mPCW, mean pulmonary capillary wedge pressure; NT-proBNP, N-terminal–pro brain natriuretic peptide; τ, time constant of left ventricular relaxation; TD, tissue Doppler. * Recent European Society of Cardiology guidelines would suggest using NT-proBNP and BNP levels of >300 and >100 pg/mL respectively. (*Adapted from* Paulus WJ, Tschope C, Sanderson JE, et al. How to diagnose diastolic heart failure: a consensus statement on the diagnosis of heart failure with normal left ventricular ejection fraction by the Heart Failure and Echocardiography Associations of the European Society of Cardiology. Eur Heart J 2007;28(20):2542.)

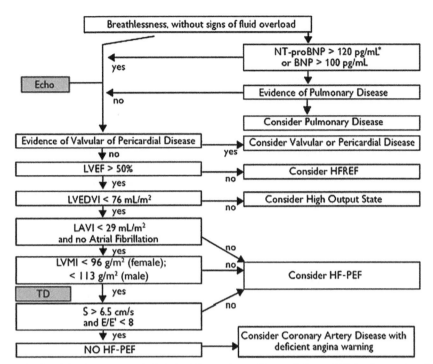

Fig. 4. Diagnostic algorithm in suspected HF-PEF without signs of heart failure. BNP, brain natriuretic peptide; E, early mitral valve flow velocity; E', early TD lengthening velocity; HF-PEF, heart failure with preserved ejection fraction; HF-REF, heart failure with reduced ejection fraction; LAVI, left atrium volume index; LVEDVI, left ventricular end-diastolic volume index; LVEF, left ventricle ejection fraction; LVMI, left ventricle mass index; NT-proBNP, N-terminal-pro brain natriuretic peptide; S, TD shortening velocity. TD, tissue Doppler. * Recent European Society of Cardiology guidelines would suggest using NT-proBNP and BNP levels of >125 and >35 pg/mL respectively. (*Adapted from*Paulus WJ, Tschope C, Sanderson JE, et al. How to diagnose diastolic heart failure: a consensus statement on the diagnosis of heart failure with normal left ventricular ejection fraction by the Heart Failure and Echocardiography Associations of the European Society of Cardiology. Eur Heart J 2007;28(20):2544; with permission.)

Summary

Careful consideration must be given when diagnosing HF-PEF, ideally using natriuretic peptides and echocardiography as described in current guidelines (**Figs. 3** and **4**).[80] Patients presenting in the outpatient setting may not have any signs of HF or echocardiographic features of HF-PEF at rest; therefore, stress echocardiography can be useful in demonstrating exercise-induced diastolic impairment, dynamic mitral regurgitation, or silent ischemia.[81] Many patients presenting with the signs and/or symptoms of HF may have an alternative diagnosis, regardless of whether they present acutely[82,83] or in the outpatient setting.[84] An alternative diagnosis, particularly HF-REF should be considered before arriving at the diagnosis of HF-PEF as this could dramatically alter treatment options available, as seen in Case 1. However, symptoms should not be solely attributed to comorbidities as patients can also have more than one condition contributing to their symptoms, as seen in Case 2. Once the diagnosis of HF-PEF has been made, focus should be given to treatment of comorbidities as there is no evidence base for treatment of HF-PEF, and comorbidities likely contribute to the morbidity and mortality associated with this condition.

REFERENCES

1. Davies M, Hobbs F, Davis R, et al. Prevalence of left-ventricular systolic dysfunction and heart failure in the Echocardiographic Heart of England Screening study: a population based study. Lancet 2001;358(9280):439–44.

2. McDonagh TA, Morrison CE, Lawrence A, et al. Symptomatic and asymptomatic left-ventricular systolic dysfunction in an urban population. Lancet 1997;350(9081):829–33.

3. Redfield MM, Jacobsen SJ, Burnett JC Jr, et al. Burden of systolic and diastolic ventricular dysfunction in the community: appreciating the scope

of the heart failure epidemic. JAMA 2003;289(2):
194–202.

4. Bleumink GS, Knetsch AM, Sturkenboom MC, et al. Quantifying the heart failure epidemic: prevalence, incidence rate, lifetime risk and prognosis of heart failure The Rotterdam Study. Eur Heart J 2004; 25(18):1614–9.

5. MacIntyre K, Capewell S, Stewart S, et al. Evidence of improving prognosis in heart failure: trends in case fatality in 66 547 patients hospitalized between 1986 and 1995. Circulation 2000;102(10):1126–31.

6. Mosterd A, Cost B, Hoes AW, et al. The prognosis of heart failure in the general population: The Rotterdam Study. Eur Heart J 2001;22(15):1318–27.

7. Bhatia RS, Tu JV, Lee DS, et al. Outcome of heart failure with preserved ejection fraction in a population-based study. N Engl J Med 2006; 355(3):260–9.

8. Owan TE, Hodge DO, Herges RM, et al. Trends in prevalence and outcome of heart failure with preserved ejection fraction. N Engl J Med 2006; 355(3):251–9.

9. Meta-analysis Global Group in Chronic Heart Failure (MAGGIC). The survival of patients with heart failure with preserved or reduced left ventricular ejection fraction: an individual patient data meta-analysis. Eur Heart J 2012;33(14):1750–7.

10. Lee DS, Gona P, Vasan RS, et al. Relation of disease pathogenesis and risk factors to heart failure with preserved or reduced ejection fraction: insights from the framingham heart study of the national heart, lung, and blood institute. Circulation 2009;119(24):3070–7.

11. Bursi F, Weston SA, Redfield MM, et al. Systolic and diastolic heart failure in the community. JAMA 2006;296(18):2209–16.

12. Ather S, Chan W, Bozkurt B, et al. Impact of noncardiac comorbidities on morbidity and mortality in a predominantly male population with heart failure and preserved versus reduced ejection fraction. J Am Coll Cardiol 2012;59(11):998–1005.

13. Taylor CJ, Roalfe AK, Iles R, et al. Ten-year prognosis of heart failure in the community: follow-up data from the Echocardiographic Heart of England Screening (ECHOES) study. Eur J Heart Fail 2012; 14(2):176–84.

14. Gottdiener JS, McClelland RL, Marshall R, et al. Outcome of congestive heart failure in elderly persons: influence of left ventricular systolic function. The Cardiovascular Health Study. Ann Intern Med 2002;137(8):631–9.

15. Devereux RB, Roman MJ, Liu JE, et al. Congestive heart failure despite normal left ventricular systolic function in a population-based sample: the Strong Heart Study. Am J Cardiol 2000;86(10):1090–6.

16. Gustafsson F, Torp-Pedersen C, Brendorp B, et al. Long-term survival in patients hospitalized with congestive heart failure: relation to preserved and reduced left ventricular systolic function. Eur Heart J 2003;24(9):863–70.

17. Lenzen MJ, Scholte op Reimer WJ, Boersma E, et al. Differences between patients with a preserved and a depressed left ventricular function: a report from the EuroHeart Failure Survey. Eur Heart J 2004;25(14):1214–20.

18. Fonarow GC, Stough WG, Abraham WT, et al. Characteristics, treatments, and outcomes of patients with preserved systolic function hospitalized for heart failure: a report from the OPTIMIZE-HF Registry. J Am Coll Cardiol 2007;50(8):768–77.

19. Yancy CW, Lopatin M, Stevenson LW, et al. Clinical presentation, management, and in-hospital outcomes of patients admitted with acute decompensated heart failure with preserved systolic function: a report from the Acute Decompensated Heart Failure National Registry (ADHERE) Database. J Am Coll Cardiol 2006;47(1):76–84.

20. Tribouilloy C, Rusinaru D, Mahjoub H, et al. Prognosis of heart failure with preserved ejection fraction: a 5 year prospective population-based study. Eur Heart J 2008;29(3):339–47.

21. Chinali M, Joffe SW, Aurigemma GP, et al. Risk factors and comorbidities in a community-wide sample of patients hospitalized with acute systolic or diastolic heart failure: the Worcester Heart Failure Study. Coron Artery Dis 2010;21(3):137–43.

22. Klapholz M, Maurer M, Lowe AM, et al. Hospitalization for heart failure in the presence of a normal left ventricular ejection fraction: results of the New York Heart Failure Registry. J Am Coll Cardiol 2004; 43(8):1432–8.

23. Steinberg BA, Zhao X, Heidenreich PA, et al. Trends in patients hospitalized with heart failure and preserved left ventricular ejection fraction: prevalence, therapies, and outcomes. Circulation 2012;126(1):65–75.

24. Masoudi FA, Havranek EP, Smith G, et al. Gender, age, and heart failure with preserved left ventricular systolic function. J Am Coll Cardiol 2003;4(2): 217–23.

25. Bishu K, Deswal A, Chen HH, et al. Biomarkers in acutely decompensated heart failure with preserved or reduced ejection fraction. Am Heart J 2012;164(5):763–70.e3.

26. Yamamoto K, Origasa H, Hori M, J-DHF Investigators. Effects of carvedilol on heart failure with preserved ejection fraction: the Japanese Diastolic Heart Failure Study (J-DHF). Eur J Heart Fail 2013;15(1):110–8.

27. Edelmann F, Wachter R, Schmidt AG, et al. Effect of spironolactone on diastolic function and exercise capacity in patients with heart failure with preserved ejection fraction: the Aldo-DHF randomized controlled trial. JAMA 2013;309(8):781–91.

28. Shah SJ, Heitner JF, Sweitzer NK, et al. Baseline characteristics of patients in the treatment of preserved cardiac function heart failure with an aldosterone antagonist trial. Circ Heart Fail 2013;6(2): 184–92.

29. Flather MD, Shibata MC, Coats AJ, et al. Randomized trial to determine the effect of nebivolol on mortality and cardiovascular hospital admission in elderly patients with heart failure (SENIORS). Eur Heart J 2005;26(3):215–25.

30. McMurray JJ, Carson PE, Komajda M, et al. Heart failure with preserved ejection fraction: clinical characteristics of 4133 patients enrolled in the I-PRESERVE trial. Eur J Heart Fail 2008;10(2): 149–56.

31. Ahmed A, Rich MW, Fleg JL, et al. Effects of digoxin on morbidity and mortality in diastolic heart failure: the ancillary digitalis investigation group trial. Circulation 2006;114(5):397–403.

32. Digitalis Investigation Group. The effect of digoxin on mortality and morbidity in patients with heart failure. N Engl J Med 1997;336(8):525–33.

33. Cleland JG, Tendera M, Adamus J, et al. The perindopril in elderly people with chronic heart failure (PEP-CHF) study. Eur Heart J 2006;27(19): 2338–45.

34. McMurray JJ, Ostergren J, Swedberg K, et al. Effects of candesartan in patients with chronic heart failure and reduced left-ventricular systolic function taking angiotensin-converting-enzyme inhibitors: the CHARM-Added trial. Lancet 2003;362(9386): 767–71.

35. Granger CB, McMurray JJ, Yusuf S, et al. Effects of candesartan in patients with chronic heart failure and reduced left-ventricular systolic function intolerant to angiotensin-converting-enzyme inhibitors: the CHARM-Alternative trial. Lancet 2003; 362(9386):772–6.

36. Yusuf S, Pfeffer MA, Swedberg K, et al. Effects of candesartan in patients with chronic heart failure and preserved left-ventricular ejection fraction: the CHARM-Preserved Trial. Lancet 2003;362(9386): 777–81.

37. Filippatos G, Teerlink JR, Farmakis D, et al. Serelaxin in acute heart failure patients with preserved left ventricular ejection fraction: results from the RELAX-AHF trial. Eur Heart J 2014;35(16):1041–50.

38. Zile MR, Baicu CF, Gaasch WH. Diastolic heart failure–abnormalities in active relaxation and passive stiffness of the left ventricle. N Engl J Med 2004; 350(19):1953–9.

39. McMurray JJ, Adamopoulos S, Anker SD, et al. ESC Guidelines for the diagnosis and treatment of acute and chronic heart failure 2012: the task force for the diagnosis and treatment of acute and chronic heart failure 2012 of the European Society of Cardiology. Developed in collaboration with the Heart Failure Association (HFA) of the ESC. Eur Heart J 2012;33(14):1787–847.

40. Hansson L, Lindholm LH, Ekbom T, et al. Randomised trial of old and new antihypertensive drugs in elderly patients: cardiovascular mortality and morbidity the Swedish Trial in Old Patients with Hypertension-2 study. Lancet 1999;354(9192): 1751–6.

41. Beckett NS, Peters R, Fletcher AE, et al. Treatment of hypertension in patients 80 years of age or older. N Engl J Med 2008;358(18):1887–98.

42. Julius S, Kjeldsen SE, Weber M, et al. Outcomes in hypertensive patients at high cardiovascular risk treated with regimens based on valsartan or amlodipine: the VALUE randomised trial. Lancet 2004; 363(9426):2022–31.

43. Dahlof B, Devereux RB, Julius S, et al. Characteristics of 9194 patients with left ventricular hypertrophy: the LIFE study. Losartan Intervention For Endpoint Reduction in Hypertension. Hypertension 1998;32(6):989–97.

44. Dahlof B, Devereux RB, Kjeldsen SE, et al. Cardiovascular morbidity and mortality in the Losartan Intervention For Endpoint reduction in hypertension study (LIFE): a randomised trial against atenolol. Lancet 2002;359(9311):995–1003.

45. Wing LM, Reid CM, Ryan P, et al. A comparison of outcomes with angiotensin-converting–enzyme inhibitors and diuretics for hypertension in the elderly. N Engl J Med 2003;348(7):583–92.

46. ALLHAT Officers and Coordinators for the ALLHAT Collaborative Research Group. The Antihypertensiveand Lipid-Lowering Treatment to Prevent Heart Attack Trial. Major outcomes in high-risk hypertensive patients randomized to angiotensin-converting enzyme inhibitor or calcium channel blocker vs diuretic: The Antihypertensive and Lipid-Lowering Treatment to Prevent Heart Attack Trial (ALLHAT). JAMA 2002;288(23):2981–97.

47. Action to Control Cardiovascular Risk in Diabetes Study Group, Gerstein HC, Miller ME, et al. Effects of intensive glucose lowering in type 2 diabetes. N Engl J Med 2008;358(24):2545–59.

48. Poole-Wilson PA, Lubsen J, Kirwan BA, et al. Effect of long-acting nifedipine on mortality and cardiovascular morbidity in patients with stable angina requiring treatment (ACTION trial): randomised controlled trial. Lancet 2004;364(9437): 849–57.

49. ACTIVE I Investigators, Yusuf S, Healey JS, et al. Irbesartan in patients with atrial fibrillation. N Engl J Med 2011;364(10):928–38.

50. Campbell RT, Jhund PS, Castagno D, et al. What have we learned about patients with heart failure and preserved ejection fraction from DIG-PEF, CHARM-preserved, and I-PRESERVE? J Am Coll Cardiol 2012;60(23):2349–56.

51. Lam CS, Roger VL, Rodeheffer RJ, et al. Cardiac structure and ventricular-vascular function in persons with heart failure and preserved ejection fraction from Olmsted County, Minnesota. Circulation 2007;115(15):1982–90.

52. Zile MR, Gottdiener JS, Hetzel SJ, et al. Prevalence and significance of alterations in cardiac structure and function in patients with heart failure and a preserved ejection fraction. Circulation 2011;124(23): 2491–501.

53. Devereux RB, Bella J, Boman K, et al. Echocardiographic left ventricular geometry in hypertensive patients with electrocardiographic left ventricular hypertrophy: The LIFE Study. Blood Press 2001; 10(2):74–82.

54. Bart BA, Goldsmith SR, Lee K, et al. Ultrafiltration in ecompensated heart failure with cardiorenal syndrome. N Engl J Med 2012;367(24):2296–304.

55. Caldwell JC, Mamas MA. Heart failure, diastolic dysfunction and atrial fibrillation; mechanistic insight of a complex inter-relationship. Heart Fail Rev 2012;17(1):27–33.

56. Naito M, David D, Michelson EL, et al. The hemodynamic consequences of cardiac arrhythmias: evaluation of the relative roles of abnormal atrioventricular sequencing, irregularity of ventricular rhythm and atrial fibrillation in a canine model. Am Heart J 1983;106(2):284–91.

57. Shantsila E, Shantsila A, Blann AD, et al. Left ventricular fibrosis in atrial fibrillation. Am J Cardiol 2013;111(7):996–1001.

58. Go AS, Hylek EM, Phillips KA, et al. Prevalence of diagnosed atrial fibrillation in adults: national implications for rhythm management and stroke prevention: the AnTicoagulation and Risk Factors in Atrial Fibrillation (ATRIA) Study. JAMA 2001;285(18): 2370–5.

59. Olsson LG, Swedberg K, Ducharme A, et al. Atrial fibrillation and risk of clinical events in chronic heart failure with and without left ventricular systolic dysfunction: results from the Candesartan in Heart failure-Assessment of Reduction in Mortality and morbidity (CHARM) program. J Am Coll Cardiol 2006;47(10): 1997–2004.

60. Konstam MA, Kramer DG, Patel AR, et al. Left ventricular remodeling in heart failure: current concepts in clinical significance and assessment. JACC Cardiovasc Imaging 2011;4(1):98–108.

61. Lieb W, Xanthakis V, Sullivan LM, et al. Longitudinal tracking of left ventricular mass over the adult life course: clinical correlates of short- and long-term change in the framingham offspring study. Circulation 2009;119(24):3085–92.

62. Cheng S, Xanthakis V, Sullivan LM, et al. Correlates of echocardiographic indices of cardiac remodeling over the adult life course: longitudinal observations from the Framingham Heart Study. Circulation 2010;122(6):570–8.

63. MacDonald MR, Petrie MC, Varyani F, et al. Impact of diabetes on outcomes in patients with low and preserved ejection fraction heart failure: an analysis of the Candesartan in Heart failure: Assessment of Reduction in Mortality and morbidity (CHARM) programme. Eur Heart J 2008;29(11): 1377–85.

64. Somers VK, White DP, Amin R, et al. Sleep apnea and cardiovascular disease: an American Heart Association/American College of Cardiology Foundation Scientific Statement from the American Heart Association Council for High Blood Pressure Research Professional Education Committee, Council on Clinical Cardiology, Stroke Council, and Council on Cardiovascular Nursing. J Am Coll Cardiol 2008;52(8):686–717.

65. Pascual M, Pascual DA, Soria F, et al. Effects of isolated obesity on systolic and diastolic left ventricular function. Heart 2003;89(10):1152–6.

66. Lam CS, Roger VL, Rodeheffer RJ, et al. Pulmonary hypertension in heart failure with preserved ejection fraction: a community-based study. J Am Coll Cardiol 2009;53(13):1119–26.

67. Hillege HL, Nitsch D, Pfeffer MA, et al. Renal function as a predictor of outcome in a broad spectrum of patients with heart failure. Circulation 2006; 113(5):671–8.

68. Ezekowitz JA, McAlister FA, Armstrong PW. Anemia is common in heart failure and is associated with poor outcomes: insights from a cohort of 12 065 patients with new-onset heart failure. Circulation 2003;107(2):223–5.

69. O'Meara E, Clayton T, McEntegart MB, et al. Clinical correlates and consequences of anemia in a broad spectrum of patients with heart failure: results of the Candesartan in Heart Failure: Assessment of Reduction in Mortality and Morbidity (CHARM) Program. Circulation 2006;113(7):986–94.

70. von Haehling S, van Veldhuisen DJ, Roughton M, et al. Anaemia among patients with heart failure and preserved or reduced ejection fraction: results from the SENIORS study. Eur J Heart Fail 2011; 13(6):656–63.

71. Anker SD, Comin Colet J, Filippatos G, et al. Ferric carboxymaltose in patients with heart failure and iron deficiency. N Engl J Med 2009;361(25): 2436–48.

72. Swedberg K, Young JB, Anand IS, et al. Treatment of anemia with darbepoetin alfa in systolic heart failure. N Engl J Med 2013;368(13):1210–9.

73. Brouwers FP, de Boer RA, van der Harst P, et al. Incidence and epidemiology of new onset heart failure with preserved vs. reduced ejection fraction in a community-based cohort: 11-year follow-up of PREVEND. Eur Heart J 2013;34(19):1424–31.

74. Ho JE, Lyass A, Lee DS, et al. Predictors of new-onset heart failure: differences in preserved versus reduced ejection fraction. Circ Heart Fail 2013;6(2): 279–86.

75. Lam CS, Lyass A, Kraigher-Krainer E, et al. Cardiac dysfunction and noncardiac dysfunction as precursors of heart failure with reduced and preserved ejection fraction in the community. Circulation 2011;124(1):24–30.

76. Solomon SD, Wang D, Finn P, et al. Effect of candesartan on cause-specific mortality in heart failure patients: the Candesartan in Heart failure Assessment of Reduction in Mortality and morbidity (CHARM) program. Circulation 2004;110(15): 2180–3.

77. McMurray J, Ostergren J, Pfeffer M, et al. Clinical features and contemporary management of patients with low and preserved ejection fraction heart failure: baseline characteristics of patients in the Candesartan in Heart failure-Assessment of Reduction in Mortality and morbidity (CHARM) programme. Eur J Heart Fail 2003;5(3):261–70.

78. Maisel A, Mueller C, Adams K Jr, et al. State of the art: using natriuretic peptide levels in clinical practice. Eur J Heart Fail 2008;10(9):824–39.

79. Galie N, Hoeper MM, Humbert M, et al. Guidelines for the diagnosis and treatment of pulmonary hypertension: the Task Force for the Diagnosis and Treatment of Pulmonary Hypertension of the European Society of Cardiology (ESC) and the European Respiratory Society (ERS), endorsed by the International Society of Heart and Lung Transplantation (ISHLT). Eur Heart J 2009;30(20):2493–537.

80. Paulus WJ, Tschope C, Sanderson JE, et al. How to diagnose diastolic heart failure: a consensus statement on the diagnosis of heart failure with normal left ventricular ejection fraction by the Heart Failure and Echocardiography Associations of the European Society of Cardiology. Eur Heart J 2007; 28(20):2539–50.

81. Penicka M, Vanderheyden M, Bartunek J. Diagnosis of heart failure with preserved ejection fraction: role of clinical Doppler echocardiography. Heart 2014;100(1):68–76.

82. Mueller C, Laule-Kilian K, Schindler C, et al. Cost-effectiveness of B-type natriuretic peptide testing in patients with acute dyspnea. Arch Intern Med 2006;166(10):1081–7.

83. Knudsen CW, Clopton P, Westheim A, et al. Predictors of elevated B-type natriuretic peptide concentrations in dyspneic patients without heart failure: an analysis from the breathing not properly multinational study. Ann Emerg Med 2005;45(6):573–80.

84. Caruana L, Petrie MC, Davie AP, et al. Do patients with suspected heart failure and preserved left ventricular systolic function suffer from "diastolic heart failure" or from misdiagnosis? A prospective descriptive study. BMJ 2000;321(7255):215–8.

Outcomes in Patients with Heart Failure with Preserved Ejection Fraction

Katrina K. Poppe, PhD[a],
Robert N. Doughty, MD, FRCP, FRACP, FCSANZ[a,b,*]

KEYWORDS

• Heart failure • Reduced ejection fraction • Preserved ejection fraction

KEY POINTS

• Patients with HF-PEF represent between 30% and 50% of all patients with HF and are a heterogenous group of patients.
• Patients with HF-PEF have better survival but similar rates of hospital admissions as those with HF-REF.
• No current therapeutic interventions seem to improve the clinical outcomes for these patients and clinical management remains focused on relief of symptoms and management of comorbidities.

INTRODUCTION

Heart failure (HF) is a significant and increasing global public health problem. In the United States, it is estimated that currently 5.1 million adult Americans have HF, with projections that this will increase to more than 8 million by 2030.[1] The diagnosis of HF continues to be associated with poor quality of life, high morbidity, and high mortality despite contemporary HF management.[2,3] Although survival for patients with HF has improved, mortality remains high, with approximately 50% dying within 5 years.[1,4] Once admitted to hospital, patients experience high rates of subsequent HF hospitalization and mortality.[2]

HF is a clinical syndrome defined *"clinically, as a syndrome in which patients have typical symptoms (eg, breathlessness, ankle swelling, and fatigue) and signs (eg, elevated jugular venous pressure, pulmonary crackles, and displaced apex beat) resulting from an abnormality of cardiac structure or function."*[5] This clinically based definition remains the encompassing definition of HF and is useful in clinical practice to identify the broad range of patients that can present with this syndrome. Importantly, indices of left ventricular (LV) systolic function, particularly LV ejection fraction (EF), are not used as criteria for this initial clinical diagnosis. The subset of HF patients with reduced EF (commonly termed HF-REF) has been extensively characterized; the pathophysiological mechanisms contributing to the progression of disease are now well understood, and therapeutic interventions, including pharmaco-based and device-based therapies, are now well established in current HF clinical practice guidelines.[5] The mortality for patients who receive all the available evidence-based therapies have been markedly reduced, with annual mortality in the large-scale clinical trials now being less than 6%.[6] Numerous new therapeutic interventions are actively being studied for patients with HF-REF, which will further refine the management of this group of patients.

[a] Department of Medicine, National Institute for Health Innovation, University of Auckland, Private Bag 92019, Auckland 1142, New Zealand; [b] Greenlane Cardiovascular Service, Auckland City Hospital, Private Bag 92024, Auckland 1142, New Zealand
* Corresponding author. Department of Medicine, Level 12, Auckland Hospital Support Building, Park Road, Auckland, New Zealand.
E-mail address: r.doughty@auckland.ac.nz

Heart Failure Clin 10 (2014) 503–510
http://dx.doi.org/10.1016/j.hfc.2014.04.012
1551-7136/14/$ – see front matter © 2014 Elsevier Inc. All rights reserved.

Role of EF in HF

LV EF has an important role in HF management because EF is an important predictor of outcome and easily identifies the group of patients with systolic impairment (ie, HF-REF), and as such, guides the delivery of evidence-based therapies.[5] However, many patients with HF have either normal or only mildly impaired EF, a group usually termed as heart failure with preserved ejection fraction or HF-PEF. The basic clinical characteristics of this group are now described: being more common among older women, with a history of hypertension, and less commonly, with a history of coronary artery disease. However, this group of patients has phenotypic heterogeneity, appears to have multiple underlying pathophysiological mechanisms, and frequently has multisystem disease.[7] Importantly, patients with HF-PEF do not appear to gain the same benefits from neurohormonal antagonists as do those with HF-REF.[8–10] As a result, further attention is being turned to the group of patients with HF-PEF.

Proportion of Patients with HF Who Have HF-PEF

Recent data from the United States have demonstrated that HF-PEF (defined here as EF $\geq 50\%$) represented 36% of all patients with HF admitted to the "Get with the Guidelines" hospitals in the United States between 2005 and 2010.[11] A further 14% of patients had a borderline EF between 40% and 49%. Thus, patients with HF with EF greater than or equal to 40% represented half of all patients admitted during that time. A Canadian study of patients with HF reported similar proportions of patients based on EF criteria, with 31% having EF greater than or equal to 50%, and a further 13% having EF 40% to 49%.[12]

The proportion of HF patients who have HF-PEF appears to be increasing over time. For example, among patients hospitalized for HF between 1986 and 2002 in Olmsted County, MN, USA, the proportion of patients with HF-PEF increased from 38% to 54%.[13] This increase was due to an increase in the absolute number of patients with HF-PEF (with the number of patients with HF-REF remaining relatively constant over that time period). Similarly, the proportion of HF patients with HF-PEF from 275 hospitals in the United States increased from 33% to 39% between 2005 and 2010.[11] It is thus clear from these and other data that HF-PEF is common, affecting between one-third to one-half of all patients with HF (depending on the cutoff of EF used to define this group of patients), and importantly, is increasing in prevalence.

CLINICAL OUTCOMES

HF has been known to be associated with high mortality and frequent hospital readmissions. During the 1980s and 1990s, hospitalizations for patients with HF initially increased in many countries and then decreased, and survival improved.[3,14,15] Data from the United States also show that survival after a diagnosis of HF has improved over time, but overall mortality remains high with approximately 50% of patients dying within 5 years.[4] One in 9 deaths in the United States has HF listed on the death certificate.[1] With the high morbidity and mortality for patients with HF, it is clinically important to understand these clinical outcomes among patients with HF-REF and HF-PEF.

In-Hospital Mortality

HF remains a common cause of hospitalization, with approximately 1 million admissions each year in the United States.[16] Hospitalization with acute decompensated HF is a high-risk time for patients with HF with the potential for serious clinical events during that in-patient stay, including death. Two large-scale registries have reported in-hospital outcome data for patients with HF-PEF compared with those with HF-REF. Data from the Acute Decompensated Heart Failure National Registry have shown that 50% of those patients admitted to hospital with acute HF had HF-PEF, although it was also notable that EF data were not available for approximately half of all the patients in this registry.[17] The in-hospital mortality was lower for patients with HF-PEF compared with those patients with HF-REF (2.8% and 3.9%, respectively, $P<.0001$). The OPTIMIZE-HF Registry (Organized Program to Initiate Lifesaving Treatment in Hospitalized Patients with Heart Failure) reported data from 48,612 patients from 259 hospital in the United States, of whom 41,267 (84.9%) had EF data available.[18] HF-PEF (here defined as EF $\geq 40\%$) accounted for 51.2% of all patients with HF. The in-hospital mortality was lower for patients with HF-PEF compared with those patients with HF-REF (2.9% and 3.9%, respectively, $P<.0001$). Notably, the in-hospital mortality was similar for those with EF >50% and those with EF 40% to 50% (2.9% and 3.0%, respectively, $P<.647$).[18] In summary, in-hospital mortality for patients with HF-PEF appears to be lower than for patients with HF-REF.

Long-Term Mortality

Over recent years, there has been uncertainty whether patients with HF-PEF have the same mortality as those with HF-REF. In 2006, 2 epidemiologic studies reported that 1-year mortality from any cause among patients with HF-PEF was 29%[13] and 22%.[12] Adjusted and unadjusted survival models from these studies reported that patients with HF-PEF were at similar risk of death from any cause as patients with HF-REF. However, one-quarter to two-thirds of patients in these studies were missing a measure of EF, introducing an important source of potential bias.

A subsequent literature-based meta-analysis of 17 prospective studies suggested that mortality was lower for patients with HF-PEF than for those with HF-REF.[19] Over a pooled mean follow-up of 4 years, there were 2468 deaths among 7688 patients with HF-PEF (32%), compared with 6831 deaths among 16,813 patients with HF-REF: odds ratio for death from any cause 0.51 (95% CI 0.48–0.55), representing a substantially lower risk of death for patients with HF-PEF. In a second analysis in this meta-analysis of similar studies, but in which EF was not consistently available, the odds ratio for death from any cause for patients with HF-PEF was 0.74 (95% CI 0.70–0.78) compared with patients with HF-REF.

Multivariable analyses, which incorporate important predictors of outcome, cannot be undertaken as part of the statistical approach within literature-based meta-analyses. Patients with HF-PEF and HF-REF are recognized as having several important differences in their clinical characteristics, many of which may have important prognostic influences. Recognizing these limitations, the Meta-analysis Global Group in Chronic Heart Failure (MAGGIC) undertook a meta-analysis using individual patient level data and outcome to examine further whether differences existed for major outcomes between patients with HF-PEF and HF-REF.[20] This meta-analysis included 50,991 patients with HF from 31 observational studies and randomized controlled trials that had not used EF as a study entry criterion. Over 3 years of follow-up, there were 2422 (23.4%) deaths among 10,347 patients with HF-PEF compared with 8332 (26.3%) deaths among 31,625 patients with HF-REF. In multivariable analyses, after adjustment for clinically important prognostic variables (including age, gender, cause of HF, a history of hypertension, diabetes, and atrial fibrillation), the hazard ratio for death from any cause for patients with HF-PEF compared with patients with HF-REF was 0.68 (95% CI 0.64–0.71) **(Fig. 1)**. Mortality for patients with EF 40% to 49% in this meta-analysis was similar to those for the HF-PEF group (EF ≥50%) **(Fig. 2)**.[20] Despite being based on a different (but overlapping) set of studies from the literature meta-

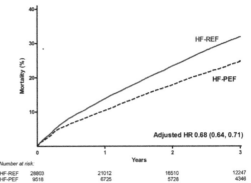

Fig. 1. Mortality for patients with HF-PEF and HF-REF in the MAGGIC meta-analysis. (*From* Meta-analysis Global Group in Chronic Heart Failure Investigators (MAGGIC). The survival of patients with heart failure with preserved or reduced left ventricular ejection fraction: an individual patient data meta-analysis. Eur Heart J 2012;33:1752; with permission.)

analysis, and necessarily using different statistical approaches, this finding reinforced that of the literature meta-analysis—that although mortality among patients with HF-PEF is high, their risk of death is clearly lower than that of patients with HF-REF.[21]

The effects of several individual prognostic factors among patients with HF-REF are well established; however, their significance among patients with HF-PEF has been uncertain. Further analyses from the MAGGIC meta-analysis have contributed to the understanding that the obesity paradox exists in HF-PEF as well as HF-REF[22]; that hyponatremia is independently predictive of death in both HF-PEF and HF-REF[23]; and that survival is better for women with HF compared with men, when adjusted for age, for both patients with HF-PEF and HF-REF.[24] Renal dysfunction is similarly important in both HF-PEF and HF-REF; however, it may be a stronger predictor of all-cause mortality in HF-REF.[25]

A risk score, based on 13 common clinical variables, was derived from the MAGGIC data set.[26] In all the HF patients in this analysis, these clinical variables could be incorporated into a simple integer score that predicted mortality over 3 years of follow-up. The risk score found that the better prognosis for patients with HF-PEF compared with those with HF-REF is more pronounced at younger ages, and that SBP was less predictive of mortality for patients with HF-PEF than in those with HF-REF.[26] External validation of the risk score in the Swedish Heart Failure Registry found that it overpredicted low risk and underpredicted high risk; however, it "demonstrated an excellent ability to categorize patients in separate risk strata."[27]

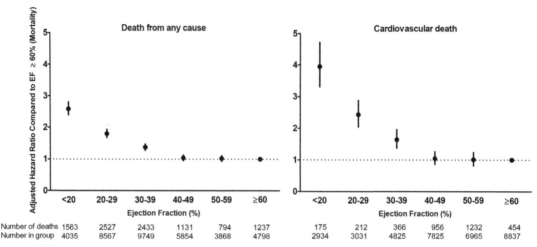

Fig. 2. Adjusted hazard ratios comparing death from any cause and cardiovascular death by groups of LV EF (with LV EF ≥60% as the reference group). (*From* Meta-analysis Global Group in Chronic Heart Failure Investigators (MAGGIC). The survival of patients with heart failure with preserved or reduced left ventricular ejection fraction: an individual patient data meta-analysis. Eur Heart J 2012;33:1753; with permission.)

A measure of EF is implicit in the differentiation of HF-PEF from HF-REF, yet it is missing in up to 70% of HF studies.[19] An exploratory analysis of the observational studies in MAGGIC found that, compared with patients with known EF, patients missing a measure of EF were older, had higher proportions of noncardiac comorbidities, and had higher proportions of other missing variables.[28] Adjusted mortality was higher than for patients with HF-PEF and similar to that of patients with HF-REF.

CAUSE OF DEATH

The extensive literature regarding patients with HF-REF has reinforced the importance of considering the cause of death among patients with HF. Sudden death and death from progressive HF are common causes of death among patients with HF-REF and appropriate evidence-based therapies[5] reduce these major causes of death among this group of patients. The trial results for patients with HF-PEF have raised many issues, including, for example, questions relating to trial design, patient inclusion criteria, and the event rates for the chosen clinical end points.[29] As a result, it is relevant to consider cause-specific mortality among those with HF-PEF. Data from the Irbesartan in Heart Failure with Preserved Ejection Fraction (I-PRESERVE) Trial have provided insights into the mechanism of death among patients with HF-PEF. In this trial, annual mortality was relatively low at 5.2%; 60% of deaths were classified as cardiovascular (with 26% sudden death, 14% HF, 5% myocardial infarction, and 9% stroke), 30% were noncardiovascular, and

10% were unknown.[30] Cardiovascular deaths are a common cause of death among patients with HF-PEF, although the proportion differs according to study design (60% of all deaths in the RCTs[30–32] and 49% of deaths in community-based observational studies[33,34]), which may reflect that observational studies often involve older patients with a wider range of comorbidities than patients in RCTs. Sudden death and death due to progressive HF appear to be less common among patients with HF-PEF compared with those with HF-REF. Further understanding of the cause of death in patients with HF-PEF will assist with the development of appropriate strategies to improve outcome for these patients.

HOSPITAL ADMISSIONS

There are more than 1 million hospital admissions each year in the United States for patients with HF, of which 71% occur among people over the age of 65 years (25% over the age of 85 years).[16] These hospital admissions account for a large proportion of the costs associated with HF.[35–37] Mortality is increased after hospitalization for HF, with greatest risk in the first month after discharge and among those with repeated hospital readmissions.[38] Thus, hospitalizations are a very important issue from a public health and patient perspective. Several studies have reported hospital admission data for patients with HF-PEF and HF-REF. Data from Canada, involving 2339 patients who survived to hospital discharge, have shown that 30-day and 1-year hospital readmission rates were similar for patients with HF-PEF compared with patients with HF-REF (30-day: 5.3% and

7.1%, respectively, $P = .66$; 1-year: 22.2% and 25.5%, respectively, $P = .09$).[12] The OPTIMIZE Registry reported that 60- to 90-day readmission rates were 29.2% for patients with HF-PEF and 29.9% for patients with HF-REF ($P = .59$). In addition, the group of patients in this Registry with EF 40% to 50% had similar readmission rates as those with EF greater than 50% (29% and 30.9%, respectively, $P = .37$).

Thus, current data suggest that hospital readmission rates after hospitalization for HF are similar for up to 1 year for patients with HF-PEF and HF-REF. However, few data are available on the frequency of readmissions and total hospital bed days, which is relevant given the high frequency of readmissions and the lower mortality for patients with HF-PEF (ie, potentially placing this group of patients in a position of having longer survival but with risk of multiple readmissions).

COMORBIDITIES IN PATIENTS WITH HF-PEF

Studies have consistently reported that the group of patients with HF-PEF appears to be older than those with HF-REF. As a consequence of this age difference, it would not be unexpected if patients with HF-PEF had more comorbid conditions than those patients with HF-REF. A report from a large cohort of predominately male Veterans from the United States has demonstrated that patients with HF-PEF had a higher prevalence of chronic lung disease, diabetes, hypertension, anemia, psychiatric disorders, obesity, peptic ulcer disease, and cancer, but lower prevalence of chronic kidney disease compared with those patients with HF-REF.[39] There was a significant increase in the proportion of patients with HF-PEF with an increasing number of comorbidities. Although overall hospital admission rates were similar between the 2 groups of HF patients, and increasing comorbidities increased the risk of all-cause hospital admission, those patients with HF-PEF had lower rates of HF hospitalization and higher rates of non-HF hospitalization compared with the patients with HF-REF.[39] These data clearly demonstrate the significant impact of comorbidities for patients with HF and also reinforce the differences between the groups of patients with HF-PEF and HF-REF. The 2012 ESC HF Guidelines recommend treatment of comorbidities as central to management for patients with HF-PEF.[5] Although this recommendation in part arises from the lack of other clinical trial data for specific treatment strategies among this group of patients with HF, recognition of the importance of comorbidities among such patients reinforces the importance of adequate management of these comorbidities.

THERAPEUTIC INTERVENTIONS FOR PATIENTS WITH HF-PEF

Therapeutic interventions for patients with HF-REF are now well established, including combined neurohormonal antagonists, directed principally at the renin-angiotensin system, sympathetic nervous system, and aldosterone. The addition of device-based therapies, including primary implantable defibrillators and cardiac resynchronization therapy, has now improved symptoms, quality of life, decreased hospitalization, and improved survival for patients with HF-REF. Unfortunately, the application of similar neurohormonal antagonists for patients with HF-PEF has not met with similar benefits.

Inhibitors of the Renin-Angiotensin System

The Candesartan in Heart failure Assessment of Reduction in Mortality and morbidity (CHARM)-Preserved trial enrolled 3023 patients with clinical HF, a prior cardiac-related hospital admission, and EF greater than 40% who were randomized to candesartan (target dose 32 mg/d) or placebo.[10] Mean follow-up was 36.3 months. There was no difference between treatment groups in the primary composite end point of cardiovascular death and HF hospitalization (unadjusted HR 0.89, $P = .118$; adjusted HR 0.86, $P = .051$).[10] The Perindopril in Elderly People with Chronic Heart Failure Study involved 850 patients 70 years or older with clinical criteria for HF and echocardiographic evidence of diastolic dysfunction (and excluding significant LV systolic impairment). Patients were randomized to receive perindopril 4 mg/d or placebo, and mean follow-up was 2.1 years. There was no statistical difference between the treatment groups for the primary composite end point of all-cause mortality and unplanned HF readmission (HR 0.919, $P = .545$).[40] The I-PRESERVE Trial involved 4128 patients 60 years of age or older with symptomatic HF and EF greater than or equal to 45%.[9] Patients were randomized to receive irbesartan 300 mg/d or placebo, and mean follow-up was 49.5 months. There was no statistical difference between the treatment groups for the primary composite end point of all-cause mortality and cardiovascular hospitalization (HR 0.95, $P = .35$).[9]

These 3 randomized, controlled trials of inhibitors of the renin-angiotensin system have been combined in a literature-based meta-analysis.[41] The pooled analysis from these 3 trials, involving 8021 patients, found no effect on all-cause mortality (OR 1.03, $P = .62$) or on HF hospitalization (OR 0.90, $P = .09$).[41] In summary, there is no clear evidence of benefit on major clinical outcomes with inhibitors of the renin-angiotensin system in patients with HF-PEF. These trial data do not preclude the use of these agents for the management of HF-PEF, where, for example, they may be used to treat comorbidities such as hypertension.

β-Blockers have not been studied extensively in patients with HF-PEF. Data from 3 trials have recently been reviewed, with no clear evidence of mortality benefit for patients with HF-PEF, although these trials only involved 1048 patients (135 deaths).[42]

Previous studies with mineralocorticoid receptor antagonists have demonstrated that these agents improve outcome among patients with HF-REF[43,44] and in patients with LV dysfunction following acute myocardial infarction.[45] This background, along with early phase mechanistic studies,[46] led to the TOP CAT (Treatment of Preserved Cardiac Function Heart Failure with an Aldosterone Antagonist) trial.[47] This study involved 3445 patients aged 50 years or older, with symptomatic HF, EF greater than or equal to 45%, and either 1 or more HF hospitalizations within 12 months or brain natriuretic peptide greater than 100 pm/mL. Patients were randomized to receive spironolactone 15 to 45 mg/d or placebo. The trial results were recently presented at the American Heart Association meeting in 2013 (Marc Pfeffer, MD, AHA November 18, 2013; Late Breaking Session) and have shown that there was no statistical difference between the treatment groups for the primary composite end point of cardiovascular death, HF readmission, or aborted cardiac arrest (HR 0.89, $P = .138$). These results are clearly of great disappointment and collectively have demonstrated that beneficial effects of neurohormonal antagonists, which are of proven benefit for patients with HF-REF, do not translate to provide similar benefits for patients with HF-PEF.

SUMMARY

In summary, HF remains a clinically defined syndrome, which can easily be categorized into 2 main groups of patients according to LV EF. Although EF has important limitations as a measure of LV systolic function, this differentiation is clinically useful. HF-PEF is a common condition, accounting for between 30% and 50% of all patients with HF, clearly depending on the EF cutoff used to define this condition. Patients with HF-PEF have lower in-hospital and lower longer-term mortality than those patients with HF-REF. Overall hospital readmission rates appear similar among patients with HF-PEF and HF-REF, confirming that the burden of disease remains high for all patients with HF. Comorbidities are frequent among patients with HF-PEF, with higher numbers of comorbid conditions being associated with a higher proportion of those who develop HF having HF-PEF and increasing the risk of hospitalization. HF-PEF represents a heterogenous group of patients, typically who are older, more commonly women with a history of hypertension, and less commonly with a history of coronary disease than patients with HF-REF. To date, there are no therapeutic interventions that appear to confer the same benefits as are seen for the pharmacologic and device-based therapies, which are now of proven value for patients with HF-REF. New therapeutic targets are urgently required for patients with HF-PEF to improve the natural history of this condition and so relieve the burden of this condition on patients and health care systems.

REFERENCES

1. Go AS, Mozaffarian D, Roger VL, et al. Heart disease and stroke statistics—2014 update: a report from the American Heart Association. Circulation 2014;129:e28–292.
2. Blackledge HM, Tomlinson J, Squire IB. Prognosis for patients newly admitted to hospital with heart failure: survival trends in 12 220 index admissions in Leicestershire 1993-2001. Heart 2003;89:615–20.
3. Schaufelberger M, Swedberg K, Köster M, et al. Decreasing one-year mortality and hospitalization rates for heart failure in Sweden: data from the Swedish hospital discharge registry 1988 to 2000. Eur Heart J 2004;25:300–7.
4. Roger VL, Weston SA, Redfield MM, et al. Trends in heart failure incidence and survival in a community-based population. JAMA 2004;292:344–50.
5. McMurray JJ, Adamopoulos S, Anker SD, et al. ESC guidelines for the diagnosis and treatment of acute and chronic heart failure 2012: the task force for the diagnosis and treatment of acute and chronic heart failure 2012 of the European Society of Cardiology. Developed in collaboration with the Heart Failure Association (HFA) of the ESC. Eur Heart J 2012; 33:1787–847.
6. Bardy GH, Lee KL, Mark DB, et al. Amiodarone or an implantable cardioverter-defibrillator for congestive heart failure. N Engl J Med 2005;352:225–37.
7. Maeder M, Kaye D. Heart failure with normal left ventricular ejection fraction. J Am Coll Cardiol 2009;53: 905–18.
8. Cleland JG, Tendera M, Adamus J, et al. Perindopril for elderly people with chronic heart failure: the PEP-CHF study. Eur J Heart Fail 1999;1:211–7.
9. Massie BM, Carson PE, McMurray JJ, et al. Irbesartan in patients with heart failure and preserved ejection fraction. N Engl J Med 2008;359: 2456–67.

10. Yusuf S, Pfeffer MA, Swedberg K, et al. Effects of candesartan in patients with chronic heart failure and preserved left-ventricular ejection fraction: the CHARM-preserved trial. Lancet 2003;362:777–81.

11. Steinberg BA, Zhao X, Heidenreich PA, et al. Trends in patients hospitalized with heart failure and preserved left ventricular ejection fraction: prevalence, therapies, and outcomes. Circulation 2012;126:65–75.

12. Bhatia RS, Tu JV, Lee DS, et al. Outcome of heart failure with preserved ejection fraction in a population-based study. N Engl J Med 2006;355:260–9.

13. Owan TE, Hodge DO, Herges RM, et al. Trends in prevalence and outcome of heart failure with preserved ejection fraction. N Engl J Med 2006;355:251–9.

14. Jhund PS, MacIntyre K, Simpson CR, et al. Long-term trends in first hospitalization for heart failure and subsequent survival between 1986 and 2003: a population study of 5.1 million people. Circulation 2009;119:515–23.

15. Shafazand M, Schaufelberger M, Lappas G, et al. Survival trends in men and women with heart failure of ischaemic and non-ischaemic origin: data for the period 1987-2003 from the Swedish hospital discharge registry. Eur Heart J 2009;30:671–8.

16. Hall MJ, Levant S, DeFrances CJ. Hospitalization for congestive heart failure: United States, 2000–2010. NCHS Data Brief 2012;108:1–8.

17. Yancy CW, Lopatin M, Stevenson LW, et al. Clinical presentation, management, and in-hospital outcomes of patients admitted with acute decompensated heart failure with preserved systolic function: a report from the Acute Decompensated Heart Failure National Registry (ADHERE) database. J Am Coll Cardiol 2006;47:76–84.

18. Fonarow GC, Stough WG, Abraham WT, et al. Characteristics, treatments, and outcomes of patients with preserved systolic function hospitalized for heart failure: a report from the OPTIMIZE-HF registry. J Am Coll Cardiol 2007;50:768–77.

19. Somaratne JB, Berry C, McMurray JJ, et al. The prognostic significance of heart failure with preserved left ventricular ejection fraction: a literature-based meta-analysis. Eur J Heart Fail 2009;11:855–62.

20. Meta-analysis Global Group in Chronic Heart Failure Investigators (MAGGIC). The survival of patients with heart failure with preserved or reduced left ventricular ejection fraction: an individual patient data meta-analysis. Eur Heart J 2012;33:1750–7.

21. Burkhoff D. Mortality in heart failure with preserved ejection fraction: an unacceptably high rate. Eur Heart J 2012;33:1718–20.

22. Padwal R, McAlister FA, McMurray JJ, et al. The obesity paradox in heart failure patients with preserved versus reduced ejection fraction: a meta-analysis of individual patient data. Int J Obes 2013. http://dx.doi.org/10.1038/ijo.2013.203.

23. Rusinaru D, Tribouilloy C, Berry C, et al. Relationship of serum sodium concentration to mortality in a wide spectrum of heart failure patients with preserved and with reduced ejection fraction: an individual patient data meta-analysis(†): Meta-Analysis Global Group in Chronic Heart Failure (MAGGIC). Eur J Heart Fail 2012;14:1139–46.

24. Martinez-Selles M, Doughty RN, Poppe K, et al. Gender and survival in patients with heart failure: interactions with diabetes and aetiology. Results from the MAGGIC individual patient meta-analysis. Eur J Heart Fail 2012;14:473–9.

25. McAlister FA, Ezekowitz J, Tarantini L, et al. Renal dysfunction in patients with heart failure with preserved versus reduced ejection fraction: impact of the new Chronic Kidney Disease-Epidemiology Collaboration Group formula. Circ Heart Fail 2012;5:309–14.

26. Pocock SJ, Ariti CA, McMurray JJ, et al. Predicting survival in heart failure: a risk score based on 39 372 patients from 30 studies. Eur Heart J 2013;34:1404–13.

27. Sartipy U, Dahlström U, Edner M, et al. Predicting survival in heart failure: validation of the MAGGIC heart failure risk score in 51 043 patients from the Swedish Heart Failure Registry. Eur J Heart Fail 2014;16:173–9.

28. Poppe KK, Squire IB, Whalley GA, et al. Known and missing left ventricular ejection fraction and survival in patients with heart failure: a MAGGIC meta-analysis report. Eur J Heart Fail 2013;15:1220–7.

29. Campbell RT, Jhund PS, Castagno D, et al. What have we learned about patients with heart failure and preserved ejection fraction from DIG-PEF, CHARM-preserved, and I-PRESERVE? J Am Coll Cardiol 2012;60:2349–56.

30. Zile MR, Gaasch WH, Anand IS, et al. Mode of death in patients with heart failure and a preserved ejection fraction: results from the Irbesartan in Heart Failure with Preserved Ejection Fraction Study (I-Preserve) trial. Circulation 2010;121:1393–405.

31. Solomon SD, Wang D, Finn P, et al. Effect of candesartan on cause-specific mortality in heart failure patients: the Candesartan in Heart failure Assessment of Reduction in Mortality and morbidity (CHARM) program. Circulation 2004;110:2180–3.

32. Solomon SD, Anavekar N, Skali H, et al. Influence of ejection fraction on cardiovascular outcomes in a broad spectrum of heart failure patients. Circulation 2005;112:3738–44.

33. Henkel D, Redfield MM, Weston S, et al. Death in heart failure: a community perspective. Circ Heart Fail 2008;1:91–7.

34. Grigorian-Shamagian L, Raviña FO, Assi EA, et al. Why and when do patients with heart failure and normal left ventricular ejection fraction die? Analysis of >600 deaths in a community long-term study. Am Heart J 2008;156:1184–90.

35. Doughty R, Yee T, Sharpe N, et al. Hospital admissions and deaths due to congestive heart failure in New Zealand, 1988-91. N Z Med J 1995;108:473–5.

36. Rydén-Bergsten T, Andersson F. The health care costs of heart failure in Sweden. J Intern Med 1999;246:275–84.

37. Stewart S, Jenkins A, Buchan S, et al. The current cost of heart failure to the National Health Service in the UK. Eur J Heart Fail 2002;4:361–71.

38. Solomon SD, Dobson J, Pocock S, et al. Influence of nonfatal hospitalization for heart failure on subsequent mortality in patients with chronic heart failure. Circulation 2007;116:1482–7.

39. Ather S, Chan W, Bozkurt B, et al. Impact of noncardiac comorbidities on morbidity and mortality in a predominantly male population with heart failure and preserved versus reduced ejection fraction. J Am Coll Cardiol 2012;59:998–1005.

40. Cleland JG, Tendera M, Adamus J, et al. The perindopril in elderly people with chronic heart failure (PEP-CHF) study. Eur Heart J 2006;27:2338–45.

41. Shah RV, Desai AS, Givertz MM. The effect of renin-angiotensin system inhibitors on mortality and heart failure hospitalization in patients with heart failure and preserved ejection fraction: a systematic review and meta-analysis. J Card Fail 2010;16:260–7.

42. van Veldhuisen DJ, McMurray JJ. Pharmacological treatment of heart failure with preserved ejection fraction: a glimpse of light at the end of the tunnel? Eur J Heart Fail 2013;15:5–8.

43. Pitt B, Remme W, Zannad F, et al. Eplerenone, a selective aldosterone blocker, in patients with left ventricular dysfunction after myocardial infarction. N Engl J Med 2003;348:1309–21.

44. Pitt B, Zannad F, Remme WJ, et al. The effect of spironolactone on morbidity and mortality in patients with severe heart failure. N Engl J Med 1999;341:709–17.

45. Zannad F, McMurray JJ, Krum H, et al. Eplerenone in patients with systolic heart failure and mild symptoms. N Engl J Med 2011;364:11–21.

46. Edelmann F, Wachter R, Schmidt AG, et al. Effect of spironolactone on diastolic function and exercise capacity in patients with heart failure with preserved ejection fraction: the Aldo-DHF randomized controlled trial. JAMA 2013;309:781–91.

47. Shah SJ, Heitner JF, Sweitzer NK, et al. Baseline characteristics of patients in the treatment of preserved cardiac function heart failure with an aldosterone antagonist trial. Circ Heart Fail 2013;6:184–92.

Clinical Trials in Patients with Heart Failure and Preserved Left Ventricular Ejection Fraction

John G.F. Cleland, MD, FRCP, FESC[a],*,
Pierpaolo Pellicori, MD[b], Riet Dierckx, MD[b]

KEYWORDS

- HFpEF • NT-proBNP • Comorbidity • Clinical trials

KEY POINTS

- Neither clinical history nor echocardiography is a reliable diagnostic method in patients with heart failure and preserved left ventricular ejection fraction (HFpEF).
- Natriuretic peptides provide a powerful diagnostic and prognostic tool in patients with HFpEF.
- Diuretics can improve symptoms and congestion.
- There is compelling but not irrefutable evidence that angiotensin-converting enzyme inhibitors improve symptoms, functional capacity, morbidity, and possibly mortality amongst patients with HFpEF.
- There is compelling but not irrefutable evidence that mineralocorticoid receptor antagonists improve outcome in patients with HFpEF and an elevated N-terminal fragment of the prohormone of brain natriuretic peptide.
- There is less evidence that digoxin or β-blockers improve the outcome of HFpEF.

INTRODUCTION

Epidemiologic reports suggest that approximately 50% of patients who have signs or symptoms of heart failure (HF) have preserved left ventricular ejection fraction (LVEF). Compared to patients with HF and a reduced LVEF (HFrEF), patients with HF and preserved LVEF (HFpEF) are older, more likely to be women, and more often have hypertension and atrial fibrillation contributing to the development of HF. Epidemiologic studies suggest that patients with HF have a similar outcome regardless of LVEF; clinical trials do not! **(Fig. 1)**.

Most clinical trials, with some notable exceptions,[1] defined HFpEF as a clinical diagnosis in the absence of a reduced LVEF. This weak definition causes problems because it does not exclude patients who have breathlessness or peripheral edema that are not primarily cardiac in origin. Treatments directed at cardiac dysfunction may be ineffective against chronic lung disease, obesity, lack of fitness, or venous insufficiency! Moreover, some of these comorbidities may be important drivers of outcome in HFpEF. The unintended consequence of excluding patients with comorbidities from clinical trials to increase their specificity for HF is a reduction in clinical event rates and loss of statistical power to show differences. The problem is further compounded by the fact that HFpEF is not one entity but many. For patients with HFrEF, using a reduced LVEF as an inclusion criterion ensures that the patient

[a] National Heart & Lung Institute, NIHR Cardiovascular Biomedical Research Unit, Royal Brompton and Harefield Hospitals NHS Trust, Imperial College, London, UK; [b] Department of Cardiology, Castle Hill Hospital, Hull and York Medical School, University of Hull, Kingston-upon-Hull, UK
* Corresponding author. Magdi Yacoub Institute, Harefield Hospital, Hill End Road, Harefield, London UB9 6JH, UK.
E-mail address: j.cleland@imperial.ac.uk

Heart Failure Clin 10 (2014) 511–523
http://dx.doi.org/10.1016/j.hfc.2014.04.011
1551-7136/14/$ – see front matter © 2014 Elsevier Inc. All rights reserved.

heartfailure.theclinics.com

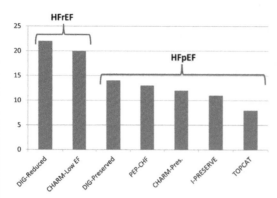

Fig. 1. Two-year mortality in patients with HFrEF and HFpEF. See text for explanation of acronyms and references.

has a cardiac problem, which may account for why clinical trials have been able to show that at least 6 interventions can reduce morbidity or mortality.[2–12] On the other hand, a normal LVEF provides no reassurance that a patient who is breathless or has swollen ankles has HF.

DIAGNOSIS AND CLASSIFICATION OF HFPEF

The diagnosis and classification of HFpEF is dealt with in detail later elsewhere in this issue, but it is appropriate to make some observations pertinent to clinical trials here. Although consensus and guidelines groups have made various recommendations for the diagnosis of HFpEF, they are relatively complex, none is universally accepted, and none has been applied to major clinical trials.[13–15] These recommendations are based on

demonstrating an elevated LV filling pressure under resting conditions. However, filling pressures may be unremarkable at rest, especially if the patient is taking diuretics, but increase steeply with volume overload or exercise.[16,17] Normal filling pressures at rest do not exclude HFpEF. Exercise capacity may not be a reliable guide either, because there are so many factors that can limit it. Natriuretic peptides are consistently powerful prognostic markers in patients with either HFrEF or HFpEF, with few exceptions,[18] and therefore provide a valuable perspective on the disease (**Fig. 2**). However, natriuretic peptides also have problems with specificity, being heavily influenced by heart rhythm and renal function, as well as myocardial function.[19,20]

The ACC/AHA guidelines for the management of HF have introduced an important distinction between those patients who have HF and those who have preserved LVEF (>40%), with 3 groups of patients being identified: "possible" HFpEF (LVEF>50%), "borderline" HFpEF (40<LVEF<49), and "improved" HFpEF (LVEF>40%) but previous evidence of HFrEF.[21] Although there is still debate about whether HFpEF and HFrEF are a continuum of the same disease or heterogeneous clusters of separate clinical entities,[22,23] the risk factors for and patient characteristics of these 2 syndromes are different.[24] The ACC/AHA guidelines also emphasize that patients with HF often have a prodromal period with a paucity of symptoms. This prodromal phase, a pathophysiology characterized by cardiomyocyte hypertrophy, an increase in myocardial collagen, and expansion of the extracellular matrix, is probably a lot longer for

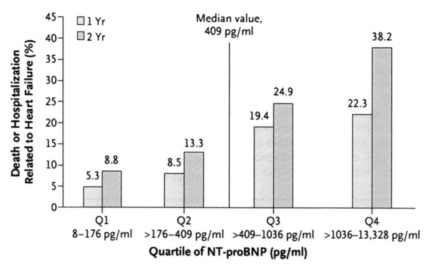

Fig. 2. Outcome according to quartiles of the plasma concentration of NT-proBNP in patients with HFpEF enrolled in the PEP-CHF study. (*From* Cleland JG, Tendera M, Adamus J, et al. The perindopril in elderly people with chronic heart failure (PEP-CHF) study. Eur Heart J 2006;27(19):2338–45; with permission.)

HFpEF than HFrEF, although symptoms may suddenly be provoked by the onset of atrial fibrillation.

Pragmatically, a combination of symptoms, use of diuretic agents to treat congestion (rather than just hypertension), left atrial dilatation, absence of substantial mitral regurgitation, and elevated plasma concentrations of natriuretic peptides (adjusted for heart rhythm, renal function, and body mass index) could be considered sufficient to secure a diagnosis of HF due to LV disease. The echocardiogram can then further inform phenotype according to LVEF, pulmonary artery pressure, and right ventricular function. More effort is required to identify different clinical phenotypes that are hidden behind the same diagnostic label and a single echocardiographic measurement of cardiac function at rest.

HARD OUTCOMES VERSUS SOFT SURROGATES

Clinically relevant outcomes should be something that patients and doctors care about. Patients who present with breathlessness and have biochemical and echocardiographic abnormalities suggesting diastolic dysfunction are often elderly, frail, and have several comorbidities. Patients with HFpEF might prefer a better quality of life and to avoid the need for hospitalization rather than seek a substantial increase in longevity. In this respect, diuretics might be considered highly effective although substantial clinical trials have not been conducted. Of course, an effective treatment of HFpEF might modify the underlying myocardial disease and thereby improve both quality of life and longevity. However, there might be a considerable delay before an intervention improves LV diastolic properties by extracellular matrix remodeling.

In summary, improvement in symptoms and reduction in morbidity may be as or more important goals for the treatment of HFpEF than a reduction in mortality. However, reduction in mortality might be a good surrogate measure of the ability of an intervention to modify disease progression and improve symptoms in the long term.

RANDOMIZED CONTROLLED TRIALS
Angiotensin-converting Enzyme Inhibitors

Only one substantial trial of angiotensin-converting enzyme (ACE) inhibitors has been conducted in HFpEF, the perindopril in elderly people with chronic heart failure (PEP-CHF) (**Fig. 3, Table 1**).[1] PEP-CHF enrolled 850 patients with HF and was unique among the large trials in requiring evidence of abnormal cardiac function.

Over the first year of follow-up, perindopril improved symptoms and distance walked in 6 minutes. A reduction in the rate of death or hospitalizations for HF was also observed with a similar relative magnitude of benefit as observed in the Studies of Left Ventricular Dysfunction (SOLVD)-treatment trial that demonstrated the benefits of enalapril in patients with HFrEF. Unfortunately, after 1 year, many patients stopped blinded therapy and, importantly, started open-label ACE inhibitors. The difference between perindopril and placebo subsequently faded. Nihilists will point out that the study failed to reach its primary endpoint and should be considered neutral. Optimists will point out the many positive aspects of the study and look for corroborative evidence.

In the Hong Kong diastolic HF study (n = 150), the use of diuretics (either loop diuretics or thiazides) quickly improved symptoms and quality of life. Addition of ramipril or irbesartan did not provide further benefit from the patients' perspective. Ramipril and irbesartan exerted similar reductions in N-terminal prohormone of brain natriuretic peptide (NT-proBNP) and improvement in cardiac function on echo.[25]

The HYVET study[26] is not, strictly speaking, a study of HFpEF but it did enroll patients who must have had a very high rate of LV diastolic dysfunction and exertional breathlessness; patients aged greater than 80 years with a systolic blood pressure of greater than 160 mm Hg. The study enrolled 3845 patients, predominantly in Europe and China, and followed them for a median of 1.8 years. Patients assigned to indapamide and perindopril (73% took the combination) had a 30% reduction in stroke, a 21% reduction in mortality, and a 64% reduction in the development of overt clinical HF on an intention-to-treat analysis (**Fig. 4**). These benefits increased to 34%, 28%, and 72%, respectively when a per-protocol analysis was applied. This trial provides corroborative evidence of the benefits of ACE inhibitors in patients with HFpEF, at least when systolic blood pressure is elevated.

Angiotensin Receptor Blockers

Apart from the Hong Kong diastolic HF study noted earlier, 2 large studies of angiotensin receptor blockers (ARBs) have been conducted (see **Fig. 3**, **Table 1**).

In the CHARM preserved trial, 3023 patients (mean age 67 years, 40% women) were randomly assigned to candesartan or placebo and followed for 37 months.[27] Eligible patients were aged greater than 18 years, had HF for more than 4 weeks, were in NYHA functional class II–IV,

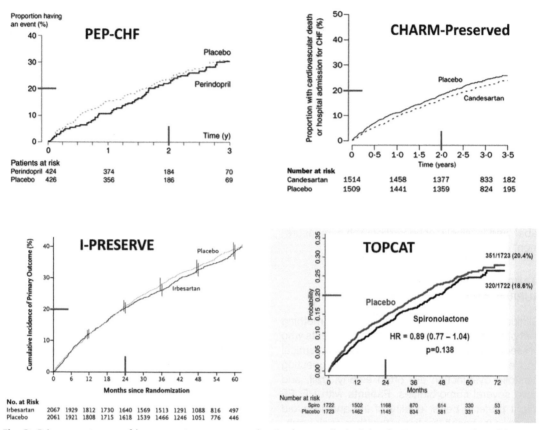

Fig. 3. Primary outcome of large, contemporary randomized controlled trials of HFpEF. Note: Red markings on the X-axes at 2 years and on the Y-axes at a 20% event rate are to assist with comparisons amongst trials. (*Data from* Refs.[1,27,29])

had a history of hospital admission for a cardiac reason, and had an LVEF greater than 40%. The primary outcome (cardiovascular death or HF admission) was neutral (22% of patients in the candesartan group vs 24% in the placebo group) (hazard ratio [HR]: 0.89, 95% confidence interval [CI] 0.77–1.03, *P* = .118); those patients randomized to candesartan had fewer hospitalizations for HF (230 vs 279; *P* = .017). Candesartan was discontinued in more patients due to hyperkalemia, worsening creatinine levels (doubled in 6% of patients on candesartan vs 3% on placebo), or hypotension. In an echo substudy of CHARM preserved, only 44% had moderate or severe diastolic dysfunction, which conferred a three-fold increased risk but it is not clear whether these patients obtained a greater benefit from candesartan.[28] Overall, CHARM suggested some benefit from ARBs.

I-PRESERVE, the largest study in HFpEF so far, randomly assigned 4128 patients (mean age 72 years, 60% women) to irbesartan or placebo and observed them for 49.5 months.[29] All patients were aged greater than 60 years, had symptoms of

HF, and an LVEF greater than 45%. Patients either had to be hospitalized for HF in the previous 6 months or have evidence of more severe HF. The primary outcome (death from any cause or hospitalization for cardiovascular cause) occurred in 36% of patients in the irbesartan group and in 37% in the placebo group (HR: 0.95 95% CI 0.86–1.05; *P* = .35). No significant differences were found between the 2 study groups for any of the other secondary outcomes. Also, there were no differences in changes in plasma NT-proBNP concentration between the 2 groups after 6 months. NT-proBNP was the strongest predictor of prognosis.[30] Further analyses suggested that patients who had only modestly elevated NT-proBNP benefitted from irbesartan but that those with grossly elevated levels did not, despite their much worse prognosis (**Fig. 5**). This suggests that there may be a "sweet spot" for therapeutic effect. Patients with too low a risk have no events and cannot benefit; patients with too high a risk will die despite intervention.[31] Detailed echocardiographic data were available in 745 patients enrolled in I-PRESERVE[32]: one-third of patients

Table 1
Outcome of randomized controlled trials of interventions acting on the renin-angiotensin-aldosterone system in patients with HFpEF (only trials with >100 patients have been reported)

Trial and Size	FU Length	Primary Outcome	Mortality	Discontinued Assigned Medication	Adverse Events
PEP-CHF[1] 850	26 mo	D-HFH Pla: 107 (25%) Per: 100 (24%) ns	Pla: 53 (12.4%) Per: 56 (13.2%)	By 18 mo Pla: 36% Per: 40%	Serious events Pla: 9 Per: 4
Hong Kong[25] 150	12 mo	QoL: improved all groups 6MWT: no change	Diur: 3 (2%) Diur + Irb: 1 (0.6%) Diur + Ram: 0	Diur: 3 Diur + Irb: 1 Diur + Ram: 6	Not reported
CHARM Preserved[27] 3023	37 mo	CVD-HFH Pla: 366 (24%) Cand: 333 (22%) ns	CVD/Non-CVD Pla: 170/74 Cand: 170/67	By 6 mo/end of study Pla: 113 (8%)/220 (18%) Cand: 157 (11%)/268 (22%)	Hypotension: 2.4% vs 1.1% ($P = .009$) Increase in creatinine: 4.8% vs 2.4% ($P<.001$) Hyperkalemia: 1.5% vs 0.9% ($P = .03$) Any: 17.8% vs 13.5% ($P = .001$)
I-PRESERVE[29] 4128	50 mo	D-CVH Pla: 763 (105 ptpy) Irb: 742 (100 ptpy) ns	Pla: 52.3 per 1000 patient-years Irb: 52.6 per 1000 patient-years $P = .07$	Pla: 14% Irb: 16%	A doubling in creatinine level occurred in 6% in Irb 4% pla ($P<.001$). 3% had K >6 mmol/L on Irb (vs 2% pla, $P = .01$).
PARAMOUNT[33] 301	36 wk	NT-proBNP lower if assigned to LCZ696 vs valsartan at 12 wk	LCZ696: 1 (0.7%) Valsartan: 2 (1.3%)		Serious events LCZ696: 22 patients (14.8%) Valsartan: 30 patients (19.7%) Angioedema in one patient assigned to LCZ696
ALDO-DHF[38] 422	12 mo	Spiro reduced E/E' but no effect on peak Vo2	Pla: 0 Spiro: 1 (<1%)	Pla: 30 (14) Spiro: 48 (23) $P = .03$	Higher incidence of worsening renal function or anemia with spiro
TOPCAT 3445	3.3 y	CVD-HFH-RCA Pla: 351 (20.4%) Spiro: 320 (18.6%) ns	Pla: 15.9% Spiro: 14.6% ns	Pla: 1 y: 14%; End: 31% Spiro: 1 y: 17%; End: 34%	Similar rate of SAE K^+ ≥5.5 greater with spiro (19% vs 9%, $P<.001$) K^+ <3.5 greater with pla (16% vs 23%, $P<.001$)

Abbreviations: Cand, Candesartan; CVD, cardiovascular death; CVH, cardiovascular hospitalization; D, death; HFH, heart failure hospitalization; Irb, irbesartan; K^+, serum potassium in mmol/L; NFMI, death and nonfatal myocardial infarction; Per, perindopril; Pla, placebo; Ram, ramipril; y, year.
Data from Refs. [1,25,27,29,33,38]

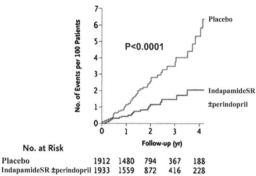

Fig. 4. HYVET: the effect of indapamide and perindo-pril compared to placebo on the development of clinically overt heart failure. (*Data from* Beckett NS, Peters R, Fletcher AE, et al. Treatment of hypertension in patients 80 years of age or older. N Engl J Med 2008;358(18):1887–98.)

did not have echocardiographic evidence of diastolic dysfunction and only 15% of patients had a more than moderately dilated left atrium (LA). Although LA enlargement and left ventricular hypertrophy provided independent prognostic information, other Doppler measurements of diastolic dysfunction, including E/E', did not.

On balance, these studies suggest that ARBs might be less effective than ACE inhibitors in patients with HFpEF.

Dual Angiotensin Receptor Blocker-Neutral Endopeptidase Inhibitors

The use of novel therapeutic molecules, like LCZ696, has shown promising results in a phase II trial (see **Table 1**).[33] Whether or not the positive effects on plasma natriuretic peptide concentrations and patients symptoms in the short term translate into better outcome on the long term has yet to be proved. However, the observed improvement in symptoms alone should be welcomed.[34,35] Recently, a large trial of LCZ in patients with HFrEF was stopped due to substantial benefit. A large outcome trial called PARAGON in patients with HFpEF and an elevated plasma concentration of natriuretic peptides is planned.

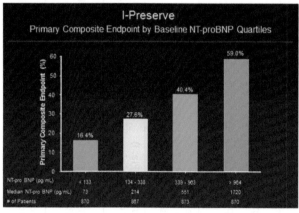

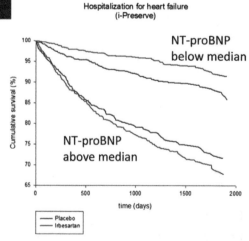

Hospitalization for heart failure
(i-Preserve)

Fig. 5. Relationship between NT-proBNP and prognosis in the I-PRESERVE trial and the effect of irbesartan above and below median NT-proBNP. (*Data from* Massie BM, Carson PE, McMurray JJ, et al. Irbesartan in patients with heart failure and preserved ejection fraction. N Engl J Med 2008;359(23):2456–67.)

Mineralocorticoid Receptor Antagonists

A series of small randomized controlled trials (RCTs)[36,37] suggested that mineralocorticoid receptor antagonists could improve some aspects of cardiac function in patients with HFpEF (see **Table 1**). In the randomized controlled Aldosterone Receptor Blockade in Diastolic Heart Failure (ALDO-DHF) trial, echocardiographic function improved in patients assigned to spironolactone (reductions in E/E′, LV end-diastolic volume, LV mass, and increases in LVEF), but this was not associated with an improvement in exercise capacity and renal function and hemoglobin declined.[38]

The larger Treatment of Preserved Cardiac Function Heart Failure with an Aldosterone Antagonist (TOPCAT) study randomized 3445 patients with HFpEF in 6 countries (US, Canada, Brazil, Argentina, Russia, Republic of Georgia) to spironolactone or placebo. The study enrolled patients with symptomatic HF, aged greater than or equal to 50 years with LVEF greater than or equal to 45% and either a hospitalization within the past year for the management of HF or elevated plasma concentrations of natriuretic peptides (BNP ≥100 pg/mL or NT-proBNP ≥360 pg/mL). Few patients in Russia or the Republic of Georgia were enrolled using the BNP criteria. Major exclusions were a glomerular filtration rate less than 30 mL/min/1.7 m2 or serum potassium greater than or equal to 5 mmol/L.

The study was neutral for its primary composite endpoint of cardiovascular mortality, aborted cardiac arrest, or hospitalization for HF. However, patients assigned to spironolactone had fewer admissions for HF, but a greater risk of hyperkalemia or worsening renal function. A prespecified subgroup analysis showed that patients enrolled using the BNP criteria, mostly patients from North America, had an event rate similar to that observed in studies of HFrEF and a 35% reduction in the primary end-point (P = .003), similar to the effects of spironolactone in HFrEF. Patients enrolled in Russia or the Republic of Georgia, based on a prior hospitalization for HF, had few events and no benefit from spironolactone. TOPCAT demonstrates that it is essential to include BNP/NT-proBNP as an entry criterion in trials of HFpEF, although the precise cut-off value for inclusion requires further exploration. Moreover, because diagnosis should always be linked to management, it provides further compelling evidence for the diagnostic importance of BNP/NT-proBNP.

β-Blockers

β-Blockers are effective in patients with HFrEF, but the evidence is less certain in patients with HFpEF (**Table 2**). In a small (n = 158) randomized study, propranolol was associated with a better cardiovascular outcome in post–myocardial infarction patients who had an LVEF greater than 40%, but had to be discontinued because of adverse effects in 14% of patients mainly because of worsening HF and hypotension.[39] In another small study (n = 97) that enrolled patients with symptoms and/or signs of HF, in sinus rhythm with an LVEF greater than 45%, carvedilol failed to improve diastolic dysfunction but did cause an increase in LA size and plasma BNP and tended to worsen symptoms.[40]

SENIORS (Study of Effects of Nebivolol Intervention on Outcomes and Rehospitalization in Seniors With Heart Failure) enrolled 2128 patients aged greater than 75 years who had either an LVEF less than 35% or a hospitalization for HF in the previous year and randomly assigned them to placebo or nebivolol. Only about 400 patients had an LVEF greater than 45%. Overall, the study showed a small reduction in the primary endpoint, death, or cardiovascular hospitalization, perhaps, in part, because of their effectiveness in reducing blood pressure, but the effect on mortality was striking in patients with LVEF less than 35%.[41] Subsequent analyses suggested no strong interaction between the benefit of nebivolol and LVEF above or below 35%,[42] but this does not entirely allay concerns that there might be no benefit in those with an LVEF greater than 45%. Also, patients with atrial fibrillation, a common comorbidity of both HFrEF and HFpEF do not appear to benefit whether or not LVEF is reduced.[43–45]

The ELANND trial enrolled 116 patients with HFpEF and evidence of diastolic dysfunction by Doppler echocardiography. Patients were randomly assigned them to placebo or nebivolol for 6 months. The 6 minute walk test improved more with placebo than with nebivolol. The authors speculated that a relative decline in exercise capacity with nebivolol may have been due to its negative chronotropic effects. No differences of effect on NT-proBNP was observed.[46] Excessive slowing of ventricular rate in HFpEF may be harmful.

Calcium Channel Blockers

Calcium antagonists are not indicated in patients with HFrEF, and probably for this reason have gained little attention in HFpEF, since the early 90s. Two small, randomized crossover studies using verapamil reported an improvement in exercise tolerance and LV diastolic function in patients with LVEF greater than 45% and hypertensive HF.[47,48] In a recent crossover trial conducted in 60 patients

Table 2
Outcome of RCTs of β-blockers, digoxin, and sildenafil in patients with HFpEF (only trials with >100 patients have been reported)

Trial and Size	FU Length	Primary Outcome	Mortality	Discontinued Assigned Medication	Adverse Events
SENIORS[41] 752 had LVEF >35%	21 mo	D-CVH Pla: 125 (34%) Neb: 110 (29%) ns	Pla: 55 (14.8%) Neb: 52 (13.7%) ns	~25% in each group	Not reported
Aronow et al,[39] 158	32 mo	D-NFMI Pro: 59% Con: 82%	Pro: 44 (56%) No Pro: 60 (76%) P = .007	Pro: 11/79 (14%)	Pro: worsening HF or hypotension in 11 patients (14%)
J-DHF[76] 245	3.2 y	CVD-HFH Pla: 34 (27.2) Carve: 29 (24.1)	Pla: 21 (16.8) Carve: 18 (15)	At end of titration, 108 patients (90%) assigned to Carve were treated with Carve	Among patients who had adverse events, Carve was discontinued in 6.
DIG-PEF[52] 988	37 mo	HFD-HFH Pla: 119 (24%) DIG: 102 (21%)	Pla: 116 (23.4%) DIG: 115 (23.4%)	Pla: 164 (33%) DIG: 159 (32%) P = .80	66 (7%) patients had suspected or confirmed DIG toxicity during routine follow-up; of them 48 occurred in DIG group (P<.001).
RELAX[60] 216	24 wk	Change In Peak Vo₂: Pla: −0.20 Sil: −0.20 ns	Pla: 0 Sil: 3	Pla: 3 (and 13 reduced dosage) Sil: 8 (and 19 reduced dosage)	AE: Pla: 78 (76%), Sil: 90 (80%) SAE: Pla 16 (16%), Sil 25 (22%) More vascular adverse events (headache, flushing, hypotension) with Sil

Abbreviations: Carve, carvedilol; CVD, cardiovascular death; CVH, cardiovascular hospitalization; D, death; DIG, digoxin; HFD, heart failure death; HFH, heart failure hospitalization; K⁺, serum potassium in mmol/L; Neb, nebivolol; NFMI, death and nonfatal myocardial infarction; Pla, placebo; Pro, propranolol; Sil, sildenafil; y, year.
Data from Refs.[39,41,52,60,76]

with AF and evidence of diastolic dysfunction (mean left atrial diameter 50 ± 7 mm and mean NT-proBNP 1039 ± 636 ng/L), diltiazem and verapamil reduced the NT-proBNP plasma levels at rest and at peak exercise compared with baseline, whereas treatment with metoprolol or carvedilol had the opposite effect.[49] Hypertension is a common cause of HF[50] and lowering blood pressure will generally improve diastolic function[51] that might be sufficient to cause remission of HF or delay or even prevent its development.

Digoxin

In the DIG (Digitalis Investigation Group) ancillary trial, 988 patients with CHF, LVEF greater than 45%, and sinus rhythm were randomized to digoxin or placebo (see **Table 2**).[52] After a mean follow-up of 37 months, patients assigned to digoxin or placebo had similar rates of the primary composite of hospitalizations for HF or cardiovascular death. However, when the analysis was restricted to the first 2 years after randomization, the effect of digoxin reduced the composite endpoint of HF-specific death or hospitalization (HR, 0.71; 95% CI, 0.52 to 0.98; P = .034), HF hospitalizations or cardiovascular mortality (HR, 0.75; 95% CI, 0.57 to 0.99; P = .044), or HF hospitalizations alone (HR, 0.66; 95% CI, 0.47 to 0.91; P = .012). In summary, there is weak evidence in favour of digoxin in patients with HFpEF but concerns about digoxin toxicity in a frail elderly population with renal dysfunction does provide a compelling case for widespread use.

Ivabradine

Several small studies have been conducted.[53,54] In a 7-day double-blind trial that included 61 patients with HFpEF, ivabradine improved peak V_{O_2} compared with control subjects, possibly by reducing the rise in LV filling pressure (E/E′ at echocardiography) during exercise.[55] A moderately large, multicentre trial has been initiated, investigating the effects of ivabradine on cardiac function, symptoms, and functional capacity.[56] Recently, animal experimental models have suggested that ivabradine may have important effects on cardiac fibroblasts and myocardial fibrosis. Ivabradine might be able to improve diastolic function through mechanisms other than heart rate reduction.[57]

Ranolazine

Several small studies have been conducted. A small, randomized, phase II study enrolled 18 patients who received ranolazine infusion followed by 2 weeks of oral treatment.[58] After 30 min of infusion, LVEDP and PCWP decreased in the ranolazine group but not in the placebo group. However, no significant echocardiographic changes were observed after infusion or at the end of the study. Furthermore, treatment with ranolazine did not alter natriuretic plasma levels or exercise capacity. A planned multicentre study has been abandoned due to low recruitment[59] and 2 ongoing trials are expected to report results in 2015.[60,61]

Sildenafil

Patients with HFpEF often develop pulmonary hypertension due to elevated left atrial pressures (see **Table 2**). Sildenafil, a phosphodiesterase-5 inhibitor, causes pulmonary vasodilation but did not alter diastolic function or pulmonary artery pressure in a multicentre trial of 216 patients with HFpEF and raised pulmonary artery pressures, nor did it result in any benefit in terms of exercise capacity or clinical status over 24 weeks.[62] Long-term, plasma concentrations of NT-proBNP and endothelin-1 increased in patients assigned to sildenafil compared with those assigned to placebo. These results contrast with a small (n = 44) one year single-centre study of sildenafil in patients with HFpEF that suggested striking benefits. The reasons for the differences between these studies is yet to be explained.[63]

Exercise Training

Impaired skeletal muscle function might contribute to exertional dyspnea and fatigue.[64] Kitzman and colleagues[65] randomized 53 elderly patients with HFpEF (mean age 70 years) to exercise training (3 days per week) or biweekly telephone calls for 16 weeks. Compared with controls, peak exercise V_{O_2} increased in those assigned to exercise, although no significant differences were observed in any echocardiographic or biochemical (BNP and norepinephrine) measurements. Similar effects of exercise training on peak V_{O_2} were also reported by Edelmann and colleagues.[66] They randomized 64 patients with HFpEF (mean age 65 years) to exercise training or usual care for 3 months. Peak V_{O_2} increased by 2.6 (1.8–3.4) ml/min/kg in those randomized to exercise, whereas no significant changes were observed in those assigned to usual care. These results were accompanied by improvement in E/E′ ratio and reversed LA remodeling in the training group as compared to the controls but not by a reduction in NT-proBNP. Furthermore, exercise training did not alter endothelial function or arterial stiffness. The increased peak V_{O_2} observed in this and other trials of exercise is probably due to improved skeletal muscle perfusion and/or oxygen utilization rather than a change in cardiac function.[67] Other substantial trials (eg, Ex-DHF-II and OPTIM-EX) have been initiated (ClinicalTrials.gov Identifier: NCT02078947).

Devices

There are no substantial trials of implantable cardiac defibrillators or cardiac resynchronization therapy in HFpEF as yet. A large trial of cardiac resynchronization therapy in patients with an LVEF in the range of 36% to 50% has recently been stopped due to poor recruitment.[68] The REDUCE-LAP-HF (REDUCE Elevated Left Atrial Pressure in Patients with HF) trial is investigating the potential of an atrial septostomy device to off-load the left atrial pressure during stress.[69] Trials of telemonitoring using noninvasive or implanted devices might help improve patient management but are confounded by the lack of effective interventions but might be used to guide diuretic therapy. Monitoring alone cannot produce clinical benefit, but the actions taken because of monitoring might.

What did We Study and What Can We do to Improve Clinical Trials?

HF is not one entity and neither is HFpEF. Many studies enrolled patients based on a clinical diagnosis, a prior history of hospitalization for what someone thought was HF, and an echocardiogram that excluded serious valve disease or HFrEF sometime in the previous 6 to 12 months.

It is likely that many patients enrolled in trials did not have HF. HFpEF may be a more paroxysmal disease than recognized so far; good treatment of hypertension may effectively cure many cases.[70,71] Excluding patients with comorbidity to try to increase diagnostic specificity for HFpEF may merely make matters worse by excluding those at high risk.[72] If the comorbidity drives the patient's clinical course, then treatment directed at cardiac dysfunction may be ineffective. Natriuretic peptides provide considerable hope for improved trial design as well as diagnosis and management in clinical practice.[20] Using echocardiographic inclusion criteria that are not associated with cardiovascular risk (such as E/E′) will result in the inclusion of patients who have little to gain in terms of improved cardiac outcomes. Other echocardiographic measurements closely associated with natriuretic peptides and adverse outcome should be explored to characterize patients and their response to treatment.[73–75] On the other hand, including patients with very high levels of NT-proBNP may identify patients who are too sick to show significant improvement from some interventions.[30,34]

SUMMARY

Although most trials have shown no favorable effects on outcome for most patients with HFpEF, there are several lessons to be learnt that should guide the direction of future RCTs. Trials should have outcomes appropriate to the needs of the patients. Often, this will not solely be mortality. Mortality should not be used as a surrogate for symptomatic efficacy. The diagnosis of HFpEF should not be based solely on clinical criteria and the absence of HFrEF. Natriuretic peptides are currently the best method for ensuring a patient has cardiac dysfunction; values of NT-proBNP greater than 250 ng/L in a patient in sinus rhythm who does not have important renal dysfunction indicates both cardiac dysfunction and an adverse prognosis. Thresholds will differ for those in atrial fibrillation or with renal dysfunction. Cardiac imaging focusing on atrial dilatation is the best alternative or corroborative test. HFpEF is heterogeneous and only some phenotypes and etiologies may respond to a particular intervention. Good diagnosis and (echocardiographic) phenotyping is essential. Comorbidity is the rule not the exception. Exclusion of patients with comorbidity is more often a sin than a virtue. Finally, ethnicity, cultural differences, and local practice might influence trial results and this must be kept in mind when planning expensive multicentre RCTs.

REFERENCES

1. Cleland JG, et al. The perindopril in elderly people with chronic heart failure (PEP-CHF) study. Eur Heart J 2006;27(19):2338–45.
2. Effects of enalapril on mortality in severe congestive heart failure. Results of the cooperative north scandinavian enalapril survival study (CONSENSUS). The CONSENSUS Trial Study Group. N Engl J Med 1987;316(23):1429–35.
3. Effect of enalapril on survival in patients with reduced left ventricular ejection fractions and congestive heart failure. The SOLVD Investigators. N Engl J Med 1991;325(5):293–302.
4. Packer M, et al. Effect of carvedilol on the morbidity of patients with severe chronic heart failure: results of the carvedilol prospective randomized cumulative survival (COPERNICUS) study. Circulation 2002;106(17):2194–9.
5. Effect of metoprolol CR/XL in chronic heart failure: metoprolol CR/XL randomised intervention trial in congestive heart failure (MERIT-HF). Lancet 1999; 353(9169):2001–7.
6. The cardiac insufficiency bisoprolol study II (CIBIS-II): a randomised trial. Lancet 1999;353(9146): 9–13.
7. Pitt B, et al. The EPHESUS trial: eplerenone in patients with heart failure due to systolic dysfunction complicating acute myocardial infarction. Eplerenone Post-AMI Heart Failure Efficacy and Survival Study. Cardiovasc Drugs Ther 2001;15(1):79–87.
8. Effectiveness of spironolactone added to an angiotensin-converting enzyme inhibitor and a loop diuretic for severe chronic congestive heart failure (the Randomized Aldactone Evaluation Study [RALES]). Am J Cardiol 1996;78(8):902–7.
9. Cleland JG, et al. Longer-term effects of cardiac resynchronization therapy on mortality in heart failure [the CArdiac REsynchronization-Heart Failure (CARE-HF) trial extension phase]. Eur Heart J 2006;27(16):1928–32.
10. Cleland JG, et al. An individual patient meta-analysis of five randomized trials assessing the effects of cardiac resynchronization therapy on morbidity and mortality in patients with symptomatic heart failure. Eur Heart J 2013;34(46):3547–56.
11. Bardy GH, et al. Amiodarone or an implantable cardioverter-defibrillator for congestive heart failure. N Engl J Med 2005;352(3):225–37.
12. Swedberg K, et al. Ivabradine and outcomes in chronic heart failure (SHIFT): a randomised placebo-controlled study. Lancet 2010;376(9744): 875–85.
13. Paulus WJ, et al. How to diagnose diastolic heart failure: a consensus statement on the diagnosis of heart failure with normal left ventricular ejection fraction by the Heart Failure and Echocardiography

Associations of the European Society of Cardiology. Eur Heart J 2007;28(20):2539–50.

14. Penicka M, et al. Heart failure with preserved ejection fraction in outpatients with unexplained dyspnea: a pressure-volume loop analysis. J Am Coll Cardiol 2010;55(16):1701–10.

15. McMurray JJ, et al. ESC guidelines for the diagnosis and treatment of acute and chronic heart failure 2012: the task force for the diagnosis and treatment of acute and chronic heart failure 2012 of the European Society of Cardiology. Developed in collaboration with the Heart Failure Association (HFA) of the ESC. Eur J Heart Fail 2012;14(8): 803–69.

16. Borlaug BA, et al. Exercise hemodynamics enhance diagnosis of early heart failure with preserved ejection fraction. Circ Heart Fail 2010;3(5): 588–95.

17. Maeder MT, et al. Hemodynamic basis of exercise limitation in patients with heart failure and normal ejection fraction. J Am Coll Cardiol 2010;56(11): 855–63.

18. Kociol RD, et al. Admission, discharge, or change in B-type natriuretic peptide and long-term outcomes: data from organized program to initiate life-saving treatment in hospitalized patients with heart failure (OPTIMIZE-HF) linked to Medicare claims. Circ Heart Fail 2011;4(5):628–36.

19. Cleland JG, et al. Plasma concentration of amino-terminal pro-brain natriuretic peptide in chronic heart failure: prediction of cardiovascular events and interaction with the effects of rosuvastatin: a report from CORONA (controlled rosuvastatin multinational trial in heart failure). J Am Coll Cardiol 2009;54(20):1850–9.

20. Cleland JG, et al. Relationship between plasma concentrations of N-terminal pro brain natriuretic peptide and the characteristics and outcome of patients with a clinical diagnosis of diastolic heart failure: a report from the PEP-CHF study. Eur J Heart Fail 2012;14(5):487–94.

21. Yancy CW, et al. 2013 ACCF/AHA guideline for the management of heart failure: executive summary: a report of the American College of Cardiology Foundation/American Heart Association task force on practice guidelines. Circulation 2013;128(16):1810–52.

22. Borlaug BA, Redfield MM. Diastolic and systolic heart failure are distinct phenotypes within the heart failure spectrum. Circulation 2011;123(18): 2006–13 [discussion: 2014].

23. De Keulenaer GW, Brutsaert DL. Systolic and diastolic heart failure are overlapping phenotypes within the heart failure spectrum. Circulation 2011;123(18):1996–2004 [discussion: 2005].

24. Brouwers FP, et al. Incidence and epidemiology of new onset heart failure with preserved vs. reduced ejection fraction in a community-based cohort:

25. Yip GW, et al. The Hong Kong diastolic heart failure study: a randomised controlled trial of diuretics, irbesartan and ramipril on quality of life, exercise capacity, left ventricular global and regional function in heart failure with a normal ejection fraction. Heart 2008;94(5):573–80.

26. Beckett NS, et al. Treatment of hypertension in patients 80 years of age or older. N Engl J Med 2008; 358(18):1887–98.

27. Yusuf S, et al. Effects of candesartan in patients with chronic heart failure and preserved left-ventricular ejection fraction: the CHARM-preserved trial. Lancet 2003;362(9386):777–81.

28. Persson H, et al. Diastolic dysfunction in heart failure with preserved systolic function: need for objective evidence: results from the CHARM echocardiographic Substudy-CHARMES. J Am Coll Cardiol 2007;49(6):687–94.

29. Massie BM, et al. Irbesartan in patients with heart failure and preserved ejection fraction. N Engl J Med 2008;359(23):2456–67.

30. Anand IS, et al. Prognostic value of baseline plasma amino-terminal pro-brain natriuretic peptide and its interactions with irbesartan treatment effects in patients with heart failure and preserved ejection fraction: findings from the I-PRESERVE trial. Circ Heart Fail 2011;4(5):569–77.

31. Cleland JG, et al. Cardiac resynchronization therapy: are modern myths preventing appropriate use? J Am Coll Cardiol 2009;53(7):608–11.

32. Zile MR, et al. Prevalence and significance of alterations in cardiac structure and function in patients with heart failure and a preserved ejection fraction. Circulation 2011;124(23):2491–501.

33. Solomon SD, et al. The angiotensin receptor neprilysin inhibitor LCZ696 in heart failure with preserved ejection fraction: a phase 2 double-blind randomised controlled trial. Lancet 2012; 380(9851):1387–95.

34. Cleland JG, Pellicori P. Defining diastolic heart failure and identifying effective therapies. JAMA 2013; 309(8):825–6.

35. Pellicori P, et al. Does speckle tracking really improve diagnosis and risk stratification in patients with HeFNEF? JACC, in press.

36. Mottram P, et al. Effect of aldosterone antagonism on myocardial dysfunction in hypertensive patients with diastolic heart failure. Circulation 2004;110(5): 558–65.

37. Deswal A, et al. Results of the randomized aldosterone antagonism in heart failure with preserved ejection fraction trial (RAAM-PEF). J Card Fail 2011;17(8):634–42.

38. Edelmann F, et al. Effect of spironolactone on diastolic function and exercise capacity in patients

11-year follow-up of PREVEND. Eur Heart J 2013; 34(19):1424–31.

with heart failure with preserved ejection fraction: the Aldo-DHF randomized controlled trial. JAMA 2013;309(8):781–91.

39. Aronow WS, Ahn C, Kronzon I. Effect of propranolol versus no propranolol on total mortality plus nonfatal myocardial infarction in older patients with prior myocardial infarction, congestive heart failure, and left ventricular ejection fraction > or = 40% treated with diuretics plus angiotensin-converting enzyme inhibitors. Am J Cardiol 1997;80(2):207–9.

40. Bergström A, et al. Effect of carvedilol on diastolic function in patients with diastolic heart failure and preserved systolic function. Results of the Swedish Doppler-echocardiographic study (SWEDIC). Eur J Heart Fail 2004;6(4):453–61.

41. Flather MD, et al. Randomized trial to determine the effect of nebivolol on mortality and cardiovascular hospital admission in elderly patients with heart failure (SENIORS). Eur Heart J 2005;26(3):215–25.

42. van Veldhuisen DJ, et al. Beta-blockade with nebivolol in elderly heart failure patients with impaired and preserved left ventricular ejection fraction: data from SENIORS (study of effects of nebivolol intervention on outcomes and rehospitalization in seniors with heart failure). J Am Coll Cardiol 2009;53(23):2150–8.

43. Mulder BA, et al. Effect of nebivolol on outcome in elderly patients with heart failure and atrial fibrillation: insights from SENIORS. Eur J Heart Fail 2012;14(10):1171–8.

44. Rienstra M, et al. Beta-blockers and outcome in heart failure and atrial fibrillationa meta-analysis. JACC Heart Fail 2013;1(1):21–8.

45. Cullington D, et al. Is heart rate important for patients with heart failure in atrial fibrillation? JACC Heart Fail 2014;2(3).

46. Conraads VM1, Metra M, Kamp O, et al. Effects of the long-term administration of nebivolol on the clinical symptoms, exercise capacity, and left ventricular function of patients with diastolic dysfunction: results of the ELANDD study. Eur J Heart Fail 2012;14(2):219–25.

47. Setaro JF, et al. Usefulness of verapamil for congestive heart failure associated with abnormal left ventricular diastolic filling and normal left ventricular systolic performance. Am J Cardiol 1990;66(12):981–6.

48. Hung MJ, et al. Effect of verapamil in elderly patients with left ventricular diastolic dysfunction as a cause of congestive heart failure. Int J Clin Pract 2002;56(1):57–62.

49. Ulimoen SR, et al. Calcium channel blockers improve exercise capacity and reduce N-terminal Pro-B-type natriuretic peptide levels compared with beta-blockers in patients with permanent atrial fibrillation. Eur Heart J 2014;35(8):517–24.

50. Levy D, et al. The progression from hypertension to congestive heart failure. JAMA 1996;275(20):1557–62.

51. Solomon SD, et al. Effect of angiotensin receptor blockade and antihypertensive drugs on diastolic function in patients with hypertension and diastolic dysfunction: a randomised trial. Lancet 2007;369(9579):2079–87.

52. Ahmed A, et al. Effects of digoxin on morbidity and mortality in diastolic heart failure: the ancillary digitalis investigation group trial. Circulation 2006;114(5):397–403.

53. Cocco G, Jerie P. Comparison between ivabradine and low-dose digoxin in the therapy of diastolic heart failure with preserved left ventricular systolic function. Clin Pract 2013;3(2).

54. Cice G, et al. Efficacy and safety of Ivabradine in hemodialysed patients with diastolic heart failure in ESC congress. 2011.

55. Kosmala W, et al. Effect of If-channel inhibition on hemodynamic status and exercise tolerance in heart failure with preserved ejection fraction: a randomized trial. J Am Coll Cardiol 2013;62(15):1330–8.

56. Effect of ivabradine versus placebo on cardiac function, exercise capacity, and neuroendocrine activation in patients with chronic heart failure with preserved left ventricular ejection fraction an 8-month, randomised double-blind, placebo controlled, international, multicentre study. EDIFY. Available at: http://apps.who.int/trialsearch/trial.aspx?trialid=EUCTR2012-002742-20-DE.

57. Navaratnarajah M, Ibrahim M, Siedlecka U, et al. Influence of ivabradine on reverse remodelling during mechanical unloading. Cardiovasc Res 2013;97(2):230–9.

58. Maier LS, et al. Ranolazine for the treatment of diastolic heart failure in patients with preserved ejection fraction: the RALI-DHF proof-of-concept study JCHF. JACC Heart Fail 2013;1(2):115–22.

59. Effect of ranolazine in heart failure patients with preserved ejection fraction. Available at: https://www.clinicaltrialsregister.eu/ctr-search/search?query=eudract_number:2011-000805-27.

60. The use of ranolazine for atrial fibrillation and diastolic heart (RAD HF). Available at: http://clinicaltrials.gov/ct2/show/NCT01887353?term=Ranolazine&rank=35.

61. The effects of ranolazine on exercise capacity in patients with heart failure with preserved ejection fraction (RAZE).

62. Redfield MM, et al. Effect of phosphodiesterase-5 inhibition on exercise capacity and clinical status in heart failure with preserved ejection fraction: a randomized clinical trial. JAMA 2013;309(12):1268–77.

63. Guazzi M, Vicenzi M, Arena R, et al. Pulmonary hypertension in heart failure with preserved ejection

fraction: a target of phosphodiesterase-5 inhibition in a 1-year study. Circulation 2011 Jul 12;124(2): 164–74.

64. Clark AL, Poole-Wilson PA, Coats AJ. Exercise limitation in chronic heart failure: central role of the periphery. J Am Coll Cardiol 1996;28(5): 1092–102.

65. Kitzman DW, et al. Exercise training in older patients with heart failure and preserved ejection fraction: a randomized, controlled, single-blind trial. Circ Heart Fail 2010;3(6):659–67.

66. Edelmann F, et al. Exercise training improves exercise capacity and diastolic function in patients with heart failure with preserved ejection fraction: results of the Ex-DHF (exercise training in diastolic heart failure) pilot study. J Am Coll Cardiol 2011; 58(17):1780–91.

67. Kitzman DW, et al. Effect of endurance exercise training on endothelial function and arterial stiffness in older patients with heart failure and preserved ejection fraction: a randomized, controlled, single-blind trial. J Am Coll Cardiol 2013;62(7):584–92.

68. MIRACLE-EF clinical study. Available at: http://clinicaltrials.gov/show/NCT01735916.

69. REDUCE LAP-HF tRIAL: a study to evaluate the DC devices, Inc. IASD™ system II to reduce elevated left atrial pressure in patients with heart failure.

Available at: http://clinicaltrials.gov/ct2/show/NCT01913613.

70. Banerjee P, et al. Diastolic heart failure. Paroxysmal or chronic? Eur J Heart Fail 2004;6(4):427–31.

71. Bulpitt CJ, et al. Results of the pilot study for the hypertension in the very elderly trial. J Hypertens 2003;21(12):2409–17.

72. Cleland JG, Taylor J, Tendera M. Prognosis in heart failure with a normal ejection fraction. N Engl J Med 2007;357(8):829–30.

73. Lam CS, et al. Pulmonary hypertension in heart failure with preserved ejection fraction: a community-based study. J Am Coll Cardiol 2009;53(13): 1119–26.

74. Pellicori P, et al. IVC diameter in patients with chronic heart failure: relationships and prognostic significance. JACC Cardiovasc Imaging 2013; 6(1):16–28.

75. Pellicori P, et al. Global longitudinal strain in patients with suspected heart failure and a normal ejection fraction: does it improve diagnosis and risk stratification? Int J Cardiovasc Imaging 2014; 30:69–79.

76. Yamamoto K, et al. Effects of carvedilol on heart failure with preserved ejection fraction: the Japanese Diastolic Heart Failure Study (J-DHF). Eur J Heart Fail 2013;15(1):110–8.

Current Therapeutic Approach in Heart Failure with Preserved Ejection Fraction

Jose Nativi-Nicolau, MD[a,b], John J. Ryan, MD[a],
James C. Fang, MD[a,b],*

KEYWORDS

- Heart failure • Diastole • Therapy

KEY POINTS

- Heart failure with preserved ejection fraction (HFpEF) is classically characterized by diastolic dysfunction, but multiple other mechanisms have been identified as potential targets for therapy.
- In HFpEF, large randomized clinical trials have failed to identify specific pharmacologic agents that improve clinical outcomes.
- The current management of HFpEF is directed to symptomatic relief of congestion with diuretics and risk factor modification.

BACKGROUND

Heart failure with preserved ejection fraction (HFpEF) is a clinical syndrome characterized by decreased exercise capacity and fluid retention in the setting of preserved left ventricular systolic function and evidence of abnormal diastolic function.[1] Left ventricular dysfunction is the hallmark mechanism,[2] but several other physiologic abnormalities are prevalent and have been independently associated with the clinical syndrome. Multiple strategies have attempted to modify these mechanisms independently (**Box 1**). Moreover, the co-morbidity burden in this population is high,[3,4] making therapeutic options a clinical challenge (**Table 1**). Compared with patients with heart failure with reduced ejection fraction (HFrEF), there is still no therapy that improves the long-term clinical outcomes in patients with HFpEF and the few

guideline-based recommendations are derived from expert opinions. However, finding therapies remains an active area of investigation; in January 2014, there were more than 40 open clinical trials in HFpEF registered in www.clinicaltrials.gov. Potential interventions are summarized in **Table 2**.

PHARMACOLOGIC THERAPY
Renin-Angiotensin System Antagonists

Patients with HFpEF have elevated plasma renin activity but to a lesser magnitude compared with patients with HFrEF.[5] The activation of the renin-angiotensin system (RAS) produces hypertension, left ventricular hypertrophy (LVH), and fibrosis, which are common pathologic findings in patients with HFpEF.[6–8] Furthermore, therapeutic blockade of the RAS system, through angiotensin-converting-enzyme (ACE) inhibitors, angiotensin

[a] Division of Cardiovascular Medicine, Department of Medicine, University of Utah Health Science Center, 50 N Medical Dr, Salt Lake City, UT 84132, USA; [b] Cardiology Section, Veterans Affairs Salt Lake City Health Care System, 500 Foothill Dr, Salt Lake City, UT 84148, USA
* Corresponding author. Division of Cardiovascular Medicine, University of Utah Health Sciences Center, 30 North 1900 East, Room 4A100, Salt Lake City, UT 84132.
E-mail address: james.fang@hsc.utah.edu

Heart Failure Clin 10 (2014) 525–538
http://dx.doi.org/10.1016/j.hfc.2014.04.007
1551-7136/14/$ – see front matter © 2014 Elsevier Inc. All rights reserved.

Box 1
Therapeutic Strategies in heart failure with preserved ejection fraction (HFpEF)

A. Targets for pharmacologic therapy

   1. Renin-angiotensin system inhibition

   2. Beta receptors blockade

   3. Aldosterone receptor blockade

   4. Calcium channel blockade

   5. Digoxin

   6. Statins

   7. Nitric oxide bioavailability

   8. Late sodium channels blockade

   9. I_f channel blockade

B. Targets for nonpharmacological therapy

   1. Devices

      a. Right atrial pacing

      b. Left atrial pacing

      c. Biventricular pacing

      d. Baroreflex activation therapy

   2. Low salt diet

   3. Exercise

---

receptor blockers (ARBs), and aldosterone blockade has improved outcomes in patients with HFrEF,[9–15] hypertension,[16] and risk factors for cardiovascular disease.[17,18] However, the results of clinical trials to date have not supported this strategy in HFpEF, despite the benefits in other cardiovascular conditions.

Three randomized clinical trials (RCTs) have evaluated the effects of RAS blockade in patients with HFpEF. The Candesartan Cilexetil in Heart Failure Assessment of Reduction in Mortality and Morbidity (CHARM)-Preserved trial compared candesartan versus placebo. After 37 months, there was no difference in the composite primary end point for cardiovascular death or heart failure readmission, but fewer patients were admitted with heart failure in the candesartan group (230 vs 279, $P = .017$). The study did not include measurements of diastolic dysfunction, and the diagnosis of HFpEF was clinically determined by the site investigator. There was a low overall death rate of 23% during the extended trial follow-up.[19]

A second trial, Perindopril in Elderly People with Chronic Heart Failure (PEP-CHF), compared perindopril versus placebo. The primary end point of all-cause mortality and heart failure admission was similar between groups. Although most patients had evidence of left atrial enlargement and

LVH (>75%), the N-terminal-pro-brain natriuretic peptide (NT-pro-BNP) was only mildly elevated and higher in the placebo group (mean 335 pg/mL in the perindopril group vs 453 pg/mL in the placebo group). The overall event rate was low (24%), limiting the power of the study. Moreover, at the end of follow-up, 35% of patients assigned to perindopril and 37% assigned to placebo were on open-label ACE-inhibitors.[20]

In the Irbesartan in Patients with Heart Failure and Preserved Ejection Fraction (I-PRESERVE) trial of irbesartan against placebo there was no statistically significant difference in the primary outcome of death from any cause or cardiovascular admission. Similar to previous trials, the HFpEF diagnosis was established by the site investigator without requiring echocardiographic documentation of diastolic dysfunction and with only modest elevations in the NT-pro-BNP (medians 360 pg/mL in the irbesartan arm vs 320 pg/mL in the placebo arm). However, compared with the previous trials, the follow-up was longer (50 months) and the event rates were higher (36%), but study-drug discontinuation remained high (34%).[21]

In contrast to the randomized data, observational studies have come to different conclusions. Lund and colleagues[22] published data from the Swedish Heart Failure Registry of 41,791 patients from 2000 to 2011. In a propensity score-matched analysis of 6658 subjects in outpatient clinics with LVEF of 40% or higher, the survival at 1 year was higher in patients treated with RAS antagonists versus untreated patients (77% vs 72% respectively, HR 0.91; 95% CI 0.85–0.98; $P = .008$). The investigators suggested that their study was more representative of HFpEF than the previous RCTs because the mean age was 79 years, with more women (53%), sicker patients (median NT-pro-BNP 2493 pg/mL), and 1-year mortality of almost 30%. However, confounding from unmeasured variables despite propensity matching is highly likely. Furthermore, the results could be attributed to the management of other concomitant conditions, such as hypertension, rather than HFpEF. Also, the medications were prescribed by different providers, including internal medicine physicians, geriatricians, cardiologists, and outpatient heart failure nurse clinicians, introducing a wide variability in practices with undefined reasons for the prescriptions (eg, hypertension, heart failure, and nephropathy).

Mujib and colleagues[23] reported the results of another propensity score analysis of 4189 patients with LVEF of 40% or higher from the Organized Program to Initiate Lifesaving Treatment in Hospitalized Patients with Heart Failure (OPTIMIZE-HF) trial linked to Medicare data. After balancing for 114 patient characteristics, the patients who were

Table 1
Registered trials in heart failure with preserved ejection fraction by 2014

Intervention/Study	Mechanism
Pharmacologic	
Amlodipine	Calcium channel blocker
Nitrites	Nitric oxide production
Isosorbide dinitrate vs isosorbide dinitrate + hydralazine	Vasodilation
Udenafil (ULTIMATE-HFpEF)	Phosphodiesterase 5 inhibitor
BAY1021189 (SOCRATES-PRESERVED)	Guanylate cyclase stimulator
Perhexiline	Mitochondrial carnitine inhibitor
Sildenafil	Pulmonary vasodilation
Diuretics + dopamine	Improvement in renal perfusion
Ranolazine (RAD-HF)	Inhibition of late sodium currents
Nifedipine	Calcium channel blocker
Ambrisentan	Endothelin blocker
Anakinra	Interleukin-1 receptor antagonist
Erythropoietin	Stimulates red-cell production
Nonpharmacological	
Exercise training	Improve endothelial dysfunction
Intracardiac defibrillators (VIP-HF)	Prevention of sudden death
Renal sympathetic denervation	Decrease sympathetic nervous system activity
Left atrial pacing (LEAD)	Improve atrial dyssynchrony
Interatrial septal device	Interatrial shunting

Abbreviations: LEAD, LEft Atrial Pacing in Diastolic Heart Failure; RAD-HF, Ranolazine for Atrial Fibrillation and Diastolic Heart Failure; SOCRATES-PRESERVED, SOluble Guanylate Cyclase stimulatoR in heArT failurE patientS with PRESERVED EF; ULTIMATE-HFpEF, Randomized Trial of Udenafil Therapy in Patients With Heart Failure With Preserved Ejection Fraction; VIP-HF, Value of ICD Implantation in Patients With Heart Failure and Preserved Ejection Fraction.

initiated on ACE inhibitors after a heart failure admission had a 9% reduction in the composite end point of all-cause mortality or heart failure admission (HR 0.91; 95% CI 0.84–0.99; $P = .028$), but without a difference in the independent end points. The variability in brands and doses of ACE inhibitors and the potential of crossovers limit the analysis.

In conclusion, the totality of observational data, randomized trials, and the current understanding of HFpEF suggest that RAS antagonism for the primary goal of improving outcomes in HFpEF at best provides modest benefits. However, such a therapeutic strategy does not appear harmful and should be considered for the treatment of appropriate concomitant common comorbidities in HFpEF.

Beta-Blockers

Similarly to patients with HFrEF, patients with HFpEF have elevated serum levels of norepinephrine,[5] suggesting a potential target for therapy. Beta-blockers have demonstrated improved

survival, left ventricular function, and myocardial remodeling in animal models of hypertension with diastolic heart failure.[24,25]

Initial retrospective data in patients with LVEF of 40% or higher suggested improved survival in patients treated with beta-blockers,[26] but this concept has being challenged in other registry analyses[27] and RCTs. The Effect of Long-term Administration of Nebivolol on clinical symptoms, exercise capacity and left ventricular function in patients with Diastolic Dysfunction (ELANDD) trial randomized 116 patients with NYHA II to III, LVEF greater than 45%, and echocardiographic evidence of diastolic dysfunction to nebivolol 10 mg daily versus placebo. After 6 months of treatment, there was no change in 6-minute walk test distance or peak oxygen uptake. The investigators suggested that the negative chronotropic effects of nebivolol could be the reason for the lack of response to exercise capacity.[28]

In the Study of the Effects of Nebivolol Intervention on Outcomes and Rehospitalisation in Seniors (SENIORS) trial of nebivolol versus placebo, there was a modest decrease in the primary composite

Table 2
Summary of large randomized clinical trials in heart failure with preserved ejection fraction

	CHARM-Preserved[19]	SENIORS[29]	PEP-CHF[20]	Ancillary DIG[87]	I-PRESERVE[21]	TOPCAT[38]
Year	2003	2004	2006	2006	2008	2013
Target daily dose	Candesartan 32 mg	Nebivolol 10 mg	Perindopril 4 mg	Digoxin (0.125–0.5 mg)	Irbesartan 300 mg	Aldactone 30 mg
Size	3023	752	850	988	4128	3445
LVEF	>40%	>35%	>40%	>45%	≥45%	≥45%
Inclusion criteria	NYHA II–IV	>70 y heart failure admission	>70 y, diagnosis of heart failure treated with diuretics, diastolic dysfunction by echo	NYHA I–IV	≥60 y, NYHA II–IV	Admission for heart failure or BNP ≥100 pg/mL or NT-pro-BNP ≥360 pg/mL
Mean age, y	67	76	76	67	72	69
Female %	40	50	55	41	60	51
Primary end point death/hospitalization HR (95% CI) P value	0.86 (0.74–1.00) P = .051	0.81 (0.63–1.04) P = .720	0.92 (0.70–1.21) P = .545	0.82 (0.63–1.07) P = .136	0.95 (0.86–1.05) P = .35	0.89 (0.77–1.04) P = .138
Secondary end point hospitalization HR (95% CI) P value	0.84 (0.70–1.00) P = .047	0.89 (0.70–1.14) P = .586	0.86 (0.61–1.20) P = .375	1.03 (0.89–1.2) P = .683		0.83 (0.69–0.99) P = .042
Death rate drug vs placebo	11% vs 11%	14% vs 15%	13% vs 12%	23% vs 23%	11% vs 11%	9% vs 10%
Hospitalization rate drug vs placebo	16% vs 18%	33% vs 35%	15% vs 17%	12% vs 15%	25% vs 26%	12% vs 14%

Abbreviations: BNP, B-natriuretic peptide; CHARM, Candesartan Cilexetil in Heart Failure Assessment of Reduction in Mortality and Morbidity; CI, confidence interval; DIG, Digitalis Investigation Group; HR, hazard ratio; I-PRESERVE, Irbesartan in Patients with Heart Failure and Preserved Ejection Fraction; LVEF, left ventricular ejection fraction; NYHA, New York Heart Association; PEP-CHF, Perindopril in Elderly People with Chronic Heart Failure; SENIORS, Study of the Effects of Nebivolol Intervention on Outcomes and Rehospitalisation in Seniors; TOPCAT, Treatment Of Preserved Cardiac function heart failure with an aldersterone anTagonist.
Data from Refs.[19–21,29,38,87]

end point of all-cause mortality or cardiovascular admission (HR 0.86; 95% CI 0.74–0.99; *P* = .039) with nebivolol. The effects of nebivolol were similar in patients with LVEF 35% or higher and less than 35%,[29,30] but only a third of patients had an LVEF greater than 35% and the trial was not powered to identify a difference in reduced versus preserved EF subgroups. The subgroup of patients with an LVEF greater than 50% was too small to draw meaningful conclusions.

The Japanese Diastolic Heart Failure (J-DHF) study compared the effects of carvedilol versus placebo in 245 patients with a clinical diagnosis of heart failure and LVEF greater than 40%. After a median follow-up of 3.2 years, there were no differences in the composite end point of cardiovascular death or heart failure admission. The study did show lower rates of the primary end point in patients who achieved standard doses (defined >7.5 mg daily) compared with controls (HR 0.54; 95% CI 0.303–0.959; *P* = .0356). However, the study was underpowered and had a low event rate of 8% compared with the expected 30%.[31]

The available evidence does not provide conclusive evidence for beta-blockade in HFpEF. Moreover, beta-blockade may exacerbate chronotropic incompetence, which is common in HFpEF. For these reasons, routine use of beta blockade for the treatment of HFpEF cannot be advocated. However, specific subgroups, such as patients with concomitant atrial fibrillation, may derive a clinical benefit from empiric beta blockade to improve diastolic filling time.

Aldosterone Receptor Blockade

Aldosterone is known to be related to diastolic mechanisms, including hypertension, LVH, and collagen accumulation.[32] Elevated serum aldosterone levels are an independent risk factor for mortality, with strong associations with stroke and sudden death in patients with coronary artery disease.[33] In patients with HFrEF, aldosterone blockade has demonstrated improved survival in patients with mild to severe symptoms when added to neurohumoral blockade with ACE inhibitors and beta-blockers.[34,35] In patients with HFpEF, serum aldosterone levels are independently associated with echocardiographic evidence of LVH, suggesting that aldosterone blockade may improve diastolic function.[36]

The Aldosterone Receptor Blockade in Diastolic Heart Failure (Aldo-DHF) trial compared spironolactone 25 mg daily versus placebo in 422 patients with LVEF of 50% or higher, echocardiographic evidence of diastolic dysfunction or atrial fibrillation, and peak Vo_2 of 25 mL/kg/min or less.[37]

At 12 months, patients on spironolactone had improved left ventricular end-diastolic filling, left ventricular mass index, and neurohumoral activation. However, there was no difference in left atrial size or in the clinical end points of exercise capacity, symptoms, or quality of life. Similar to previous HFpEF trials, the population was healthier (87% NYHA II), had low NT-pro-BNP levels (median 153 ng/L), and few comorbidities (5% with atrial fibrillation). However at 12 months there was significant decrease in the systolic and diastolic blood pressure, which may support blood pressure control in this population.[37]

The Treatment Of Preserved Cardiac function heart failure with an aldersterone anTagonist (TOPCAT) trial was designed to address clinical outcomes of aldosterone blockade in HFpEF. A total of 3445 patients with LVEF of 45% or higher and at least 1 admission for heart failure in the preceding 12 months (or BNP ≥100 pg/mL or NT-pro-BNP ≥360 pg/mL if no hospitalization) were randomized to spironolactone (target dose of 30 mg daily) or placebo. After an average follow-up of 3.5 years, there was no difference in the primary end point of cardiovascular death, heart failure admission, or surviving a cardiac arrest (HR 0.89; 95% CI 0.77–1.04; *P* = .138). There was a reduction in the secondary end point of heart failure readmissions (12% in spironolactone group vs 14.2% in the placebo group, HR 0.83; 95% CI 0.69–0.99; *P* = .042). This finding may not have been surprising in that spironolactone has a diuretic effect, albeit modest.[38]

Unfortunately, the trial evidence to date does not allow firm conclusions regarding the routine use of spironolactone in HFpEF. If aldosterone blockade is considered in the continuum of heart failure syndromes, its diuretic effect appreciated, and its role in the myocardial and vascular fibrosis is considered, it would appear reasonable to consider its selective use in HFpEF, potentially to reduce heart failure hospitalization.

Sildenafil

A paradigm of microvascular dysfunction and abnormal cyclic guanosine monophosphate (cGMP) signaling has been proposed as an underlying mechanism for HFpEF. Paulus proposes that concomitant comorbidities promote inflammation and lead to decreased nitric oxide (NO) bioavailability in the endothelium (**Fig. 1**). The decrease in NO affects cGMP-dependent protein kinase G signaling in the myocyte with subsequent hypertrophy and stiffness.[39,40] Animal and human models also have demonstrated upregulation of the myocyte phosphodiesterase type 5 (PDE5) expression in failing and hypertrophied right

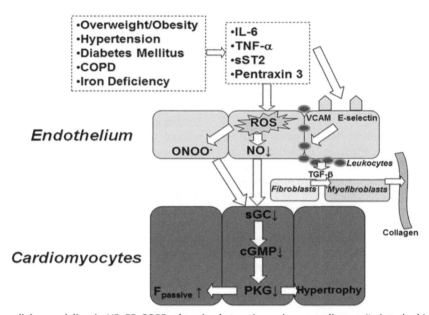

Fig. 1. Myocardial remodeling in HFpEF. COPD, chronic obstructive pulmonary disease; IL, interleukin; PKG, protein Kinase G; ROS, reactive oxygen species; sST2, soluble ST2; sGC, Soluble guanylate cyclase; TGF, transforming growth factor; TNF, tumor necrosis factor; VCAM, vascular cell adhesion molecule. (*From* Paulus WJ. A novel paradigm for heart failure with preserved ejection fraction: comorbidities drive myocardial dysfunction and remodeling through coronary microvascular endothelial inflammation. J Am Coll Cardiol 2013;62(4):264; with permission.)

ventricles and exacerbate the decrease in NO availability.[41,42] Blocking the catabolism of cGMP with phosphodiesterase inhibition can decrease cellular and chamber hypertrophy,[43,44] enhance right ventricular contractility,[41,42] improve calcium handling,[44] and decrease sympathetic activity.[45] In patients with pulmonary arterial hypertension, the PDE5 inhibitor, sildenafil, has demonstrated improvement in exercise capacity and pulmonary hemodynamics.[46,47]

Two randomized clinical trials have used the PDE5 inhibitor, sildenafil, for the treatment of HFpEF. In a study of 44 patients by Guazzi and colleagues,[48] patients with echocardiographic evidence of diastolic dysfunction, LVEF of 50% or higher, and pulmonary artery systolic pressure greater than 40 mm Hg were randomized to sildenafil 50 mg 3 times a day or placebo. At 12 months, sildenafil decreased pulmonary artery pressure and resistance and improved right ventricular function and dimension. However, this population had severe elevation in right ventricular afterload with a mean transpulmonary gradient of greater than 15 mm Hg and pulmonary vascular resistance of greater than 3 Wood units. The patients in this study also had severe right ventricular dysfunction with a mean central venous pressure

of 23 mm Hg and central venous pressure to wedge pressure ratio of greater than 1. These are not common hemodynamic profiles for patients with HFpEF,[49,50] and right ventricular unloading could potentially be the main reason for the improvements seen.

The PhosphdiesteRasE-5 Inhibition to Improve CLinical Status and EXercise Capacity in Diastolic Heart Failure (RELAX) trial enrolled a total of 216 outpatients with heart failure, LVEF of 50% or higher, elevated NT-pro-BNP or elevated filling pressures, and reduced exercise capacity. Patients were randomized to sildenafil 20 mg 3 times daily for 12 weeks followed by 60 mg 3 times daily for 12 weeks versus placebo.[51] The participants were representative of a typical HFpEF population with mean age of 69 years, 48% women, and 53% with moderate heart failure symptoms. Comorbidities were common (85% hypertension, 51% atrial fibrillation, 55% stage 3/4 kidney disease) and there was significant diastolic dysfunction (median NT-pro-BNP 700 pg/mL, median left atrial volume index 43 mL/m^2). At 24 weeks, there was no difference between groups in any end point, including peak oxygen consumption, 6-minute walk distance, quality of life, diastolic function, or left ventricular remodeling.

Neprilysin Inhibition

Natriuretic peptides are known to have potent natriuretic and vasodilatory effects. Through cGMP signaling, they also have antiadrenergic and antihypertrophic effects.[52,53] Neprilysin is an endopeptidase that degrades several peptides, including atrial natriuretic peptide and B-natriuretic peptide.[54] Neprilysin inhibition has been identified as a potential pharmacologic therapy to decrease fibrosis and with potential benefits for patients with HFpEF. In HFrEF, the combination of ACE and neprilysin inhibition in a single agent using omapatrilat improved functional class, LVEF, blood pressure,[55] and readmission rates compared with lisinopril.[56] A similar strategy using omapatrilat improved diastolic function in preclinical studies,[57] although clinical outcomes were unclear. However, the drug was ultimately not approved because of side effects, especially angioedema.

The Prospective Comparison of LCZ696 (an ARB/neprilysin inhibitor) with an ARB on Management of Heart Failure with Preserved Ejection Fraction (PARAMOUNT) phase II trial, randomized 301 patients with NYHA II to III, LVEF of 45% or higher, and NT-pro-BNP greater than 400 pg/mL to LCZ696 200 mg twice daily versus valsartan 160 mg twice daily. LCZ96 was well tolerated and significantly decreased NT-pro-BNP levels (783–605 pg/mL) compared with valsartan (862 pg/mL to 835 pg/mL) at 12 weeks ($P<.05$).[58] These results were encouraging enough to develop the PARAGON-HF trial to address the impact of LCZ696 on clinical outcomes. However, as of this writing, the trial was suspended by the sponsor for unclear reasons (ClinicalTrials.gov Identifier: NCT01920711).

Statins

Several observational studies have suggested the beneficial effects of statins in patients with HFpEF. The EuroHeart Failure Survey in 3148 patients with LVEF of 40% or higher showed a decrease in all-cause mortality in patients treated with statins.[59] Fukuta and colleagues,[60] in a observational analysis of 137 patients with heart failure and LVEF of 50% or higher, showed better survival in patients treated with statins (HR 0.20; 95% CI 0.06–0.62; $P = .005$) after adjusting for hypertension, diabetes mellitus, coronary artery disease, and serum creatinine. Shah and colleagues,[61] in a large US cohort of 13,533 patients with recent admissions for heart failure and LVEF greater than 50%, showed significant improvements in mortality in patients treated with statins (relative risk [RR] 0.73, 95% CI 0.68–0.79) after adjusting for total cholesterol level, coronary artery disease, diabetes, hypertension, and age. In contrast, randomized data in HFrEF have not confirmed the benefits of statins in heart failure. For example, in the randomized Gruppo Italiano per lo Studio della Sopravvivenza nell'Infarto Miocardico–Heart Failure (GISSI-HF) and Controlled Rosuvastatin Multinational Trial in Heart Failure (CORONA) trials of HFrEF, the potent statin, rosuvastatin did not improve the primary end point.[62] A recent meta-analysis of 11 studies with 17,985 patients with HFpEF showed that statin use was associated with a 40% reduction in mortality.[63] However, at present, there is no published prospective randomized study of statins in patients with HFpEF and no clear indication for statin therapy for the primary purpose of improving clinical outcomes in heart failure.

A variety of other miscellaneous agents have been studied in small mechanistic investigations (**Table 3**) but have not yet been subjected to large prospective randomized trials. The one notable exception is digoxin, which was hypothesized to improve autonomic balance in HFpEF. However, in a large prespecified substudy of the Digitalis Investigation Group (DIG) trial, digoxin failed to make a significant clinical impact.

NONPHARMACOLOGICAL THERAPY
Low-Salt Diet

Experimental models of hypertension have demonstrated that diets with high salt content induce severe hypertension, LVH, and diastolic dysfunction.[64,65] In patients with HFpEF, elevated dietary salt intake correlates with elevated BNP levels.[66] Hummel and colleagues[67,68] studied 13 patients with hypertension, LVEF of 50% or higher, and evidence of diastolic dysfunction (by catheterization, echocardiography, or elevated neurohormones). The subjects treated with the sodium-restricted Dietary Approaches to Stop Hypertension diet (DASH/SRD) for 21 days had improved systemic blood pressure, oxidative stress, diastolic function, arterial elastance, and ventricular-arterial coupling.

Exercise

The effect of endurance exercise training was evaluated in 63 patients with HFpEF with a mean age of 70 years. Patients were randomized to 16 weeks of exercise training versus attention control (including frequent phone calls and reminders). Endurance training increased peak V_{O_2} (15.8 ± 3.3 mL/kg/min vs 13.8 ± 3.1 mL/kg/min, $P = .0001$) and quality of life. However, measurements of endothelial function with brachial artery flow mediated dilation

Table 3
Clinical trials of miscellaneous agents in heart failure with preserved ejection fraction

Agent	Published	Inclusion Criteria	N	Study Type	Outcome
Verapamil[88]	1990	LVEF >45% Abnormal diastolic filling	20	Crossover trial against placebo	Increased exercise capacity Improved diastolic function
Verapamil[89]	2002	Normal LVEF NYHA II–III	15	Crossover trial	Increased exercise capacity Improved diastolic function
Digoxin[87]	2006	LVEF >45%	988	Randomized controlled trial	No difference in mortality or readmission
Ranolazine[90]	2013	LVEF >50% Abnormal diastolic filling	20	Randomized controlled trial	No change in exercise tolerance
Ivabradine[91]	2013	LVEF >50% Abnormal diastolic filling	61	Randomized controlled trial	Increased exercise capacity Improved diastolic function

Abbreviations: LVEF, left ventricular ejection fraction; NYHA, New York Heart Association.
Data from Refs.[87–91]

and measurements of arterial stiffness with carotid arterial distensibility were unchanged. This study suggests that the beneficial effects of exercise training on exercise capacity may be mediated by mechanisms other than improvements in endothelial dysfunction and arterial stiffness.[69] The Exercise Training in Diastolic Heart Failure-Pilot Study (Ex-DHF) randomized 64 patients with HFpEF to supervised endurance/resistance training in addition to usual care or to usual care alone. After 3 months the patients in the training arm had increased peak Vo_2 from 16.1 ± 4.9 ml/min/kg to 18.7 ± 5.4 ml/min/kg; $P<.001$ with concomitant improvements in the physical dimensions of quality of life. Based on these studies, physical activity and exercise training appears safe in this patient population may be considered.[70]

Pacing

Patients with HFpEF have chronotropic incompetence, which contributes to decreased exercise capacity.[71,72] The Restoration of Chronotropic Competence in Heart Failure Patients with Normal Ejection Fraction (RESET) study was a prospective, multicenter, double-blind randomized crossover trial to evaluate atrial rate adaptive pacing in patients with admissions for heart failure or elevated natriuretic peptide and LVEF of 50% or higher (ClinicalTrials.gov Identifier: NCT00670111). However, the study was terminated because of difficulty in enrollment.[73]

Preliminary studies have demonstrated that some patients with HFpEF have interatrial conduction delays.[74] Left atrial pacing through the coronary sinus has been evaluated in 6 patients with interatrial conduction delay (p wave >120 ms in lead II), short left atrioventricular interval during electrophysiological studies, and restrictive echocardiographic pattern in a crossover study. After 3 months, there was significant improvement in the mean 6-minute walk distance (240 ± 25 m vs 190 ± 15 m, $P<.05$), and diastolic function. Interestingly, after 1 week of turning off the left atrial pacing, exercise capacity decreased. The LEft Atrial Pacing in Diastolic Heart Failure (LEAD) study is expected to enroll patients with diastolic heart failure and atrial dyssynchrony and compare the effects of left atrial pacing in a larger cohort of patients (ClinicalTrials.gov Identifier: NCT01618981).

Several observational studies have demonstrated the presence of echocardiographic mechanical dyssynchrony in patients with HFpEF.[75–78] Patients with HFpEF and worse dyssynchrony also have wider QRS interval, higher left ventricular mass indices, and lower mitral annular relaxation velocities.[79] There are no specific studies of cardiac resynchronization in patients with HFpEF, but in a subgroup analysis of the PROSPECT study, 86 patients with NYHA III to IV with LVEF greater than 35% and QRS greater than 130 ms had similar improvements in clinical scores compared with the patients with LVEF less than 35% after 6 months. The Pacing for Heart Failure With Preserved Ejection Fraction study will evaluate the effects of a new pacing method (fusion pacing) delivered by a cardiac resynchronization therapy-defibrillator device in patients with HFpEF (LVEF >50%) and evidence of regional mechanical delay of 65 ms or more (ClinicalTrials.gov Identifier: NCT01045291). The study completed enrollment in 2013.

Baroreflex Activation Therapy

Chronic activation of the baroreflex in the carotid sinus with electrical impulses from a pulse generator has been tested in patients with resistant hypertension.[80] The stimulation of the baroreceptors produces a negative feedback in the autonomic nervous system with inhibition of the sympathetic system and activation of the parasympathetic system with subsequent bradycardia and vasodilation. The Rheos Diastolic Heart Failure trial has tested this device in patients with LVEF of 45% or higher and clinical heart failure with elevated BNP or NT-pro-BNP (ClinicalTrials.gov Identifier: NCT00718939). The study completed enrollment in 2012 but the results have yet to be reported.

CONTEMPORARY THERAPEUTIC APPROACH

Current guidelines are emblematic of the challenge clinicians face in the management of HFpEF. For example, the American College of Cardiology Foundation/American Heart Association Heart Failure Guidelines recommend symptomatic relief with diuretics and risk factor control, including hypertension, coronary artery disease, and atrial fibrillation.[1] Of note, almost all of these recommendations come from expert opinions (Level of Evidence C) (**Table 4**). A practical approach to management is described in **Box 2**. The therapeutic approach starts with the identification of other conditions that can present with dyspnea/edema and preserved systolic function and mimic HFpEF (eg, constriction, cor pulmonale, restrictive heart disease). If diagnostic certainty persists, additional testing, such as right heart catheterization or cardiopulmonary exercise testing, can be illuminating.

Once HFpEF is confirmed, management should be directed toward symptomatic relief of congestion and treatment of concomitant conditions, such as hypertension, atrial fibrillation,[80] and chronotropic incompetence (see **Box 2**). Patients with HFpEF are known to have an exaggerated hypertensive response to exercise,[71] suggesting an important role for blood pressure control.[81] Atrial fibrillation in patients with HFpEF is associated with higher markers of neurohormonal activation, impaired systolic and diastolic function and decreased exercise capacity.[82] Treatment of atrial fibrillation should include a consideration of rhythm control (eg, with ablation[83] and/or antiarrhythmic therapy) in addition to a rate control strategy (eg, see recent 2014 AHA/ACC/HRS guidelines).[84] Chronotropic incompetence is often underappreciated as a cause of exercise intolerance in HFPEF and can be exacerbated by agents such as beta-blockers, calcium channel blockers, and amiodarone. In some rare circumstances, revascularization may even be of benefit in HFpEF.[85] In addition, the European Society of Cardiology Guidelines emphasize the recognition and optimal treatment of other comorbities such as diabetes, obesity, renal insufficiency, chronic obstructive pulmonary disease, obstructive sleep apnea and anemia.[86]

Ultimately, judicious decongestion with diuretics remains the cornerstone of HFPEF management in order to provide symptomatic relief. It is important

Table 4
Recommendations of therapy for patients with HFpEF

Recommendations	COR	LOE
Systolic and diastolic blood pressure should be controlled according to published clinical practice guidelines	I	B
Diuretics should be used for relief of symptoms due to volume overload	I	C
Coronary revascularization for patients with CAD in whom angina or demonstrable myocardial ischemia is present despite GDMT	IIa	C
Management of AF according to published clinical practice guidelines for HFpEF to improve symptomatic HF	IIa	C
Use of beta-blocking agents, ACE inhibitors, and ARBs for hypertension in HFpEF	IIa	C
ARBs might be considered to decrease hospitalization in HFpEF	IIb	B
Nutritional supplementation is not recommended in HFpEF	III: No Benefit	C

Abbreviations: ACE, angiotensin-converting enzyme; AF, atrial fibrillation; ARBs, angiotensin-receptor blockers; CAD, coronary artery disease; COR, Class of Recommendation; GDMT, guideline-directed medical therapy; HF, heart failure; HFpEF, heart failure with preserved ejection fraction; LOE, Level of Evidence.
From Yancy CW, Jessup M, Bozkurt B, et al. 2013 ACCF/AHA guideline for the management of heart failure: a report of the American College of Cardiology Foundation/American Heart Association Task Force on practice guidelines. Circulation 2013;128(16):e240–327; with permission.

> **Box 2**
> **Contemporary treatment of HFpEF**
>
> 1. Exclude conditions that mimic HFpEF (eg, restriction, constriction, pulmonary arterial hypertension, cor pulmonale).
> 2. Consider other diagnostic testing as needed (eg, brain natriuretic peptide, echocardiogram, right heart catheterization, cardiopulmonary exercise test).
> 3. Identify and treat hypertension and inadequate blood pressure response to exercise.
> 4. Identify chronotrophic incompetence during stress test and consider adjusting removing or decreasing bradycardic agents.
> 5. Identify and treat atrial fibrillation.
> 6. Identify and treat coronary artery disease and ischemia.
> 7. Identify and treat other comorbidities, eg, diabetes, obesity, renal insufficiency, chronic obstructive pulmonary disease, obstructive sleep apnea, and anemia.
> 8. Judicious use of diuretics, with particular attention to overdiuresis.
> 9. Lifestyle modifications, eg, salt and fluid restriction, weight loss, physical activity, and exercise.

to note that patients with HFpEF may have decreased end-diastolic volumes, and modest decreases in preload can result in precipitous declines in stroke volume and cardiac output leading to hypotension and renal insufficiency. In light of the TOPCAT trial results, it is important to at least consider the use of spironolactone as a diuretic choice. Until more evidence is gathered, the diuretic endpoint should primarily be directed at symptom relief rather than a surrogate endpoint such as a biomarker or filling pressure.

Although nitrates can be considered on an empiric basis, there is insufficient evidence to advocate for their routine use. Physical activity and exercise are advocated in all patients with heart failure for its potential effects in exercise capacity and quality of life.

SUMMARY

In contrast to patients with HFrEF, attempts to identify therapies to improve the outcomes in patients with HFpEF have been unsuccessful. Methodological challenges of the previous studies include a lack of uniform criteria to define HFpEF and low event rates. Patients with HFrEF share a common pathophysiology of neurohumoral activation that is a clear target for therapies. In contrast, patients with HFpEF have multiple underlying mechanisms behind their clinical presentation, creating a challenge to identify a single therapeutic target. The current management of HFpEF is directed to symptomatic relief of congestion with diuretics and risk factor modification. Several mechanisms are under investigation as potential targets for therapy to improve the outcomes of this heterogeneous population.

REFERENCES

1. Yancy CW, Jessup M, Bozkurt B, et al. 2013 ACCF/AHA guideline for the management of heart failure: a report of the American College of Cardiology Foundation/American Heart Association Task Force on Practice Guidelines. J Am Coll Cardiol 2013;62(16):e147–239.
2. Zile MR, Baicu CF, Gaasch WH. Diastolic heart failure—abnormalities in active relaxation and passive stiffness of the left ventricle. N Engl J Med 2004;350(19):1953–9.
3. Owan TE, Hodge DO, Herges RM, et al. Secular trends in renal dysfunction and outcomes in hospitalized heart failure patients. J Card Fail 2006;12(4):257–62.
4. Owan TE, Hodge DO, Herges RM, et al. Trends in prevalence and outcome of heart failure with preserved ejection fraction. N Engl J Med 2006;355(3):251–9.
5. Benedict CR, Johnstone DE, Weiner DH, et al. Relation of neurohumoral activation to clinical variables and degree of ventricular dysfunction: a report from the Registry of Studies of Left Ventricular Dysfunction. SOLVD Investigators. J Am Coll Cardiol 1994;23(6):1410–20.
6. Devereux RB, Pickering TG, Cody RJ, et al. Relation of renin-angiotensin system activity to left ventricular hypertrophy and function in experimental and human hypertension. J Clin Hypertens 1987;3(1):87–103.
7. Hogg K, McMurray J. Neurohumoral pathways in heart failure with preserved systolic function. Prog Cardiovasc Dis 2005;47(6):357–66.
8. Wright JW, Mizutani S, Harding JW. Pathways involved in the transition from hypertension to hypertrophy to heart failure. Treatment strategies. Heart Fail Rev 2008;13(3):367–75.
9. Effects of enalapril on mortality in severe congestive heart failure. Results of the Cooperative North Scandinavian Enalapril Survival Study (CONSENSUS). The CONSENSUS Trial Study Group. N Engl J Med 1987;316(23):1429–35.
10. Effect of enalapril on survival in patients with reduced left ventricular ejection fractions and

congestive heart failure. The SOLVD Investigators. N Engl J Med 1991;325(5):293–302.

11. Effect of enalapril on mortality and the development of heart failure in asymptomatic patients with reduced left ventricular ejection fractions. The SOLVD Investigators. N Engl J Med 1992;327(10): 685–91.

12. Cohn JN, Johnson G, Ziesche S, et al. A comparison of enalapril with hydralazine-isosorbide dinitrate in the treatment of chronic congestive heart failure. N Engl J Med 1991; 325(5):303–10.

13. Pfeffer MA, Braunwald E, Moye LA, et al. Effect of captopril on mortality and morbidity in patients with left ventricular dysfunction after myocardial infarction. Results of the survival and ventricular enlargement trial. The SAVE Investigators. N Engl J Med 1992;327(10):669–77.

14. Cohn JN, Tognoni G, Valsartan Heart I. Failure trial, a randomized trial of the angiotensin-receptor blocker valsartan in chronic heart failure. N Engl J Med 2001;345(23):1667–75.

15. Granger CB, McMurray JJ, Yusuf S, et al. Effects of candesartan in patients with chronic heart failure and reduced left-ventricular systolic function intolerant to angiotensin-converting-enzyme inhibitors: the CHARM-Alternative trial. Lancet 2003; 362(9386):772–6.

16. Dahlof B, Devereux RB, Kjeldsen SE, et al. Cardiovascular morbidity and mortality in the Losartan Intervention For Endpoint reduction in hypertension study (LIFE): a randomised trial against atenolol. Lancet 2002;359(9311):995–1003.

17. Yusuf S, Sleight P, Pogue J, et al. Effects of an angiotensin-converting-enzyme inhibitor, ramipril, on cardiovascular events in high-risk patients. The Heart Outcomes Prevention Evaluation Study Investigators. N Engl J Med 2000;342(3):145–53.

18. Fox KM, EURopean trial On reduction of cardiac events with Perindopril in stable coronary Artery disease Investigators. Efficacy of perindopril in reduction of cardiovascular events among patients with stable coronary artery disease: randomised, double-blind, placebo-controlled, multicentre trial (the EUROPA study). Lancet 2003;362(9386):782–8.

19. Yusuf S, Pfeffer MA, Swedberg K, et al. Effects of candesartan in patients with chronic heart failure and preserved left-ventricular ejection fraction: the CHARM-Preserved Trial. Lancet 2003;362(9386): 777–81.

20. Cleland JG, Tendera M, Adamus J, et al. The perindopril in elderly people with chronic heart failure (PEP-CHF) study. Eur Heart J 2006;27(19):2338–45.

21. Massie BM, Carson PE, McMurray JJ, et al. Irbesartan in patients with heart failure and preserved ejection fraction. N Engl J Med 2008;359(23): 2456–67.

22. Lund LH, Benson L, Dahlstrom U, et al. Association between use of renin-angiotensin system antagonists and mortality in patients with heart failure and preserved ejection fraction. JAMA 2012; 308(20):2108–17.

23. Mujib M, Patel K, Fonarow GC, et al. Angiotensin-converting enzyme inhibitors and outcomes in heart failure and preserved ejection fraction. Am J Med 2013;126(5):401–10.

24. Kobayashi M, Machida N, Mitsuishi M, et al. Beta-blocker improves survival, left ventricular function, and myocardial remodeling in hypertensive rats with diastolic heart failure. Am J Hypertens 2004; 17(12 Pt 1):1112–9.

25. Nishio M, Sakata Y, Mano T, et al. Beneficial effects of bisoprolol on the survival of hypertensive diastolic heart failure model rats. Eur J Heart Fail 2008;10(5):446–53.

26. Dobre D, van Veldhuisen DJ, DeJongste MJ, et al. Prescription of beta-blockers in patients with advanced heart failure and preserved left ventricular ejection fraction. Clinical implications and survival. Eur J Heart Fail 2007;9(3):280–6.

27. Hernandez AF, Hammill BG, O'Connor CM, et al. Clinical effectiveness of beta-blockers in heart failure: findings from the OPTIMIZE-HF (Organized Program to Initiate Lifesaving Treatment in Hospitalized Patients with Heart Failure) Registry. J Am Coll Cardiol 2009;53(2):184–92.

28. Conraads VM, Metra M, Kamp O, et al. Effects of the long-term administration of nebivolol on the clinical symptoms, exercise capacity, and left ventricular function of patients with diastolic dysfunction: results of the ELANDD study. Eur J Heart Fail 2012; 14(2):219–25.

29. Flather MD, Shibata MC, Coats AJ, et al. Randomized trial to determine the effect of nebivolol on mortality and cardiovascular hospital admission in elderly patients with heart failure (SENIORS). Eur Heart J 2005;26(3):215–25.

30. van Veldhuisen DJ, Cohen-Solal A, Bohm M, et al. Beta-blockade with nebivolol in elderly heart failure patients with impaired and preserved left ventricular ejection fraction: data from SENIORS (Study of Effects of Nebivolol Intervention on Outcomes and Rehospitalization in Seniors With Heart Failure). J Am Coll Cardiol 2009;53(23):2150–8.

31. Yamamoto K, Origasa H, Hori M, et al. Effects of carvedilol on heart failure with preserved ejection fraction: the Japanese Diastolic Heart Failure Study (J-DHF). Eur J Heart Fail 2013;15(1):110–8.

32. Brilla CG, Weber KT. Mineralocorticoid excess, dietary sodium, and myocardial fibrosis. J Lab Clin Med 1992;120(6):893–901.

33. Tomaschitz A, Pilz S, Ritz E, et al. Plasma aldosterone levels are associated with increased cardiovascular mortality: the Ludwigshafen Risk and

Cardiovascular Health (LURIC) study. Eur Heart J 2010;31(10):1237–47.

34. Pitt B, Zannad F, Remme WJ, et al. The effect of spironolactone on morbidity and mortality in patients with severe heart failure. Randomized Aldactone Evaluation Study Investigators. N Engl J Med 1999;341(10):709–17.

35. Zannad F, McMurray JJ, Krum H, et al. Eplerenone in patients with systolic heart failure and mild symptoms. N Engl J Med 2011;364(1):11–21.

36. Edelmann F, Tomaschitz A, Wachter R, et al. Serum aldosterone and its relationship to left ventricular structure and geometry in patients with preserved left ventricular ejection fraction. Eur Heart J 2012; 33(2):203–12.

37. Edelmann F, Wachter R, Schmidt AG, et al. Effect of spironolactone on diastolic function and exercise capacity in patients with heart failure with preserved ejection fraction: the Aldo-DHF randomized controlled trial. JAMA 2013;309(8):781–91.

38. Stiles Steve. Aldo-antagonist falls short but impresses in preserved-EF heart failure: TOPCAT. 2013. Available at: http://www.medscape.com/viewarticle/814622.

39. Paulus WJ, Tschope C. A novel paradigm for heart failure with preserved ejection fraction: comorbidities drive myocardial dysfunction and remodeling through coronary microvascular endothelial inflammation. J Am Coll Cardiol 2013;62(4): 263–71.

40. Greene SJ, Gheorghiade M, Borlaug BA, et al. The cGMP signaling pathway as a therapeutic target in heart failure with preserved ejection fraction. J Am Heart Assoc 2013;2(6):e000536.

41. Nagendran J, Archer SL, Soliman D, et al. Phosphodiesterase type 5 is highly expressed in the hypertrophied human right ventricle, and acute inhibition of phosphodiesterase type 5 improves contractility. Circulation 2007;116(3):238–48.

42. Shan X, Quaile MP, Monk JK, et al. Differential expression of PDE5 in failing and nonfailing human myocardium. Circ Heart Fail 2012;5(1): 79–86.

43. Takimoto E, Champion HC, Li M, et al. Chronic inhibition of cyclic GMP phosphodiesterase 5A prevents and reverses cardiac hypertrophy. Nat Med 2005;11(2):214–22.

44. Nagayama T, Hsu S, Zhang M, et al. Sildenafil stops progressive chamber, cellular, and molecular remodeling and improves calcium handling and function in hearts with pre-existing advanced hypertrophy caused by pressure overload. J Am Coll Cardiol 2009;53(2):207–15.

45. Al-Hesayen A, Floras JS, Parker JD. The effects of intravenous sildenafil on hemodynamics and cardiac sympathetic activity in chronic human heart failure. Eur J Heart Fail 2006;8(8):864–8.

46. Galie N, Ghofrani HA, Torbicki A, et al. Sildenafil citrate therapy for pulmonary arterial hypertension. N Engl J Med 2005;353(20):2148–57.

47. Rubin LJ, Badesch DB, Fleming TR, et al. Long-term treatment with sildenafil citrate in pulmonary arterial hypertension: the SUPER-2 study. Chest 2011;140(5):1274–83.

48. Guazzi M, Vicenzi M, Arena R, et al. Pulmonary hypertension in heart failure with preserved ejection fraction: a target of phosphodiesterase-5 inhibition in a 1-year study. Circulation 2011; 124(2):164–74.

49. Schwartzenberg S, Redfield MM, From AM, et al. Effects of vasodilation in heart failure with preserved or reduced ejection fraction implications of distinct pathophysiologies on response to therapy. J Am Coll Cardiol 2012;59(5):442–51.

50. Drazner MH, Prasad A, Ayers C, et al. The relationship of right- and left-sided filling pressures in patients with heart failure and a preserved ejection fraction. Circ Heart Fail 2010;3(2):202–6.

51. Redfield MM, Chen HH, Borlaug BA, et al. Effect of phosphodiesterase-5 inhibition on exercise capacity and clinical status in heart failure with preserved ejection fraction: a randomized clinical trial. JAMA 2013;309(12):1268–77.

52. Gardner DG, Chen S, Glenn DJ, et al. Molecular biology of the natriuretic peptide system: implications for physiology and hypertension. Hypertension 2007;49(3):419–26.

53. Potter LR, Abbey-Hosch S, Dickey DM. Natriuretic peptides, their receptors, and cyclic guanosine monophosphate-dependent signaling functions. Endocr Rev 2006;27(1):47–72.

54. Gu J, Noe A, Chandra P, et al. Pharmacokinetics and pharmacodynamics of LCZ696, a novel dual-acting angiotensin receptor-neprilysin inhibitor (ARNi). J Clin Pharmacol 2010;50(4):401–14.

55. McClean DR, Ikram H, Garlick AH, et al. The clinical, cardiac, renal, arterial and neurohormonal effects of omapatrilat, a vasopeptidase inhibitor, in patients with chronic heart failure. J Am Coll Cardiol 2000;36(2):479–86.

56. Eisenstein EL, Nelson CL, Simon TA, et al. Vasopeptidase inhibitor reduces in-hospital costs for patients with congestive heart failure: results from the IMPRESS trial. Inhibition of Metallo Protease by BMS-186716 in a Randomized Exercise and Symptoms Study in Subjects With Heart Failure. Am Heart J 2002;143(6):1112–7.

57. Gronholm T, Cheng ZJ, Palojoki E, et al. Vasopeptidase inhibition has beneficial cardiac effects in spontaneously diabetic Goto-Kakizaki rats. Eur J Pharmacol 2005;519(3):267–76.

58. Solomon SD, Zile M, Pieske B, et al. The angiotensin receptor neprilysin inhibitor LCZ696 in heart failure with preserved ejection fraction: a phase 2

double-blind randomised controlled trial. Lancet 2012;380(9851):1387–95.

59. Lenzen MJ, Scholte op Reimer WJ, Boersma E, et al. Differences between patients with a preserved and a depressed left ventricular function: a report from the EuroHeart Failure Survey. Eur Heart J 2004;25(14):1214–20.

60. Fukuta H, Sane DC, Brucks S, et al. Statin therapy may be associated with lower mortality in patients with diastolic heart failure: a preliminary report. Circulation 2005;112(3):357–63.

61. Shah R, Wang Y, Foody JM. Effect of statins, angiotensin-converting enzyme inhibitors, and beta blockers on survival in patients >or=65 years of age with heart failure and preserved left ventricular systolic function. Am J Cardiol 2008;101(2):217–22.

62. Florkowski CM, Molyneux SL, George PM. Rosuvastatin in older patients with systolic heart failure. N Engl J Med 2008;358(12):1301 [author reply: 1301].

63. Liu G, Xin-Xin Zheng, Yan-Lu Xu, et al. Meta-analysis of the effect of statins on mortality in patients with preserved ejection fraction. Am J Cardiol 2014;113(7):1198–204.

64. Klotz S, Hay I, Zhang G, et al. Development of heart failure in chronic hypertensive Dahl rats: focus on heart failure with preserved ejection fraction. Hypertension 2006;47(5):901–11.

65. Matsui H, Ando K, Kawarazaki H, et al. Salt excess causes left ventricular diastolic dysfunction in rats with metabolic disorder. Hypertension 2008;52(2):287–94.

66. Sadanaga T, Ando K, Hirota S, et al. B-type natriuretic peptide levels are decreased by reducing dietary salt intake in patients with compensated heart failure with preserved ejection fraction. Intern Med J 2013;43(6):663–7.

67. Hummel SL, Seymour EM, Brook RD, et al. Low-sodium dietary approaches to stop hypertension diet reduces blood pressure, arterial stiffness, and oxidative stress in hypertensive heart failure with preserved ejection fraction. Hypertension 2012;60(5):1200–6.

68. Hummel SL, Seymour EM, Brook RD, et al. Low-sodium DASH diet improves diastolic function and ventricular-arterial coupling in hypertensive heart failure with preserved ejection fraction. Circ Heart Fail 2013;6(6):1165–71.

69. Kitzman DW, Brubaker PH, Herrington DM, et al. Effect of endurance exercise training on endothelial function and arterial stiffness in older patients with heart failure and preserved ejection fraction: a randomized, controlled, single-blind trial. J Am Coll Cardiol 2013;62(7):584–92.

70. Edelmann F, Gelbrich G, Dungen HD, et al. Exercise training improves exercise capacity and diastolic function in patients with heart failure with preserved ejection fraction: results of the Ex-DHF (Exercise training in Diastolic Heart Failure) pilot study. J Am Coll Cardiol 2011;58:1780–91.

71. Borlaug BA, Melenovsky V, Russell SD, et al. Impaired chronotropic and vasodilator reserves limit exercise capacity in patients with heart failure and a preserved ejection fraction. Circulation 2006;114(20):2138–47.

72. Brubaker PH, Joo KC, Stewart KP, et al. Chronotropic incompetence and its contribution to exercise intolerance in older heart failure patients. J Cardiopulm Rehabil 2006;26(2):86–9.

73. Kass DA, Kitzman DW, Alvarez GE. The restoration of chronotropic competence in heart failure patients with normal ejection fraction (RESET) study: rationale and design. J Card Fail 2010;16(1):17–24.

74. Eicher JC, Laurent G, Mathe A, et al. Atrial dyssynchrony syndrome: an overlooked phenomenon and a potential cause of 'diastolic' heart failure. Eur J Heart Fail 2012;14(3):248–58.

75. Phan TT, Abozguia K, Shivu GN, et al. Myocardial contractile inefficiency and dyssynchrony in heart failure with preserved ejection fraction and narrow QRS complex. J Am Soc Echocardiogr 2010;23(2):201–6.

76. Morris DA, Vaz Perez A, Blaschke F, et al. Myocardial systolic and diastolic consequences of left ventricular mechanical dyssynchrony in heart failure with normal left ventricular ejection fraction. Eur Heart J Cardiovasc Imaging 2012;13(7):556–67.

77. De Sutter J, Van de Veire NR, Muyldermans L, et al. Prevalence of mechanical dyssynchrony in patients with heart failure and preserved left ventricular function (a report from the Belgian Multicenter Registry on dyssynchrony). Am J Cardiol 2005;96(11):1543–8.

78. Yu CM, Zhang Q, Yip GW, et al. Diastolic and systolic asynchrony in patients with diastolic heart failure: a common but ignored condition. J Am Coll Cardiol 2007;49(1):97–105.

79. Santos AB, Kraigher-Krainer E, Bello N, et al. Left ventricular dyssynchrony in patients with heart failure and preserved ejection fraction. Eur Heart J 2014;35(1):42–7.

80. Bisognano JD, Bakris G, Nadim MK, et al. Baroreflex activation therapy lowers blood pressure in patients with resistant hypertension: results from the double-blind, randomized, placebo-controlled rheos pivotal trial. J Am Coll Cardiol 2011;58(7):765–73.

81. James PA, Oparil S, Carter BL, et al. 2014 evidence-based guideline for the management of high blood pressure in adults: report from the panel members appointed to the Eighth Joint National Committee (JNC 8). JAMA 2014;311:507–20.

82. Zakeri R, Borlaug BA, McNulty SE, et al. Impact of atrial fibrillation on exercise capacity in heart failure with preserved ejection fraction: a RELAX trial ancillary study. Circ Heart Fail 2014;7:123–30.

83. Machino-Ohtsuka T, Seo Y, Ishizu T, et al. Efficacy, safety, and outcomes of catheter ablation of atrial fibrillation in patients with heart failure with preserved ejection fraction. J Am Coll Cardiol 2013; 62(20):1857–65.

84. Fuster V, Ryden LE, Cannom DS, et al. 2011 ACCF/AHA/HRS focused updates incorporated into the ACC/AHA/ESC 2006 Guidelines for the management of patients with atrial fibrillation: a report of the American College of Cardiology Foundation/American Heart Association Task Force on Practice Guidelines developed in partnership with the European Society of Cardiology and in collaboration with the European Heart Rhythm Association and the Heart Rhythm Society. J Am Coll Cardiol 2011;57:e101–98.

85. Hwang SJ, Melenovsky V, Borlaug BA. Implications of Coronary Artery Disease in Heart Failure with preserved Ejection Fraction. J Am Coll Cardiol 2014.

86. McMurray JJ, Adamopoulos S, Anker SD, et al. ESC guidelines for the diagnosis and treatment of acute and chronic heart failure 2012: The Task Force for the Diagnosis and Treatment of Acute and Chronic Heart Failure 2012 of the European Society of Cardiology. Developed in collaboration with the Heart Failure Association (HFA) of the ESC. Eur J Heart Fail 2012;14:803–69.

87. Ahmed A, Rich MW, Fleg JL, et al. Effects of digoxin on morbidity and mortality in diastolic heart failure: the ancillary digitalis investigation group trial. Circulation 2006;114:397–403.

88. Setaro JF, Zaret BL, Schulman DS, et al. Usefulness of verapamil for congestive heart failure associated with abnormal left ventricular diastolic filling and normal left ventricular systolic performance. Am J Cardiol 1990;66:981–6.

89. Hung MJ, Cherng WJ, Kuo LT, et al. Effect of verapamil in elderly patients with left ventricular diastolic dysfunction as a cause of congestive heart failure. Int J Clin Pract 2002;56:57–62.

90. Maier LS, Layug B, Karwatowska-Prokopczuk E, et al. RAnoLazIne for the treatment of diastolic heart failure in patients with preserved ejection fraction: the RALI-DHF proof-of-concept study. JACC Heart Fail 2013;1:115–22.

91. Kosmala W, Holland DJ, Rojek A, et al. Effect of If-channel inhibition on hemodynamic status and exercise tolerance in heart failure with preserved ejection fraction: a randomized trial. J Am Coll Cardiol 2013;62:1330–8.

Index

Note: Page numbers of article titles are in **boldface** type.

Heart Failure Clin 10 (2014) 539–542
http://dx.doi.org/10.1016/S1551-7136(14)00046-4
1551-7136/14/$ – see front matter © 2014 Elsevier Inc. All rights reserved.

heartfailure.theclinics.com

Moving?

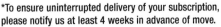

Make sure your subscription moves with you!

To notify us of your new address, find your **Clinics Account Number** (located on your mailing label above your name), and contact customer service at:

Email: **journalscustomerservice-usa@elsevier.com**

800-654-2452 (subscribers in the U.S. & Canada)
314-447-8871 (subscribers outside of the U.S. & Canada)

Fax number: **314-447-8029**

Elsevier Health Sciences Division
Subscription Customer Service
3251 Riverport Lane
Maryland Heights, MO 63043

*To ensure uninterrupted delivery of your subscription, please notify us at least 4 weeks in advance of move.

ELSEVIER

Printed and bound by CPI Group (UK) Ltd, Croydon, CR0 4YY

03/10/2024

01040382-0013